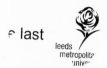

Audiology in Education

D1514167

Audiology in Education

Edited by
Wendy McCracken and Siobhán Laoide-Kemp

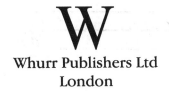

Whurr Publishers Ltd
London

First published 1997
by Whurr Publishers Ltd
19B Compton Terrace,
London N1 2UN,
England

British Library Cataloguing in Publication Data
A catalogue record for this book is available from the
British Library.

ISBN 1 861560 17 6 ✓

Printed and bound in the UK by Athenaeum Press Ltd,
Gateshead, Tyne & Wear

Contents

Contributors

David Adams
ENT Consultant and Senior Lecturer at Queen's University, Belfast, Northern Ireland, UK.

Sue Archbold
M Phil Coordinator, Director of Rehabilitation, Nottingham Paediatric Cochlear Implant Programme, and Chairperson of the Audiology and Educational Technology Committee of the National Executive Council of the British Association of Teachers of the Deaf, UK.

Margaret Baldwin
Principal Audiological Scientist in the London Districts of Redbridge and Waltham Forest, UK.

Fred Berg
Researcher in room acoustics and sound equipment, and Professor Emeritus of the Department of Communicative Disorders and Deaf Education at Utah State University, Logan, USA.

Russell Brett
Teacher of the Deaf and Educational Audiologist, leading a team of peripatetic teachers of the deaf in Wigan, UK.

Gwen Carr
Teacher of the Deaf and Head of the Service for Sensory Impaired Children in Stockport, UK.

Frans Coninx
Professor, Department for the Education and Rehabilitation of the Hearing Impaired, University of Cologne, Germany, and Director of Research and Development, Instituut voor Doven, St Michielsgestel, The Netherlands.

Allison Joshua
Senior Lecturer, Special Education Department, University of Jos, Nigeria. Formerly Research Fellow in Audiology and Honorary Tutor in Audiology, Centre for Audiology, Education of the Deaf and Speech Pathology, University of Manchester, UK.

Siobhán Laoide–Kemp
Senior Audiologist and Visiting Teacher of the Deaf in Ireland. Department of Education, Marlborough Street, Dublin, Ireland.

Dawna Lewis
Senior Audiologist, **Boys Town** National Research Hospital, Omaha, Nebraska, USA.

Sue Lewis
Education Officer for the Ewing Foundation, The Centre for Audiology, Education of the Deaf and Speech Pathology, University of Manchester, UK.

David Lyon
Consultant, Educational Audiologist and Private Practice Clinical Audiologist, Atlantic, Canada.

Wendy McCracken
Lecturer in the Education of the Deaf, Centre for Audiology, Education of the Deaf and Speech Pathology, University of Manchester, UK.

John Mick Moore
Executive Director, Special Services Department of the Puget Sound Educational Service District, Seattle, Washington, USA.

Martin Smith
Head of Services for Hearing-Impaired and Visually-Impaired Children in Dorset, UK.

Lynn Stewart
Speech and Language Therapist, and Manager of the Special Needs Team of Speech and Language Therapists of Homefirst Community Trust, Northern Ireland, UK.

Peter Watkin
Head of Audiology Services in the London Districts of Redbridge and Waltham Forest, and Governor of Hawkswood School, UK.

Foreword

Audiological assessment, observation, support and information for children with deafness (I use this term to cover all degrees of hearing impairment) takes place not only in hospitals and health care settings, but in homes and schools as well. Detailed and accurate audiological profiling is built up from a number of important components: clinical tests; clinical verification of device appropriateness (e.g., hearing aids and cochlear implants); performance monitoring in home and school; evaluation of responsiveness, listening, communication, preferences in home and school settings; ecological aspects of home/school acoustics, family dynamics, behaviour, and their interactions with device management. There is ample evidence that for habilitation to be successful it is crucial to place the child and family at the centre of service provision and service. Ongoing monitoring contributes to the many detailed decisions which need to be made on the basis of the whole child in the home and school context.

The notion that regular hospital or clinical–based audiological assessment is sufficient to determine all audiological management decisions is based on too narrow a view of audiology, and serves the child and family poorly. While first–class health–based audiology services are essential—though in the 1990s still, sadly, by no means always available—they are insufficient on their own. Children with hearing impairment spend relatively little time in the artificial clinical environment, and most of their time in the acoustically, linguistically, educationally and socially challenging environments of home and school. How they function, how they progress, how teachers and parents can be fully involved in habilitative management and monitoring, are issues that are crucial to the child and family, and ultimately to outcomes.

This view of paediatric audiology—that it spans family, education and health contexts and environments—has a strong tradition in the UK, largely due to the early influence of the Ewings at the University of Manchester. Although their names became associated with a particular philosophical approach to deaf education, their great contribution was to emphasise the family and educational context of audiological care. Thus the 1957 text *Educational Guidance and the Deaf Child* (Manchester University Press, A. Ewing Ed.) is a classic and very early example of the synergy of educational and health–based audiology, ranging as it does from early screening tests to hearing aid management, classroom acoustics and (what was then called) parent guidance.

McCracken and Laoide–Kemp carry on that tradition. The need for high quality texts in the field of educational audiology is considerable and largely unmet, and their book will help to fill an important gap for Teachers of the Deaf, Educational Audiologists and other professionals and parents in this area. We need Teachers of the Deaf and audiologists—often called educational audiologists—who work with the child and family 'on location', in home and school. Sometimes, for instance, in the USA, clinical audiologists work in educational settings; elsewhere, in the UK for example, Teachers of the Deaf with a Masters qualification in audiology, effectively combine the educational and audiological perspectives. This book is a much needed and timely addition to the literature in this area.

J M Bamford
March 1997

Introduction

Exciting and valuable developments have taken place in the field of audiology within the last 10 years. Opportunities for earlier and more effective listening experiences for all deaf children are greater than they have ever been before. The challenge for all professionals involved in this field is to be aware of the choices which need to be made available to these children through their parents and teachers. This demands a multi-disciplinary approach. We present the reader with a book which has been produced as a result of close collaboration between contributors drawn from a wide range of disciplines. All share the belief that close professional co-operation is central to meeting the diverse needs of deaf children. As technology develops and educational systems evolve, this becomes increasingly important.

The teacher of the deaf bears the responsibility of working closely with deaf children and their families as well as with teachers, social workers and specialist clinical colleagues. A sound knowledge base is essential if he/she is to advocate effectively on behalf of the deaf child. This book aims to provide this theoretical base. It is written primarily for teachers of the deaf, and is divided into three sections. Each section is designed to inform and encourage the reader to extend his/her knowledge base and to explore new ideas by using the comprehensive bibliography at the end of each section. A core book list at the end of the book provides the reader with an 'essential reading list'.

Audiology in Education has been designed to provide information in an accessible and thought provoking way. It will also be a very useful text on many levels for professionals from a variety of backgrounds, including teachers in the mainstream, educational audiologists, paediatric habilitators, audiological scientists, audiological physicians, speech therapists and social workers for the deaf.

Section A
Information and
Interpretation

Introduction

The teacher of the deaf must understand the effect of a diagnosis of deafness within a family setting. For any parent, this is the time when a range of questions will need to be answered. A teacher of the deaf has responsibility for interpreting and explaining a range of audiological information previously imparted in a clinical setting. The security of the home environment provides the parents with the opportunity to consider, reflect and discuss this information. Teachers of the deaf must be conversant with audiological procedures and be able to interpret and impart test results accurately. This is a partnership. While the teacher of the deaf will report ongoing progress and potential problems back to the clinical setting, the teacher should also be prepared to ask for clarification and advice.

Information will need to be explained to other teachers and co-professionals. Within the context of special learning needs in children, the teacher's role may become more pivotal in providing additional and complementary diagnostic information. This section provides a comprehensive background for the teacher of the deaf, which will ensure that information exchanged between parents, schools, clinics and co-professionals will prove beneficial to all concerned, and lead to the most appropriate management of each deaf child.

Chapter 1
Diagnostic Procedures

M BALDWIN AND P M WATKIN

Introduction

This chapter presents the tests of hearing commonly used with children. The emphasis is on interpretation of test results. The tests generally measure the child's impairment of hearing, that is, the loss of sensitivity to sound. Others indicate the pathology causing this loss of sensitivity. Whilst these two domains are essential in a diagnostic clinic, they may not adequately describe the child's difficulties in performing auditory tasks. Such measures of hearing disability are often restricted to tests of speech discrimination in the quiet. Problems with discriminating speech in noise, auditory attention, sound localisation, etc., often have to be assumed from the measures of impairment. Whilst there is an obvious relationship between the domains, the effects of hearing loss are individually variable (see Figure 1.1). Disability depends on communication strategy and environment. Educational disability thus requires an evaluation undertaken in the classroom or home. An integrated approach to paediatric assessment is therefore essential, with teachers specialising in this field of endeavour able to evaluate the implications of the diagnostic test results, the way they relate to each other, and their limitations. It is worth recalling that hearing is the perception of sound. It has long been established that the auditory cortex has little effect on the ability to hear pure tones (Kryter and Ades, 1943, cited by Northern and Downs, 1991) — and yet how often are children still labelled by audiogram descriptors?

Before considering individual tests it is worth defining some common semantics. Procedures are classified as subjective or objective - the latter test involuntary physiological activity. Despite their technical sophistication, they require subjective interpretation, which is often difficult. Subjective tests are based on voluntary responses and require modification according to age. Initially, they consist of observations of the child's responses, and are referred to as the *behavioural hearing tests*. However, all subjective tests are in fact behavioural. To enable an

3

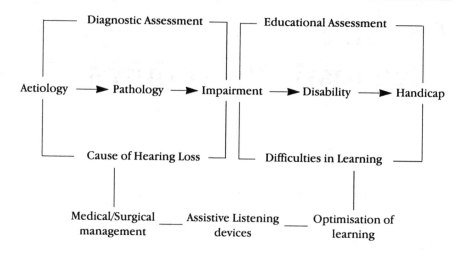

Figure 1.1 The relationship between diagnostic and educational audiology

evaluation of educational disability, hearing assessment must define the loss of sensitivity to a range of sounds. This requires a test battery approach whereby diagnostically useful information is integrated from several different types of test. The order of discussion facilitates this approach. It does not imply a hierarchy of worth, and the seemingly simpler tests should not be undervalued. This complementary relationship of the different tests is illustrated in the case studies.

Pure-tone audiometry

Until the audiometer was introduced in the early part of the present century, audiometry was undertaken with sets of tuning forks of different pitch. Koenig (1832-1901) tested a very wide range of tones with a set of 150 forks (Hinchcliffe, 1981). Although tuning forks remain clinically useful, the introduction of the audiometer has allowed this measurement of hearing for pure tones to be standardised. Audiometers deliver pure tones of calibrated pitch (frequency measured in Hertz, Hz) and loudness (intensity measured in decibels, dB).

Decibel scales are often misunderstood and misinterpreted and therefore require further explanation at this point. The decibel is a logarithmic ratio used to measure the intensity or power of a sound. It is convenient to measure the sound in this way as the range of audible sound is extensive, ranging from 20-200,000,000 microPascals (μP). Table 1.1 shows the relationship between the logarithmic decibel scale and sound pressure measurements made in μP. For each 20 decibel increase, the sound pressure increases 10 times. Physical measurements of sound intensity are therefore made in dBSPL (dB sound pressure level) with an internationally agreed reference point of 20 μP, corresponding to the threshold of 'normal' hearing at 1 kHz.

Table 1.1 Sound pressure levels measured in dBSPL and μP

microPascals	dBSPL	Example of sound
200,000,000	140	Rocket taking off
20,000,000	120	Aircraft taking off
2,000,000	100	Pneumatic drill
200,000	80	Noise inside a lorry
20,000	60	Conversational speech
2,000	40	Quiet speech
200	20	Birdsong
20	0	1 kHz pure-tone just audible

There are a variety of decibel scales used in many applications of sound intensity measurement, each having a different reference zero. It is therefore important to recognise which scale is being used. In audiology the three most commonly used scales are dBSPL, dBA and dBHL (dB hearing level). The human ear is most sensitive to frequencies between 500 Hz and 4 kHz. In other words, more sound energy is required for us to hear low frequency sounds below 500 Hz and high frequency sounds above 4 kHz. In pure-tone audiometry, normal hearing thresholds measured in dBSPL would vary with frequency. A reference level has therefore been defined whereby 0 dBHL represents normal hearing at each audiometric frequency (based on the hearing of otologically normal adults). It is possible to convert dBHL to dBSPL by using appropriate conversion factors as seen in Table 1.2.

Table 1.2 Conversion factors from dBHL and dBA to dBSPL

Frequency	dBHL to dBSPL (TDH39/MX41AR cushion)	dBA to dBSPL
250	+25.5	+9
500	+11.5	+3
1000	+7	0
2000	+9	−1
4000	+9.5	−1
8000	+13	+1

In audiology, free-field sound measurements are made in dBSPL or in dBA using a sound level meter (SLM). The 'A' weighting scale on an SLM is also designed to reflect the sensitivity of the human ear and the reference level varies with frequency. A minimal level of 30 dBA represents normal hearing across the frequency range in free-field measurements of hearing. Confusion can arise, for example, if results of an infant distraction test presented in dBA are considered to be comparable with audiometric thresholds measured in dBHL. The effects of room acoustics, position of the sound source and the use of frequency modulated (warble) tones cannot be disregarded when comparing free-field with closed circuit measurements. Conversion factors from dBA or dBSPL to dBHL have been suggested by several authors and these are summarised in Table 1.3. The variability inherent between the figures demonstrates the difficulties involved in converting free-field measurements to an approximation of the closed circuit measurements. Free-field measurements are therefore most usefully presented in the decibel scale on which they were measured.

Table 1.3 Conversion factors from free-field measurements made in dBA and dBSPL to dBHL

Frequency	250	500	1000	2000	4000
dBA to dBHL					
Chiveralls (1974)	−15	−11	−7	−8	−8
Nolan (1978)	−17	−8.5	−7	−10	−10.5
Lutman and McCormick (1987)	−3	−3	−4	−2	+3
dBSPL to dBHL					
(45 degrees azimuth)					
Morgan et al (1979)	+20	+8	+4	+4	−4.5

The term pure-tone audiometry applied to this cohort refers almost exclusively to the assessment of hearing sensitivity. This is measured by the quietest sounds that can be heard with this level being termed the *threshold of hearing*. It is more precisely defined as the point at which the pure tone is audible in 50% of presentations. The air conduction threshold is measured for tones delivered by headphones placed on the ears; the bone conduction threshold is measured for tones delivered by a vibrator placed on the mastoid bone. The thresholds are graphically plotted on the audiogram with the intensity in dBHL on the Y-axis, and the frequencies from 125 Hz to 8 kHz being marked at octave intervals on the X-axis. The standard audiogram format (BSA, 1989) is illustrated in Figure 1.2.

The measurement of hearing threshold

There are several procedures for measuring hearing threshold. They elicit slightly different results, but the procedure that has been accepted as standard is the Hughson-Westlake technique (1944) described by Carhart and Jerger (1959). This can be found in detail in BSA recommended procedures (1981b). It is also known as the '10 down - 5 up' procedure.

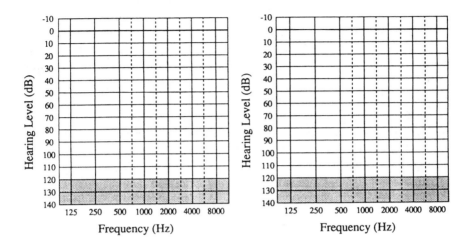

Figure 1.2 The pure-tone audiogram (BSA, 1989)

A 1 kHz pure tone is presented at 40 dB above expected threshold and the subject is asked to respond, usually by pressing a button. When a clear response is obtained, the sound level is decreased in 10 dB steps until there is no longer a response. The intensity of the tone is then increased in 5 dB steps until a positive response is again achieved. This point is checked by decreasing 10 dB and once more increasing in 5 dB steps. The subject's threshold is the quietest level at which there is a response in at least half of the ascending trials, with a minimum of two responses at this level.

This procedure is repeated at 2000, 4000, 8000, 500, 250 Hz for each ear. The subjective impression of threshold is the point of uncertainty. Thresholds can vary on repeat testing, particularly if they are undertaken by different testers employing different audiometers. Test-retest variability can be as much as 15 dB at any one frequency (Brasier, 1974). Young children also exhibit test-retest variability and there are some difficulties in assessing normal values of hearing threshold in this age group. It is not surprising therefore that children respond at levels slightly above threshold and various studies have shown an improvement in threshold with increasing age. However, any apparent 'improvement' must be dependent upon test technique and attention raising, rather than increased auditory acuity. In any event such improvements are small.

Interpretation of the audiogram

The audiogram provides information about both the degree and type of hearing loss. Tones delivered by the headphones pass through the outer and middle ears before being transduced by the inner ear. Thus air conduction thresholds are affected by dysfunction in any part of the ear, and measure the total degree of hearing loss. The audiometric degree of hearing loss may be described, for convenience, using the terms agreed by the BSA and BATOD (1988). They are detailed in Table 1.4. The audiometric descriptors are based on the pure-tone thresholds averaged between 250 Hz and 4 kHz, and thus it is often useful to employ an additional descriptor of configuration, e.g., a profound high frequency hearing loss, or a mild mid frequency impairment. However the caution that "the descriptors do not imply a classification of function or educational attainment or potential" should be noted. The terms describe the audiogram and not the child.

Table 1.4 Descriptors for pure-tone audiograms (BSA and BATOD, 1988)

Degree of hearing loss	hearing level (dBHL)
Normal	0-19
Mild	20-40
Moderate	41-70
Severe	71-95
Profound	95+

Tones delivered by the bone conductor are transmitted directly to the cochlea. The bone conduction thresholds are affected when there is a loss of inner ear hearing. By measuring both the air and bone conduction thresholds the type of hearing loss may be defined. The difference between the air and bone conduction thresholds reveals the presence of an 'air–bone gap'. An air–bone gap of 15 dB or more is considered significant.

- A conductive hearing loss is present when bone conduction is normal and air conduction thresholds are impaired.
- A sensorineural hearing loss is present when both air and bone conduction thresholds are equally impaired.
- A mixed hearing loss is present when both the air and bone conduction thresholds are impaired, and there is an additional superimposed air–bone gap.

This use of both air and bone conduction to define the type of hearing loss is illustrated in Figure 1.3.

Examples of simple unmasked audiograms, illustrating types and degrees of loss are illustrated in Figure 1.4. Before these are inspected, the symbols currently recommended (BSA, 1989) for use in pure-tone audiometry require consideration. These are detailed in Figure 1.5. It is, however, worth noting that this symbol system is not universally employed, and the legend should be carefully checked before reading an audiogram.

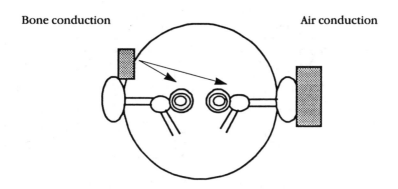

Figure 1.3 The use of air and bone conduction to define the type of hearing loss

Vibrotactile thresholds

Interpretation of the audiogram also requires consideration of the intensity level at which an individual might feel the vibration of the sound stimulus. These vibrotactile thresholds vary between individuals but the usual range at different frequencies is detailed in Table 1.5 (Boothroyd and Cawkwell, 1970).

Vibrotactile thresholds for bone conduction at 250 Hz must be considered a possibility at 20 dBHL. Audiogram 'c' illustrated in Figure 1.4 could be misinterpreted as a mixed hearing loss. Such artefacts caused by tactile rather than auditory stimulation are not found above 1 kHz. However even at these higher frequencies, problems of interpretation are caused by the output limitation of bone vibrators. In many audiometers, bone conductor output is limited to 70 dB. This limitation, plus the tactile artefacts present up to 1 kHz, restricts the ability of pure-tone audiometry to define the presence of a conductive component to a severe hearing loss. Further tests are necessary to assess whether there is a middle ear component to such losses.

Table 1.5 Vibrotactile thresholds at different frequencies

Frequency (Hz)	250	500	1000	2000	4000
Air conduction threshold (dBHL)	80-110	100-120	120-130	-	-
Bone conduction threshold (dBHL)	20-40	55-70	80-85	-	-

Masking in pure-tone audiometry

The audiograms illustrated in Figure 1.4 were all unmasked. However, further inspection demonstrates that the hearing losses illustrated are symmetrical between the ears. When account is also taken of the vibrotactile thresholds, there is an absence of a significant air–bone gap.

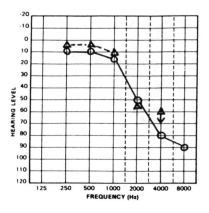
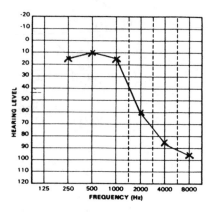

Audiogram 'a' - A severe high frequency sensorineural hearing loss in both ears.

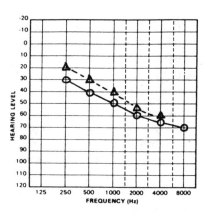
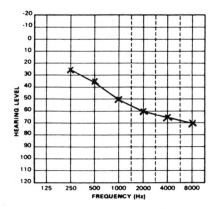

Audiogram 'b' - A mild to moderate sensorineural hearing loss in both ears.

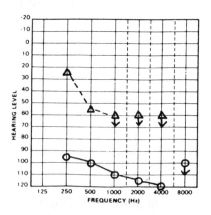
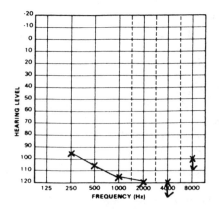

Audiogram 'c' - A profound sensorineural hearing loss in both ears.

Figure 1.4 Some examples of simple unmasked audiograms

		RIGHT EAR	LEFT EAR
A/C	unmasked or masked (true threshold)	○	✕
A/C	unmasked – possible shadow threshold	●	⊼
A/C	masked – no change after masking	◓	⋏
B/C	unmasked	△	△
B/C	masked	[	]

Figure 1.5 The symbols currently recommended for use in pure-tone audiometry (BSA, 1989)

Problems occur with both air and bone conduction threshold measurements when there is a difference in hearing between the ears. These problems will be discussed in turn.

Masking in air conduction testing

When the pure-tone stimulus is transmitted to the ear by air conduction via the headphones, the sound energy causes the skull to vibrate and the sound can cross the skull to the opposite cochlea. The sound energy that is lost as it crosses the skull is known as **interaural attenuation**. The sound energy lost varies from 40 to 85 dB using the standard air conduction headphones (Smith and Markides, 1981). Thus a tone of 40 dB delivered to an ear being tested may just be heard by a normally sensitive cochlea in the opposite non-test ear (Figure 1.6a), and a false response may be obtained. Louder tones delivered to the test ear may be heard at suprathreshold levels in the opposite ear (Figure 1.6b).

The fact that the response comes from the better hearing cochlea of the non-test ear would not be apparent, and such cross-over of the stimulus can give a complete shadow curve audiogram. This shadow curve has in fact been obtained from the non-test ear. A hearing loss in the test ear may thus be readily disguised. An example of such a shadow curve can be seen in Figure 1.7.

This problem is remedied by the application of an effective masking noise to the better hearing non-test ear. The application of continuous narrow-band masking noise to the non-test ear prevents the tone that has crossed over from being heard. **Masking is needed during air conduction testing at any frequency where there is a difference of 40 dB or more between the air conduction threshold of the poorer hearing test ear and the bone conduction threshold of the non-test ear.**

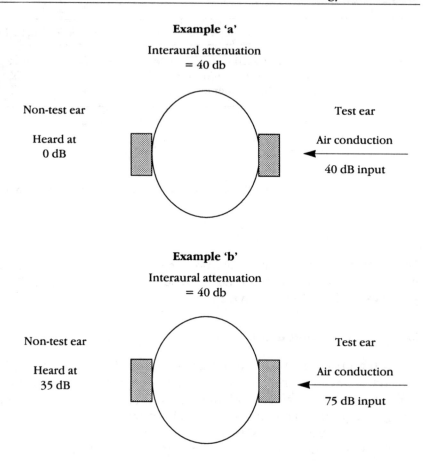

Example 'a'

Interaural attenuation
= 40 db

Non-test ear   Test ear

Heard at   Air conduction
0 dB
                                                              40 dB input

Example 'b'

Interaural attenuation
= 40 db

Non-test ear   Test ear

Heard at   Air conduction
35 dB
                                                              75 dB input

Figure 1.6 Illustration of interaural attenuation in air conduction testing

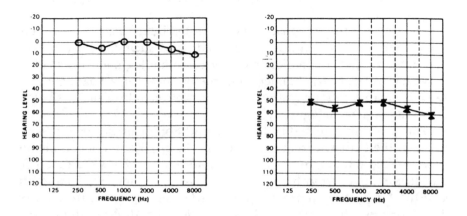

Figure 1.7 An example of a possible shadow curve on the left with normal hearing in the right ear

It is important that the correct amount of masking is used, and although procedural details are not discussed, they are fully detailed in the BSA recommendations (1986). However, tests which require masking need to be identified as such – without the application of masking in the audiogram illustrated in Figure 1.7, it is not possible to know the true hearing level in the left ear. After correctly masking the non-test ear, a profound hearing loss on the left could be revealed as shown in Figure 1.8.

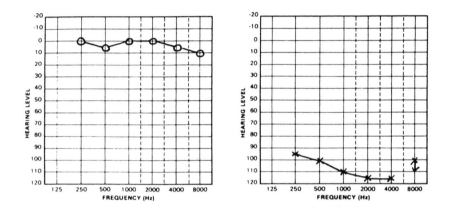

Figure 1.8 Profound deafness revealed in the left ear following masking

Alternatively, masking may make no difference as shown in Figure 1.9. The different symbols used in Figures 1.7, 1.8 and 1.9 illustrate how masking has been used.

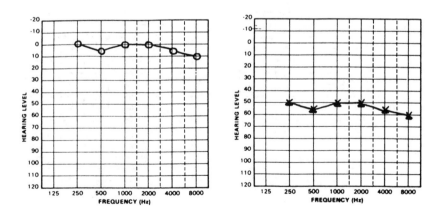

Figure 1.9 A moderate hearing loss is confirmed following masking

Masking in bone conduction testing

The interpretation of bone conduction thresholds which have been unmasked is even more open to error. Interaural attenuation in bone conduction varies between individuals and with frequency. However, there may be minimal attenuation in some children, and a bone vibrator placed on one mastoid may stimulate both cochleae equally (Figure 1.10).

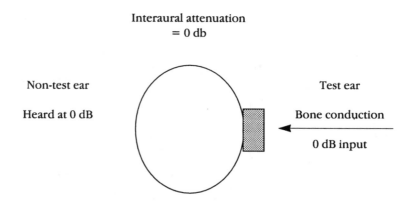

Figure 1.10 Illustration of interaural attenuation in bone conduction testing

Figure 1.11 illustrates an audiogram with a mild loss in one ear. Unmasked bone conduction only tells us that there is one normally hearing cochlea, and this could be in either ear. Because both cochleae may be stimulated by a bone vibrator placed on either ear it is reasonable to assume that the inner ear hearing of the ear under test can only be measured if masking has been applied to the non-test ear.

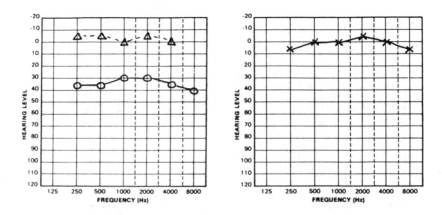

Figure 1.11 An example of a mild hearing loss on the right with normal hearing on the left and unmasked bone conduction

However it is not always necessary to mask when measuring bone conduction thresholds, and masking is only required if the test ear could show a greater impairment of inner ear function. This situation is only present when there is a significant air–bone gap in the test ear. **Masking is needed during bone conduction testing at any frequency where there is an air–bone gap with the unmasked bone conduction threshold being greater than 10 dB better than the air conduction threshold.** In this example masking the better hearing ear may reveal the mild unilateral loss to be sensorineural as shown in Figure 1.12.

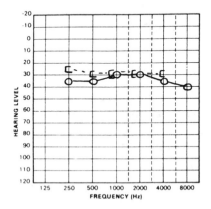 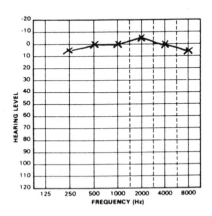

Figure 1.12 A mild sensorineural hearing loss in the right ear demonstrated by the application of masking to the left ear

Masking dilemmas

Masking is therefore essential to evaluate hearing correctly. However, an important limitation of pure-tone audiometry is that masking dilemmas may occur and these may prevent the measurement of the true hearing thresholds. Masking dilemmas result from over-masking. Such dilemmas are by no means rare in paediatric practice and an example of an audiogram where over-masking would occur can be seen in Figure 1.13. Applying the rules noted above, both air and bone conduction thresholds require masking to be applied to the non-test ear. However the masking levels will need to be very high to be audible and could then cross over to the cochlea of the test ear. If the cochlea in the test ear has normal sensitivity, the threshold in this ear is affected because of over-masking. Discrepant results may therefore be obtained and true thresholds may be difficult to establish when there is a large bilateral conductive hearing loss.

In Figure 1.13 it is possible that the child has no hearing at all in one ear, with normal cochlear function and a large conductive loss present in the hearing ear. Unfortunately, audiometry cannot determine which is the dead ear.

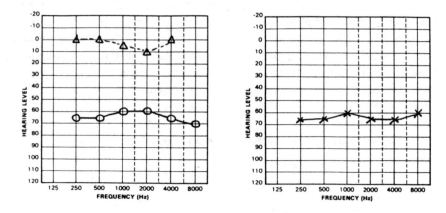

Figure 1.13 An example of an audiogram presenting a masking dilemma

To reduce the problem of over-masking, insert earphones may be used to deliver the masking noise. These may significantly reduce the cross over of masking noise to the test ear (Killion et al., 1985). Alternative audiometric tests such as the modified Rainville procedure may also assist with such dilemmas (Rainville, 1959; Jerger and Tillman, 1960), but they are difficult to use with children. Other examinations within the test battery are required to establish pathology.

It is important that such difficulties in measuring hearing threshold are fully appreciated as there is likely to be an impairment/disability mismatch. Those involved in real life assessments should recognise the presence of such mismatches. Masking dilemmas also illustrate an additional and equally important principle; pure-tone audiometry cannot always establish with certainty the level of impairment in both ears. However, children themselves after the age of 7 years increasingly recognise the presence of a dead ear (Watkin et al., 1990). Talking to the child may be the simplest (and possibly the only) way of resolving such dilemmas.

Play audiometry

Once a child is able to respond to sounds by performing a task, pure-tone audiometry should be possible through play. Initially the child needs to be conditioned to respond appropriately to the tones. In the younger child such conditioning is more readily achieved by employing stimuli within a calibrated sound field. The frequency modulation afforded by warble tones provides a more consistent intensity level in a sound field (Walker et al., 1984). The intensity level at a set position within the sound field is measured for each test frequency using a sound level meter. Unfortunately, difficulties in precise positioning and other variables may necessitate the measurement of sound levels at the child's ear during the test. However, generally this simply adds to procedural confusion.

Decibel scales have been dealt with elsewhere, but for sound field measurements dBA or dBSPL are used. The dBA scale is most commonly used in clinical practice to measure the results of play audiometry. There are no national or international standards, but the ASHA (1991) report, which is the outcome of a working group set up to look at sound field calibration, recommended the use of dBSPL.

Conditioning a young child within a sound field can be readily undertaken by a tester working alone. The test should flow naturally from the other behavioural hearing tests undertaken, and most children aged 30 months and over should be able to comply with the test procedures. However, if the test is to progress to the measurement of reliable pure-tone thresholds, it is the authors' experience that two testers working together gain optimal results. The test set-up is illustrated in Figures 1.14 and 1.15.

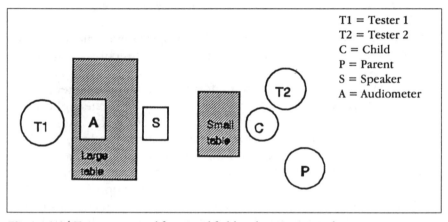

Figure 1.14 Test set-up used for sound field and pure-tone audiometry

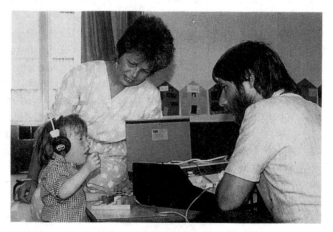

Figure 1.15 Photograph of a child performing play audiometry

Tester 1 (T1) operates the audiometer with the second tester (T2) sitting with the child at a small table on his level. The parent should be allowed to remain close to the child. A variety of toys which facilitate the observation of a conditioned response to the sound stimuli should be available, for example, balls on stick, pegs in board, men in boat, etc. T2 gains a rapport with the child through the toys, and conditions appropriate play responses to the stimuli, such as "When the little man makes a noise we put him in the boat". This chapter provides only the briefest glimpse into the techniques involved. However two practical errors are so often encountered as to be worthy of note:

- Verbal explanations should be kept to a minimum. A short viewing of the video "A Word in Your Ear" (1992) convinces that ferrets can be readily conditioned to respond to sounds without the use of language.
- The initial sounds which are employed to teach the child the procedure must be comfortably above the hearing threshold.

When the child is able to respond appropriately to the signal, the sound level can be reduced to threshold and a 'free-field' audiogram obtained.

Sound field testing only reveals information about the better hearing ear and the child should be encouraged to wear the headphones. A single headphone can be used and the child asked to "listen on the telephone". Each ear can be tested separately if the headphone is held firmly against the ear. The child may then be willing to accept the headset. In a similar way the bone conductor can be held against the mastoid without the use of the headband. A flexible approach is needed. If the free-field results were normal, most information may be gained by testing the 1 kHz response in each ear first to exclude a unilateral hearing loss. If, on the other hand, the free-field results demonstrated a moderate or severe hearing loss, it might be most useful to start with bone conduction to determine the nature of the hearing loss. T1 has to compromise between speed and accuracy, as the child's attention may be short-lived. Descending in 20 dB steps is acceptable and employing the '10 down 5 up' procedure to check below a threshold of 20 dBHL is generally less useful than obtaining thresholds to a wider variety of frequencies. Longer intervals between tone presentations should be used to check for reliability. Initially a three-point audiogram is attempted, and if the child continues to be attentive, the remaining frequencies can be tested. Testers require experience and effective teamwork to get the best results from the child. The two testers can bring different skills to the situation and even the most 'difficult to test' children should produce reliable masked audiograms well before school entry. Despite the discussed limitations, the achievement of a reliable pure-tone audiogram is a milestone in the management of the hearing-impaired child.

Pure-tone sweep testing

Although the current chapter concerns the diagnostic testing of hearing, it is necessary for teachers to be aware of the hearing screening tests undertaken at school entry or during the first year of primary education. The test recommended by the Joint Working Party on Child Health Surveillance (Hall, 1996) is a modified pure-tone audiogram performed at fixed intensity level. This method of pure-tone audiometry is known as the 'sweep test'. Even in districts where the methods of identifying hearing loss in early childhood have demonstrable success, the school sweep test is still necessary to identify those children with unilateral sensorineural deafness, and those with milder losses (Watkin, 1991). A small number of the latter will be sensorineural in type, but the overwhelming majority of children identified by such screens suffer from otitis media with effusion (OME). Difficulties arise with the test because the criteria for failure depend mainly on the environmental noise within the school. If excessively stringent criteria are chosen, the majority of children fail the test. Thus in many schools a sweep through the frequencies at 25 or even 30 dBHL is undertaken, and diagnostic assessment may be initiated only when there is failure at more than one frequency. Inevitably such a test cannot be very sensitive and those children with a very mild loss remain unidentified by the procedure. If there remains any suspicion that a child's hearing is impaired, the child should be referred for a diagnostic assessment, irrespective of the results of the school screen.

Visual reinforcement audiometry

Over the last 30 years, visual reinforcement audiometry (VRA) has been developed as a behavioural technique widely used for testing the hearing of infants and young children. It can be employed clinically to measure the hearing thresholds of 6 month old infants, with the upper range extending to the age when play audiometry becomes possible. The technique is appropriate for children who are not developmentally ready to be 'conditioned' to respond to stimuli by performing an appropriate play task. It is undoubtedly a powerful audiological tool, which is now becoming more widely used. This procedure is discussed in detail by Coninx and Moore in Chapter 3. Procedural details have been presented in detail by Bamford and McSporran (1993). The test set-up is illustrated in Figure 1.16.

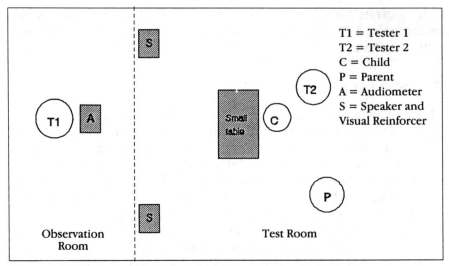

Figure 1.16 Test set-up used for visual reinforcement audiology

The sound stimuli can also be presented in different ways:

- via standard headphones,
- via a bone conductor,
- via insert earphones (tubephones),
- through the child's own earmoulds in hearing aid evaluation.

VRA and insert earphones

It is possible to assess each ear separately using VRA, and herein lies its advantage over the behavioural hearing tests undertaken at this age. The ears can be audiologically separated for VRA by continuing to use the speaker in the sound field, whilst applying narrow band masking to the non-test ear via an ear insert. However, if it is possible to apply masking through an insert earphone, such an intrusion may also be tolerated for delivering a tonal stimulus. Standard headphones could be used, but are poorly tolerated even by many older children.

The use of insert earphones to undertake VRA has been described in detail by Bamford and McSporran (1993). They have been shown to be comparable to standard TDH headphones when calibrated for the audiometer in use (Borton et al., 1989; Frank and Vavrek, 1992). Correction factors must be applied to convert the dial setting of the audiometer to dBSPL at the child's ear. These are provided by the manufacturer, but more precise measurements can be made by calculating the correction factors using a hearing aid test box and HA2 (2cc) coupler. Insert earphones provide frequency specific information about each ear and their use with VRA allows the plotting of an audiogram even in children as young as 5 to 7 months (Talbott, 1987).

The earphones include a foam eartip which is inserted into the child's external auditory canal. The eartip is connected to a sound transducer by a tube, and the transducers for both ears are clipped to the child's clothes. For the child already wearing hearing aids, it is possible to attach the earmoulds directly to the tube conveying sound from the transducer. This is usually readily accepted by the child who is used to wearing earmoulds, enabling the audiologist to work towards obtaining ear-specific information at an early age.

Another advantage is in hearing aid selection and evaluation. It is possible to measure the dBSPL in the child's ear canal with a probe tube microphone at each threshold estimate, and this can be used to select gain and maximum output targets (Seewald, 1992).

The behavioural hearing tests

Behavioural observation audiometry

Behavioural observation audiometry (BOA) is an assessment of behavioural reaction to sound under structured conditions. It is generally employed with infants under 6 months of age, or with developmentally delayed children who are not sitting and cannot be tested by the infant distraction test or VRA (Thompson and Weber, 1974). It is most important to appreciate that, unlike most other tests, BOA measures auditory responsiveness and is not a test of threshold. It relies on a sound stimulus triggering an observable reaction from the child. The behavioural response has to be subjectively time locked to the stimulus.

Various responses to sound occur in early infancy. BOA employs human observation of responses; the types of behaviour that may be observed are:

- increased or decreased sucking movements,
- stilling to the sound or quietening if vocalising,
- eye-widening or eye-blinking,
- eye movement or inclination of the head towards the direction of the sound,
- arousal from sleep,
- increased movement of limbs.

The responsiveness of the child varies with age and the stimulus used. Speech is the most effective stimulus, and bands of noise are more effective than pure tones (Thompson and Thompson, 1972; Eisenberg, 1983). This increased responsiveness with increased bandwidth presents a dilemma with the infant distraction test and is further discussed within that section. Northern and Down's auditory behaviour index (1984) usefully summarises the expected response of infants to noisemakers, warble tones and speech. Responses are observable to speech at significantly quieter levels than to tones in the first 4 months of life. The infant's responsiveness to quieter stimuli increases with increasing age. The expected responses also change with age. Thus the eye-widening, stirring response of a neonate develops into a rudimentary head turn by 4 months, and into direct localisation of sound on the horizontal plane by 7 months.

However, observation of auditory behaviour is subject to many difficulties. The response is influenced by the arousal state and habituates rapidly. There is thus poor test-retest repeatability. Thompson and Weber (1974) examined this intrasubject variability. They found that the responsiveness to sound rapidly reduced with repeated presentation. Thus BOA is only possible for a very limited number of sound presentations. This limits its clinical usefulness. They also examined the variability of response between different babies and found enormous intersubject variability. This was as much as 65 dBSPL in babies aged from 3 to 5 months — once again severely restricting clinical usefulness.

Another problem is the observer's subjective interpretation of the 'response'. Gans and Flexer (1982) demonstrated bias when testing multiply handicapped children with this technique. Gans (1987) and Gans and Gans (1993) described a modified BOA procedure in which the child was videotaped during the test session. Sound and no-sound trials were presented through a loudspeaker using synthesised speech and narrow-band noise at known intensity levels. The stimulus was masked out on play-back so the judges were blind to the presence or absence of the sound. The behavioural changes were judged for certainty by two examiners using a six-point scale adapted from Bench et al. (1976). This technique decreases the subjectivity of the procedure and was useful in the assessment of profoundly multiply handicapped children (Gans and Gans, 1993).

The auropalpebral reflex (APR)

One of the behavioural observations that can usefully be made is to elicit the APR. As early as 1946, Froeschels and Beebe described it as the cochleopalpebral reflex. The APR is an involuntary eye-blink in response to a loud auditory signal, but it is often combined with a much larger startle response and even a head jerk. It can be readily observed in most normally hearing babies, children and indeed adults, in response to a loud "Ba!" usually presented at 80 dBA. When absent, increasing the stimulus may elicit a response. Usually two testers are employed, one to make the sound about 6 inches behind the baby's ear with the mouth covered, and the other to observe the baby's reaction. The baby should initially be in a relaxed state on the parent's lap, and the parent should be warned about the ensuing stimulus and advised not to react if possible. The observer may need to attenuate the sound by blocking her ears to prevent her own involuntary eye-blink! The test is usually carried out on each side separately, but habituation occurs quite quickly and repeated attempts to elicit a response are not worthwhile.

The information the APR provides is limited:

- If the APR is present at normal levels the infant could still have a mild or moderate recruiting hearing loss, or indeed a high frequency hearing loss.
- In cases of conductive hearing loss it may be absent or a louder stimulus may be required.
- It is absent in severe or profound deafness.
- It has been noted that in some infants with neurological damage the APR is consistently absent (Froding, 1960; Tucker and Battacharya, 1992).

As in other neonatal behavioural observations, the ability to elicit an APR is highly dependent upon the pre-stimulus state of the baby. It may therefore be difficult to elicit even in a normally hearing neonate.

BOA including APR is usefully employed during the first half of infancy and in the behavioural assessment of multiply handicapped children who are not developmentally able to perform in distraction testing or VRA. The latter group of children may need to be assessed over an extended period of time and in an environment which is familiar to them where they are relaxed. The visiting teacher of the deaf may be able usefully to assess the child either at home or in school using voice sounds, music or familiar sound stimuli. For example it may be possible to observe a stilling or quieting to a musical toy at home, and although the stimulus is broad-band (i.e., not frequency specific), it can give useful information that may not be readily available in the clinic setting.

To reduce observer subjectivity, conditions need to be controlled and it is clearly helpful to make use of video recording. However, the fact that BOA does not allow for threshold measurement is inherent and unassailable. Reliable and repeatable responses are difficult to obtain, and the difficulties experienced by professional observers of auditory behaviour in early infancy explain why deafness is so long hidden from some parents.

The infant distraction test

The infant distraction test is one of several techniques suitable for testing auditory behaviour during the second half of infancy. Some 25 years after the initial description (Ewing and Ewing, 1944), it was adopted as a universal screen by community child health services throughout the UK. Simple in concept, but deceptively difficult to apply sensitively, the test has provoked considerable debate.

The test is based on the infant's maturing auditory behaviour. By 7 months' developmental age, sounds are localised at ear level on the horizontal plane. This, combined with postural maturation and development of vision and social behaviour, facilitates the undertaking of the test during the second half of infancy. Although sound localisation has started to develop before this age, the technique is less specific before 7 months of age. Sound localisation can also be assessed after infancy and the test is still useful in the second year of life. However, test techniques have to be adapted in the latter case.

Auditory behaviour is dependent upon the relationship of the different aspects of development, and the test cannot measure hearing in isolation. Within a screening context, this has made the test of variable validity. However it remains a powerful diagnostic tool when properly applied by paediatric audiologists. Problems of test methodology have been perceptively investigated by McCormick, and further details should be sought by those undertaking the test (McCormick, 1988). The following is a brief procedural account.

The test set-up is illustrated in Figure 1.17. Two trained testers are required. The infant is seated on the parent's knee, facing forward in an erect position, allowing full head turns toward the sound source. The distracter is situated in the front and has the role of controlling the infant's attention. Offering the required level of distraction without engrossing the infant requires practice and experience. Ideally the distracter should be positioned behind a low table and should persuade the baby to focus attention on a small object on the table. The object is covered. The tester positioned behind the mother presents the sound stimulus during a brief window of opportunity which follows the baby's loss of interest in the covered object. The localisation response is observed by the distracter. Although the sound stimulus will not be localised at every presentation, valid responses must be repeatable and false turns eliminated with 'no-sound trials'. In a screening programme, responses should be to sound stimuli at a 'minimal level' of 30 dBA, whereas in a diagnostic clinic the threshold of localisation is measured.

The test stimuli employed have changed over the years and since the early methodological descriptions. Traditionally noisemakers and voice have been used in a screening situation, and many consider that infants are more responsive to these sounds. The frequency composition of the various stimuli are detailed in Table 1.6. There are some disadvantages in using such stimuli both for screening and measurement of hearing threshold. Those screening infant hearing have to ensure that the sounds presented are at the 'minimal level', and frequency specificity is lost when localisation thresholds are measured with the use of increased sound intensities.

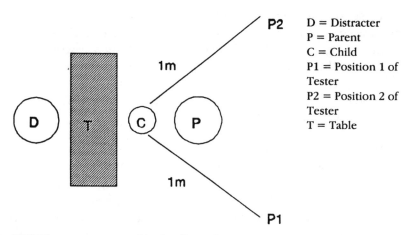

Figure 1.17 The test set-up used in the distraction test

McCormick considers that using a hand held warble tone generator provides a more accurate stimulus of known intensity and frequency. This is unarguably the case. However there is some debate about the responsiveness of infants to such tones. Northern and Downs' auditory behaviour index (see section on BOA) states that infants of 7—9 months localise noisemakers at 30–40 dBSPL and warble tones at 45 dBHL. Mendel (1968), and subsequently Eisenberg (1983) confirmed that bandwidth and patterning are two of the characteristics of the stimuli that affect behavioural responses to sound in infancy. McCormick (1988) considers that increased responsiveness to the traditional noisemakers is in fact due to loss of frequency specificity. In practice, both sound sources offer advantages, and in diagnostic clinics both are used.

Table 1.6 The frequency specificity of traditional sound stimuli employed in the infant distraction test

Stimuli used in the IDT: frequency composition at 30 dBA in Hz.	
"oo"	less than 500 Hz
Sibilant "s"	more than 3 kHz
G chime bar	1600 Hz
C chime bar	512 Hz
Manchester Rattle	8-10 kHz

Although a seemingly simple test to carry out it requires training and experience to be used effectively, the test procedure having to be stringently adhered to as simple procedural errors can be costly. Testers have to be vigilant to avoid:

- Presenting the sound stimulus within the baby's peripheral vision.
- Presenting the sounds at incorrect levels.

- Presenting sounds of undefined or broad-band frequency.
- Casting shadows that can alert the baby to the tester's presence.
- Attracting the baby by other sensory stimuli such as strong perfume.
- Cueing the presence of the tester by visual communication between the tester and distracter.
- Positioning the baby in front of a reflective surface where he can see the tester.

Despite methodological improvements, the distraction test has not been sensitive as a screen (Martin et al., 1981; Brown et al., 1989; Robertson et al., 1995). However, problems other than the test itself have often significantly contributed to the poor performance. Martin et al. measured the age of identification of deafness in the UK when the distraction screen was not being employed universally, Brown et al. recorded the failure of the screen when district coverage was barely above 50%, and Robertson et al. noted the complex interplay of different factors contributing to impaired screen sensitivity. The screen can undoubtedly be successful (McCormick et al., 1984; Watkin, 1991), but even so it is salutary to read parental comments about its worth (NDCS, 1983; Robinson, 1987).

Test difficulties arise from the infant's increasing state of 'purposeful alertness'. Hearing is integrated with the other senses of vision, olfaction and touch. It is impossible for the infant to ignore these cues and unless procedure is strictly adhered to, inadvertent presentation of these stimuli invalidates the test result. A fundamental difficulty is the visual insatiability of the hearing impaired infant. Inevitably the greatest test experience has been with hearing babies, and this population has sensory development that can be appropriately assessed by the test. Those babies with impaired hearing continually visually search, and use all sensory inputs to detect seemingly imperceptible cues. This makes the test much more difficult to apply to the targeted population. Thus, half a century after its initial description, improvements in test methodology are still being made.

Co-operative tests

The 'co-operative' test was another behavioural test first described by Ewing and Ewing (1944). Like other similar procedures employed at this age, the child's developing use of language is utilised. Using simple toys, the child is encouraged to follow commands such as "give this to Mummy", "give it to teddy" and "put in on the table". Usually three commands are established at conversational voice level with additional visual cues being available to the child. The tester's voice is then reduced to a level of 40 dBA and the commands given out of vision. If the child does not respond, the voice level is raised and the response level is measured on a sound level meter in dBA. The test is completed by distraction testing for mid and high frequency stimuli with the child remaining in the same position.

Although simple in essence, the test requires a high level of skill in handling children. Most audiologists continue to search in vain for the co-operative 2 year old. It has therefore fallen from favour and is not very often used in diagnostic assessment, because more useful information is obtained by sound field testing. The test, along with assessment of response to other commands, can be a useful precursor to other procedures and is simple to implement if used casually. When rapport is being gained with the child (usually whilst the parent is giving the history), the commands can be given without it appearing to be a distinct and separate test procedure. Additionally in the 2 year old who habituates rapidly to VRA and who cannot yet condition for performance testing, the co-operative test may reveal a limited amount of information, which may still be of diagnostic importance.

The performance test

The Ewings also described the performance test – known colloquially as the 'go-game'. The technique is appropriately employed with children aged from 27 to 30 months. In this test the child is conditioned to perform a play task to a verbal stimulus "go!". Suitable play tasks are detailed in the section on play audiometry. The child is conditioned in vision with an initial voice level of 60 dBA. This can be done simply by demonstration and the test is therefore useful where language difficulties complicate the test routine. When the child is conditioned and responding reliably to the stimulus, the tester's voice level should be reduced to 35 dBA and visual clues removed. Any facial movement could give a visual clue and therefore this test is best undertaken with the tester positioned at an angle of 45 degrees and 3 feet behind the child. The test may be undertaken from either side, although this does not necessarily audiologically separate the ears. If there is no response, the voice level is raised until the threshold of response is obtained. It is measured on a sound level meter. High frequency responses can be assessed using the same technique and by 'conditioning' the child to respond to a sibilant 's'. This can be achieved by saying "when the snake says 's' put the man in the boat". As in all tests, the responses obtained should be repeatable.

The test has little place in the diagnostic clinics of today. As a general rule, if the child is developmentally ready for the 'go-game', conditioning to other auditory stimuli will be possible – and much more informative. However the test facilitates a seamless delivery of diagnostic tests, and allows 'play audiometry' to flow naturally from the simpler Behavioural Hearing Tests. Performance testing with voice as the stimulus can also be useful if peripatetic teachers of the hearing-impaired and parents work on conditioning at home prior to the child's clinic appointment, when free-field or pure-tone audiometry will be undertaken. Certainly the test has the singular advantage of not requiring any test equipment, other than suitable toys that are commonly found in most homes.

Tests of speech perception

Since the sensitivity of a child's hearing will largely be judged by both parents and teachers on the ability to discriminate speech, the inclusion in every diagnostic assessment of a test of hearing for speech has high face validity. Traditionally such tests have been considered to assess speech discrimination, but more accurately, they test for speech recognition or perception.

The tests are valued because a primary function of the auditory system is speech perception, and therefore the use of speech stimuli seems more appropriate than psycho-acoustic tests employing tones. It is clear that measures of speech perception ability should employ speech as the signal (Boothroyd, 1991). However, the isolated monosyllabic tests usually employed as part of a routine diagnostic assessment are constrained in such a way that great weight is given to the peripheral hearing mechanism and very little to the central processes involved (Fry, 1961). A variety of speech tests are widely available. An all-purpose speech test does not exist and tests should be selected according to their purpose.

The purposes of speech testing

Speech tests are employed for a variety of reasons:

- Confirmation of the degree of hearing loss is required in paediatric practice where threshold uncertainty may exist. Speech is a meaningful stimulus for demonstrating the presence of the degree of impairment to parents, and this makes it a mandatory component of paediatric assessment.
- Identifying the type of hearing loss requires a test battery approach including the use of speech as a stimulus. Although there is considerable overlap, speech recognition generally differs according to whether the auditory dysfunction is conductive, sensory, neural or resulting from a disorder of central processing.
- Response to speech stimuli also assists in identifying non-organic hearing loss (NOHL). The incidence in children over the age of 7 years who were referred for diagnostic testing has been reported to be as high as 18% (Baldwin and Watkin, 1992). Although Barr's

presentation of NOHL is now over 35 years old (Barr, 1960), the case histories and discussion remain relevant today. Although it may be due to attention seeking behaviour, there is frequently deep psychological stress either within the home or school. Brooks and Geoghegan (1992) emphasised the long standing and deep seated psychological difficulties that may be present. Interestingly nearly all surveys have included children who were fitted with hearing aids or who required educational provision for their hearing loss. This itself demonstrates the diagnostic difficulties encountered.

- Educational and social handicap is dependent upon the disability in communication encountered in a variety of real world environments. Successful educational habilitation requires a realistic assessment of hearing disability as well as the measures of impairment available from diagnostic tests. Similarly hearing aid evaluation requires assessment of benefits or difficulties in real world communication.
- Auditory training requires systematic analysis of specific problem areas in speech recognition. A qualitative assessment of the individual speech features is required, with longitudinal analysis of error patterns. Although it has always clearly been a prerequisite for successful auditory training, such tests of feature perception have gained greater impetus with the habilitation offered to cochlear implantees.

Speech test variables

The principles behind the variables offered by different speech tests are outlined. These test principles are illustrated in Appendix A with reference to tests available and in current use in the UK; some of the tests used in North America are summarised in Appendix B. Individual test procedures are not described in detail.

Redundancy present in the test

Speech is a complex acoustic stimulus. Whilst the pure-tone audiogram measures hearing by frequency and intensity, the speech signal is three dimensional, requiring an additional assessment of temporal resolution. The frequently represented speech banana relates frequency to intensity but ignores the time domain. The fact that speech is not simply a sequence of discrete sounds poses problems in assessing the perception of the acoustic cues present. Additionally, perception of everyday speech is dependent on other cues used in parallel and simultaneously (Cutting and Pisoni, 1978).

Language is governed by rules of structure:

- The phoneme is the minimum information bearing unit of the speech stimulus. Phonological rules govern their combination as words.

- The arrangement of words in sentences is governed by the rules of syntax, and meaning is extracted by applying semantic rules.
- Additionally contextual and visual cues are invariably employed in the normal perception of speech (Summerfield and Foster, 1983).

There is thus a hierarchy of cues which allow deductions to be made even if the acoustic information is degraded by a reduced stimulus or the presence of background noise. With the message being conveyed simultaneously in these different ways, many of the cues available in everyday speech are redundant. The way in which the test material is constrained offers more or less redundancy to the listener. This constitutes one of the main test variables. The level of redundancy is also dependent upon the subject's knowledge of the test language. If the vocabulary employed in a test is outside a child's experience, the availability of cues is relatively reduced. To reduce the influence of perceptual abilities unrelated to hearing, items should be within the child's vocabulary. The hierarchy of increasing redundancy for the different tests is displayed in Appendix B3.

Test types

Tests of feature perception

These employ minimum redundancy to determine the use of specific acoustic cues. Test constraints facilitate analytical speech testing. Synthetic tests (e.g. THRIFT, Boothroyd, 1986) are being increasingly employed to measure speech features.

Monosyllable speech tests

These are less constrained than the tests designed to measure feature perception, but their reduced redundancy also dispenses with the higher linguistic levels.

The **Arthur Boothroyd (AB) lists** (Boothroyd, 1968) employing consonant-vowel-consonant (CVC) words. Redundancy in monosyllabic recognition may be further reduced by using nonsense syllables. However, children try to make sense of nonsense (Watson, 1957). The reader will understand well this dilemma.

The **Four-Alternative Auditory Feature (FAAF)** (Foster and Haggard, 1987) test is only usable with older children. The Two-Alternative Picture Pointing test (TAPP) (Haggard et al., 1984) is similar in concept to the FAAF. The test vocabulary is suitable for use with 5 year olds.

The **toy discrimination tests** of Kendal and McCormick employ words within the vocabulary of pre-school children. They facilitate speech testing on children aged from 30 months, and in some cases below. However, the vocabulary of even these simple tests has a degree of cultural bias.

The **E2L test** (Bellman and Marcuson, 1991) has been devised for use with children where English is a second language.

The **Manchester junior word lists** (Watson, 1957) employ words suitable for use with junior aged school children. Although Arthur Boothroyd (AB) word lists are often employed with children from around 6 or 7 years of age, a considerable number of the words are outside the usual vocabulary of children of this age. Watson (1957) also devised the **Manchester picture test**, allowing for the testing of more linguistically compromised children of this age.

The **Fry phonemically balanced word lists** (Fry, 1961) consist of 10 lists of 35 words. The test time required to administer these phonemically balanced lists precludes their use even with older children. Phonemic 'balancing' requires the frequency of the vowels and consonants contained in the tests to conform to the frequency distribution of sounds present in current English. Such phonemic balancing is not possible with limited test material and is thus not fully achieved in those tests employed with children. However the monosyllable tests are not intended to measure real life disability in the hearing of speech, and the need for them to be phonemically balanced is reduced.

Sentence tests

These provide a stimulus containing higher redundancy. They are thus more appropriate for assessing disability at a higher linguistic level. The use of continuous speech does not allow for ease of scoring. However sentence tests are usefully employed with children.

The **BKB sentence lists** (Bench, Kowal and Bamford, 1979) were based on the vocabulary and grammar of hearing-impaired children aged from 8 to 15 years. A simplified picture related BKB test is also available for children below 8 years.

Speech in noise tests

These add a further dimension useful for the more realistic assessment of hearing disability. The noise should have energy present across the speech spectrum. The amalgamation of speech from several speakers to form speech babble has high validity, but the difference between the speech signal and the babble differs across the frequency spectrum, and a single signal to noise (S/N) ratio is thus difficult to define.

Noise generated to have a spectrum similar to the long term speech spectrum facilitates the measurement of the S/N ration. Steady noise is also less likely to mask speech than noise which is intensity modulated.

The BKB sentence lists have been recorded against such modulated speech-spectrum-shaped noise as the **Sentence Identification in Noise Test**. The FAAF and **Two-Alternative Picture Pointing (TAPP)** tests are also used against such a noise background. An **automated McCormick toy test** (Palmer et al., 1991) allows speech testing against a noise background for pre-school children.

Audio-visual material

This is probably the most realistic predictor of disability in everyday communication. Live voice presentation with lip reading allows this, but there are problems inherent in such presentation, which are discussed below. The presentation of stimuli by video cassette allows greater test standardisation.

The **Four-Alternative Disability and Speechreading Test (FADAST)** (Summerfield and Foster, 1983) is similar to the FAAF test, but with the speaker displayed on screen. The **BKB lists** have also been recorded for audio-visual presentation (Rosen and Corcoran, 1982).

Subject response

Tests are also differentially constrained by the response format. The simplest, least constrained format is for the child to be instructed to repeat what was heard, guessing if necessary. Such tests have an open response format. Both the AB monosyllable word lists and the BKB sentences employ an open response format. There are obvious advantages in knowing what was heard by the child, but there are also disadvantages:

- Children will often try to grasp for meaning when a word is misheard. They may not say what they actually heard, especially if it does not seem appropriate or contextually correct (for instance, they may have heard dick for dig, but remain silent).
- Additionally many of the children who would be most usefully tested have delayed language development and errors of speech production.
- The tester has to hear the response clearly when there is an open choice.

These problems of interaction between tester and tested are overcome by using multiple choice tests. Such tests have a closed response format with the child selecting from a set of allowed responses. With older children and adults it is possible to eliminate the variable of tester hearing by asking the subject to complete a pro-forma worksheet. This format is usually employed with the Four-Alternative Auditory

Feature (FAAF) test. As the test name implies, the subject has a closed choice of four alternative monosyllables, and self recording is available to the subject. The FAAF test illustrates well an advantage of close response testing. The responses are restricted and this facilitates analysis of error type. However, using written response introduces another variable and is not useful with younger children. Closing the availability of response is achieved with this age group by using pictures as in the Manchester Picture (MP) Test and the Two-Alternative Picture Pointing (TAPP) test. Unfortunately, when the choice of response is so constrained, guessing inevitably takes place and chance may contaminate the result. The BKB sentences have also been produced in picture related closed set format. With pre-school children, toy tests are also employed to close the response availability. In such tests the child is asked to point to the named toy.

Method of presentation

Presentation of the test material is governed by the purpose of the test and the age of the child.

Live voice presentation decreases test reliability, but is generally used in the toy discrimination and picture recognition tests undertaken with young children. The use of a sound level meter is required to measure the level of speech used. Unless the effect of adding lip reading is required, stringent measures are needed to ensure that visual cues are not presented in such live voice tests. To facilitate this, an automated McCormick toy test is now available with speaker presentation of digitally stored speech waveforms.

Recorded speech tests allow for uniformity of presentation, through use of calibrated equipment. Generated noise can also be added to the recordings to facilitate presentation at defined signal to noise ratios. Green (1987) cites several studies which demonstrate that handicap resulting from hearing loss is more highly correlated with free-field presentation of speech stimuli.

Headphone presentation is often employed with older children, with separation of the ears by the application where necessary of wide-band masking. The use of effective masking is further detailed by Evans (1987). The AB word lists are usually employed this way, although they can if required be presented in a sound field or even if necessary by live voice.

Reliability and scoring

The reliability of speech tests is only partly dependent upon the method of presentation. Test materials themselves result in inherent variability in reliability. Increased reliability is proportional to the quantity of material to be recognised. In children this requires balancing with the ability of the child to participate and complete the test reliably.

The number of items to be scored can be increased in shorter word lists by scoring the phonemes rather than the words. Thus, although the AB word lists each consist of 10 monosyllables, these are split into their three phonemes for scoring.

Each list is scored as a percentage of 30 phonemes rather than 10 words. Thus;

ship heard as ship = three points,
ship heard as tip = two points,
ship heard as pit = one point.

The child's memory and cognitive ability have a surprisingly large effect if test items are repeated. Separate lists within a single test are therefore used. The lists should be equivalent in terms of difficulty and phonemic content. The 15 lists included in the AB word lists are isophonemic, each list having the same phonemic content. However, all the lists are not considered to be equally difficult and lists 9, 10 and 15 are often omitted (Markides, 1978). List equivalence is even more difficult to obtain with sentence tests. The Manchester Sentence Test suffers particularly from this lack of sentence standardisation.

The reliability of tests, properly presented and with equivalent lists, is of vital importance in assessing improvements following rehabilitation. Such improvements should show statistically different results before and after intervention. Green (1987) demonstrated that minimal differences between before and after tests have to be large if a single test list is employed. Thus, if a 50% discrimination score is achieved, a change in the score following intervention is only significant if the new score is either above 73% or below 27%. Similar critical differences are also present for the FAAF and BKB tests.

Recording the results

As in all the variables associated with different speech tests, the method of response scoring depends upon the purpose for which the test is being employed. With the simple closed set toy or picture tests, the voice level necessary for the child to obtain a near maximum discrimination score (MDS) is usually employed. McCormick considers that the quietest level which achieves an 80% score should be recorded when his test materials are used. A criterion just below the MDS is used because there is a wide range of voice level that will achieve a score of 100%. Greater precision is achieved by choosing a discrimination score criterion below this ceiling effect. There is also a floor effect once discrimination falls to zero. For this reason many tests record the level at which a 50% score is achieved (Lutman and Clark, 1986).

Such scoring methods are also usual when speech is presented against background noise. It would be useful if the signal to noise ratio (SNR) could be fixed and the speech level simply increased until the speech reception threshold (SRT) is achieved. However, because degradation of the signal by noise has a rapidly deleterious effect in the hearing impaired, it is not possible to use the same SNR for all tests. This problem has been overcome by the use of adaptive tests whereby the SNR is varied during the test. The result is then scored as the SNR necessary to achieve a 50% correct score. For a description of the speech audiogram refer to Appendix B1.

Speech audiometry has a limited, but specific, role as a diagnostic procedure. Low redundancy material is advantageously used. However, it is clearly an error to use such constrained material for the meaningful assessment of communication disability. It is also of very limited use for analysis of error patterns, for verification, or for auditory training and other rehabilitative measures. These areas are of paramount importance for those involved in the education of a child who has a hearing impairment.

Otoadmittance measurements

Routine audiological assessment now invariably includes an objective test of middle ear function. Within the schema of assessing pathology, impairment and disability, several objective tests measuring within the pathology domain now exist. These include reflectometry (Teele and Teele, 1984), tympanic membrane displacement (Marchbanks and Martin, 1984), sonotubometry (Jonathan et al., 1986) and otoadmittance or impedance audiometry. The latter tests are now routinely used and they will be further detailed in this chapter. However, it is worth recalling that following the initial reports (Metz, 1946) there was a high resistance to clinical acceptance. Although the physical basis of the tests is now readily accessible to the interested (Berlin and Cullen, 1980), terminology was initially confusing. Differences between admittance and impedance, meters and bridges, quotients of stiffness and products of mass, and the use of equivalent units of measurement made clinicians wary. Confusions still exist.

Terminology

Acoustic impedance can be conceptualised as the hindrance to the flow of sound through the mechanisms of the middle ear. **Otoadmittance** is a measure of the efficiency with which the sound flows through the middle ear. It is the inverse of impedance. The term **impedance audiometry** has gained widespread usage, but in fact nearly all instruments are now automated otoadmittance meters. This term is therefore gaining in acceptance and will be used within this text.

The efficiency with which different sounds flow through the ear is frequency dependent. Different middle ear mechanisms resist the passage of different frequencies. The admittance to a 226 Hz tone is generally measured because the ease with which this frequency passes through the ear reflects the stiffness of the middle ear ossicles and the tympanic membrane. Sound passes through the middle ear most efficiently when the ossicles and tympanic membrane are readily mobile and compliant.

The **compliance** of the middle ear is a measure of the mobility of the middle ear structures and this directly reflects the ability of the ear to admit sound. Clearly sounds can only be heard once they have been admitted to the ear. Hence the importance of measuring otoadmittance.

The admittance meter

The components of the admittance meter

The acoustic admittance meter consists of three components linked together by a single probe inserted with an airtight seal in the external ear. The components are illustrated in Figure 1.18. They consist of:

- an oscillator producing a sound,
- a pump to vary the air pressure in the ear canal,
- a sound level meter to measure the SPL in the canal.

The principle underpinning the test is that the sound is fed into the external canal and kept at a constant intensity (usually 85 dBSPL) whilst the air pressure in the ear canal is altered by the pump. Although admittance of a variety of tones can be measured, a 226 Hz probe tone is usually employed. If the sound level in the external canal falls, this reduction is measured by the sound level meter and to keep the sound in the canal constantly at 85 dBSPL, more sound has to be fed in from the oscillator. The amount of sound that has to be fed in from the oscillator directly reflects the amount of sound that has been admitted to the middle ear.

The units of measurement

Admittance measurements thus record the two variables of pressure in the external ear canal and the amount of sound that has to be fed in to balance the sound that has been lost through its admission to the middle ear.

Measures of compliance

It has already been noted that the amount of sound flowing into the middle ear directly reflects its compliance. Compliance can thus be measured directly as the amount of sound requiring to be fed into the

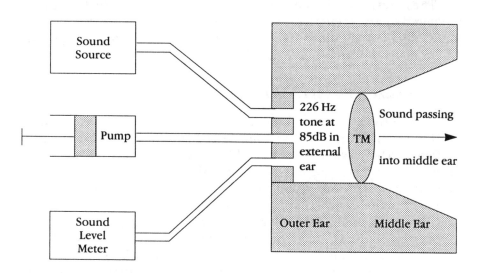

Figure 1.18 The components of an acoustic admittance meter

external canal from the oscillator. Units equivalent to measures of sound level are usually employed to measure the compliance. These require clarification. It is clear that a sound of the same intensity introduced into two dissimilar rooms will result in a higher sound pressure level in the smaller room. The sound pressure level is inversely proportional to the size of any hard walled cavity. Thus it is possible to calibrate the sound level in the external canal in terms of the volume of a hard walled cavity that would give the same sound pressure level if the same sound intensity was introduced. In this way, compliance values are calibrated as an equivalent volume in millilitres.

Measures of pressure in the ear canal

The pressure in the external canal can be altered by the pump. Pressure measurements are in conventional units of daPa. Changes in the admittance of sound to the middle ear that occur with different pressures in the external ear canal are the basis of the clinical otoadmittance tests.

Clinical otoadmittance tests

The facility to measure the efficiency with which sound is admitted to the ear is clinically employed in several tests: the ear canal volume can be measured medial to the probe tip. Tympanometry measures the mobility of the tympanic membrane and middle ear mechanism at different middle ear pressures. The acoustic reflex test determines the level of sound stimulation that results in contraction of the stapedial muscle.

These tests will be dealt with in turn. Other tests such as those required to assess eustachian tube function have been omitted, but are fully detailed in more extensive texts (e.g., *Clinical Impedance Audiometry*, edited by Jerger and Northern, 1980).

Measurement of the ear canal volume

With the probe inserted in the ear canal, the pressure is increased to +200 daPa. This flexes the ear drum inwards and the middle ear system is stiffened. The probe tone delivered into the ear canal is reflected back from the immobile tympanic membrane. The sound pressure in this hard walled cavity is measured and converted into an equivalent volume. This is the absolute cavity size of the ear canal minus the ear canal volume (ECV). Clearly this volume will vary with age. In a young child or infant it is often 0.5cc or less, increasing towards the adult value of 2cc with age.

The measurement of ECV can give valuable information. If the tympanic membrane is perforated, or a ventilating tube (a grommet) is in place, the tone will flow into the middle ear. Provided that the eustachian tube is closed, a sound pressure level will be achieved in the enlarged cavity. The volume measurement will reflect the increased cavity size and ECV may be as large as 6cc. However, even with a perforated tympanic membrane or with a grommet in situ, the ECV in an infant may barely exceed 1cc, reflecting the much smaller middle ear space. If the eustachian tube is patent, sound will continue to flow and a cavity size will not be measurable. Automated meters now recognise this and record that 'no seal' has been achieved. Clearly measurements of ECV are clinically useful, but interpretation requires judgement.

Tympanometry

Tympanometry is the most widely used admittance test. It measures the changes in the compliance of the tympanic membrane induced by changing the pressure in the ear canal. The result is graphically displayed with the compliance on the Y-axis and pressure on the X-axis (Figure 1.19).

Initially the pressure in the external canal is increased to +200 daPa. This is point 'a' in Figure 1.19. With the tympanic membrane stiffened, the compliance is low, and all further changes in the compliance are measured relative to this point. The compliance is thus considered as zero at point 'a'. The pressure in the ear canal is then reduced by the pump. When there is no pressure difference across the ear drum, the pressure in the canal reflects the middle ear pressure. At this point the tympanic membrane and middle ear ossicles are fully mobile, and sound is maximally admitted to the middle ear. The compliance thus increases to its maximum value - point 'b' in Figure 1.19. The pressure recorded

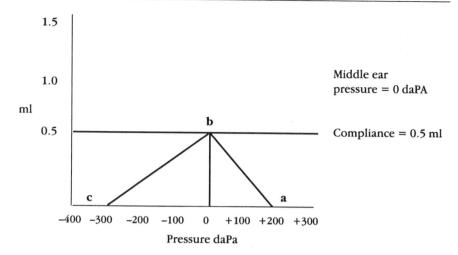

Figure 1.19 An example of a normal tympanogram showing how middle ear pressure and tympanic membrane compliance are measured

on the X-axis at this point of maximal compliance reflects the pressure in the middle ear cavity. The pressure is then reduced to –400 daPa. Once again the ear drum is increasingly stretched, this time with outward flexion. Again sound is increasingly reflected into the canal with little being admitted into the middle ear. The compliance thus once again decreases to zero (point 'c' in Figure 1.19). The British Society of Audiology recommended procedures may be referred to for further procedural details (BSA, 1992).

The above description belies the simplicity of the automated screening tests. Such instruments are designed to yield rapid results with the probe hand held and sealed against the orifice of the external auditory meatus. Pressures are automatically set, and with pressure sweep rates up to 200 daPa/sec, the test is completed in seconds.

An example of a tympanogram recorded by an automatic admittance meter is illustrated in Figure 1.20. The ECV, compliance and middle ear pressure are conveniently displayed.

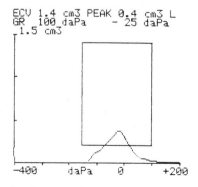

Figure 1.20 An example of a normal tympanogram recorded from a GSI 38 admittance meter

Condition	Tympanometric Features	Tympanogram

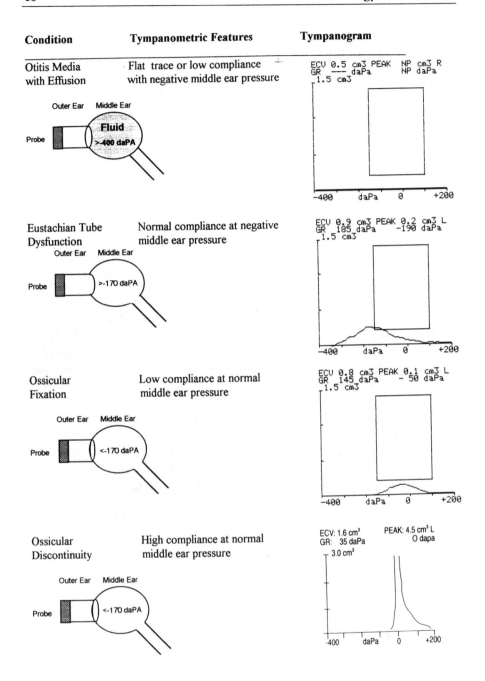

Otitis Media with Effusion — Flat trace or low compliance with negative middle ear pressure

Eustachian Tube Dysfunction — Normal compliance at negative middle ear pressure

Ossicular Fixation — Low compliance at normal middle ear pressure

Ossicular Discontinuity — High compliance at normal middle ear pressure

Figure 1.21 Tympanometric features of paediatric otological conditions

Condition	Tympanometric features	Tympanogram

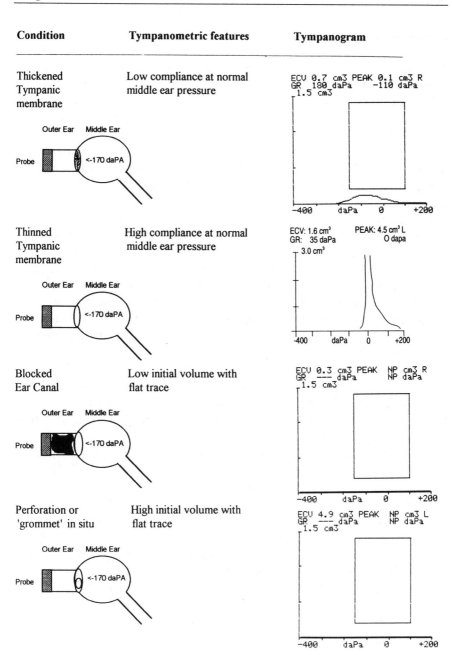

Thickened Tympanic membrane — Low compliance at normal middle ear pressure

ECV 0.7 cm3 PEAK 0.1 cm3 R
GR 180 daPa −110 daPa

Thinned Tympanic membrane — High compliance at normal middle ear pressure

ECV: 1.6 cm³ PEAK: 4.5 cm³ L
GR: 35 daPa O dapa

Blocked Ear Canal — Low initial volume with flat trace

ECV 0.3 cm3 PEAK NP cm3 R
GR −−− daPa NP daPa

Perforation or 'grommet' in situ — High initial volume with flat trace

ECV 4.9 cm3 PEAK NP cm3 L
GR −−− daPa NP daPa

Figure 1.21 (cont)

Interpretation of tympanograms

The admission of sound into the middle ear, as displayed by the tympanogram, reveals valuable clinical information in many different middle ear pathologies. Some of these patterns are displayed in Figure 1.21. Such patterns may be categorised according to the Jerger classification (Jerger, 1970). The gradient of the compliance curve may also be detailed. However it is probably just as informative to describe the tympanogram simply in terms of compliance and middle ear pressure. Interpreting the values of these measures poses some difficulties, irrespective of the descriptive convention.

Normal values of middle ear pressure vary with age. In adults with normally aerated middle ear clefts, the peak compliance occurs within a pressure range from +50 to –50 daPa. Brooks (1968) found that middle ear pressures were lower in children, with a normal pressure being as low as –170 daPa. Such a negative middle ear pressure signifies the presence of eustachian tube dysfunction, and even though this may be a common finding in children, it can affect hearing – as any air traveller will testify.

Normal values of compliance also vary with age. They are usually considered to be abnormal if they fall outside the range 0.2cc – 1.8cc. There is however considerable overlap between normal and abnormal ears, and compliance considered in isolation may mislead.

In children, tympanometry is most commonly employed to identify the presence of otitis media with effusion (OME). The tympanogram is usually completely flat with a compliance of less than 0.1cc. However when the compliance peaks at the lower end of the normal range, this may or may not signify the presence of an effusion. A flat tympanogram may be attributable to scarring of the tympanic membrane (tympanosclerosis) or other pathologies stiffening the middle ear mechanism and a reduced compliance in children does not simply equate with the presence of OME. It would be predicted that ossicular fixation would result in a reduced compliance, but perversely very often the tympanometric pattern is entirely normal. Although it is possible to define normal compliance values, middle ears frequently exhibit more than one pathology. It is the more peripheral middle ear abnormality which dominates the picture and this may obscure an underlying pathology. Absolute reliance on tympanometry in clinical isolation is therefore not possible.

Acoustic reflex testing

Another routinely used test of acoustic admittance is the measurement of the acoustic or stapedial reflex. This diagnostically important test requires basic understanding of the reflex arc illustrated in Figure 1.24. Sound presented to the ear is carried by the ossicles to the cochlea where the signal is transduced for transmission along the auditory nerve to nuclei in both sides of the brainstem. Sound of sufficient intensity results in stimulation of the facial nerve to both ears and this causes the stapedial muscles attached to the crus of the stapes to contract. The ossicular chains are stiffened, reducing sound admittance in both ears. Because sound stimulation of one ear results in a bilateral stiffening of the middle ear mechanism, the reduction in admittance may be recorded from either ear. Thus in ipsilateral testing the change in admittance is recorded in the same ear as that stimulated by the sound. For contralateral testing the admittance changes are measured in the ear opposite to that being stimulated (Figure 1.22).

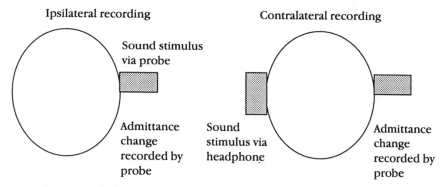

Figure 1.22 Stapedial reflex recording methods

The stiffening of the ossicles results in a downward deflection in the compliance measured in the probe ear. The strength of the reflex is intensity dependent with pure tones of around 85 dBHL (±5 dB) eliciting the reflex in the normal ear (Lutman, 1987). Stapedial reflex thresholds recorded for pure tones from 500Hz to 4 kHz are illustrated in Figure 1.23 from a manually operated diagnostic machine and also from an automatic otoadmittance meter.

Broad-band noise and speech elicit the reflex at quieter levels and this difference has been used in the past as a predictor of hearing loss (Hall, 1980). However, the importance of reflex measurement lies in the diagnostic information revealed about both the stimulated and probe ears. These effects are summarised in Figure 1.24.

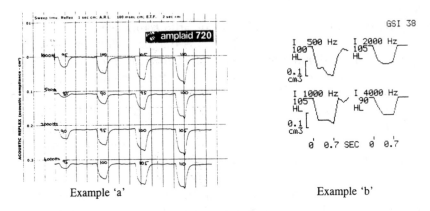

Figure 1.23 Two examples of acoustic reflex threshold measurement

The probe ear gives information about the facial nerve and middle ear mechanism in that ear:

- Any pathology which stiffens the middle ear mechanism will reduce and usually abolish the reflex in that ear.
- Although the compliance is characteristically increased in ossicular discontinuity, the effect of the stapedial muscle contraction will not be conveyed to the ear drum, and once again the reflex will typically be absent.
- The reflex is absent in facial nerve palsy.

The stimulated ear gives information about the type and degree of hearing loss in that ear – irrespective of the ear recording the change in admittance:

- The threshold of the reflex is increased in direct relation to the degree of impairment when there is a conductive loss in the stimulated ear. Thus if the stimulated ear has a 40 dB conductive loss, the reflex would be elicited at 125 dB – beyond the level of many admittance machines.
- The threshold of the reflex does not increase in direct relation to the degree of hearing loss when there is a cochlear loss in the stimulated ear. Thus if the stimulated ear has a 40 dB cochlear loss, the reflex would be elicited at 95 dB. This reduction in the 'span' between the threshold of hearing and the reflex threshold provides a measure of the recruitment in the stimulated ear. Its absence may signify the presence of retrocochlear pathology in the stimulated ear.
- Brainstem pathology may result in reflex abnormalities. The most recognisable reflex pattern caused by a lesion in the centre of the brainstem is the presence of normal ipsilateral reflexes in both ears

with the absence of contralateral reflexes. Examination of Figure 1.24 will clarify the reason for this. However such reflex patterns are rare.

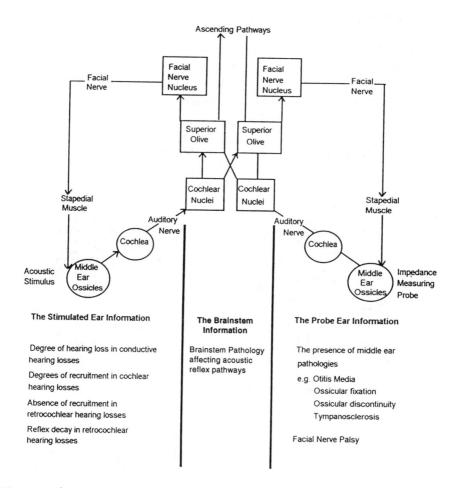

Figure 1.24 The acoustic stapedial reflex pathways

Figure 1.25 illustrates a pure-tone audiogram with a mild conductive loss in the left ear. Such a loss is typically seen in OME. Acoustic reflexes were recorded both ipsilaterally and contralaterally. It is standard convention to record the reflex for the stimulated ear and this practice is used below with the right contralateral reflex being obtained with the right ear stimulated and the probe in the left ear:

- With the probe in the right ear and the tone in the right, ipsilateral reflexes (IR) are recorded at normal levels.
- With the probe in the right ear and the tone in the left, contralateral reflexes (CR) are recorded at a raised level, as the stimulus intensity has to be increased proportional to the degree of conductive hearing loss.

- With the probe in the left ear and the tone in the left, ipsilateral reflexes (IR) are absent because the conductive pathology in the left ear has already reduced the middle ear compliance and this prevents any further decrease in the admittance resulting from the contraction of the stapedial muscle.
- With the probe in the left ear and the tone in the right, contralateral reflexes (CR) are absent because despite the normal hearing in the right ear, the middle ear pathology present in the left once again prevents any further change in admittance in that ear.

Acoustic stapedial reflexes are thus a useful and objective test for assessing the presence of middle ear pathology, the degree of hearing loss, and the presence or absence of recruitment.

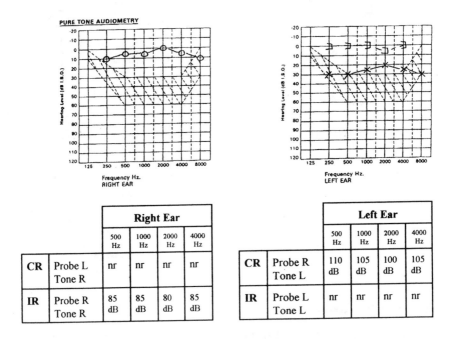

		Right Ear			
		500 Hz	1000 Hz	2000 Hz	4000 Hz
CR	Probe L Tone R	nr	nr	nr	nr
IR	Probe R Tone R	85 dB	85 dB	80 dB	85 dB

		Left Ear			
		500 Hz	1000 Hz	2000 Hz	4000 Hz
CR	Probe R Tone L	110 dB	105 dB	100 dB	105 dB
IR	Probe L Tone L	nr	nr	nr	nr

Figure 1.25 PTA and stapedial reflex measurements

Auditory brainstem response

Auditory brainstem response (ABR) is an objective test of hearing. It is one of a number of electro-physiological tests which are collectively known as electric response audiometry (ERA). The other tests will not be described here as they are not used routinely in the investigation of hearing threshold in children. ABR may also be referred to as BSER, brainstem electric response or brainstem evoked response. The term ABR is preferred.

ABR provides information about hearing threshold without a consciously made response from the child. To be reliably undertaken, the electrical activity of the brain (EEG) must be quiet as in natural sleep or during general anaesthesia. It is therefore readily undertaken on babies under 4 or 5 months of age where behavioural tests to threshold are not possible. It can also assist in the objective assessment of older children including those with multiple handicaps, but sedation or general anaesthesia may be required.

Surface electrodes must be attached to the scalp to record electrical activity from the brain (EEG) as in Figure 1.26. Click stimuli are presented through a headphone triggering electrical activity along the auditory pathway up to the brainstem. The electrical activity occurs at a specific time from the onset of the click, and is said to be time-locked to the stimulus. By repeatedly collecting these time-locked responses, the random brain activity (EEG) can be averaged out using computer averaging techniques, and the response to the sound extracted. In threshold assessments, 1000–2000 clicks are presented, and the response builds up in the form of a waveform (Figure 1.27).

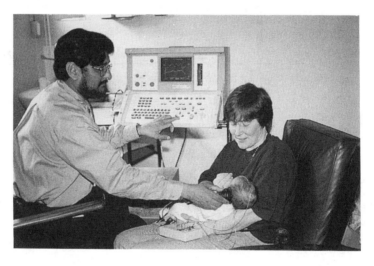

Figure 1.26 Photograph of the test set-up for the auditory brainstem response

Jewett and Williston (1971) first classified the waveform, labelling its seven peaks I to VII. They also recommended that positive values are plotted upwards. It is surprising that 25 years later some centres plot positive waves downwards. This reverses the appearance of the ABR with peaks becoming troughs. It is difficult to justify this inversion of the trace, and within this text the recommended convention is employed. In Figure 1.27 waves I to V have been labelled according to this convention with the negative wave after wave VII being labelled the

SN10. This is the slow negative response occurring at around 10 ms after the onset of the stimulus (Hashimoto, 1992). The seven peaks and the SN10 are thought to originate from the discharge of nerve fibres at the main relay nuclei along the auditory pathway from the ear to the auditory cortex. The anatomical origin of the waveform is shown in Figure 1.28.

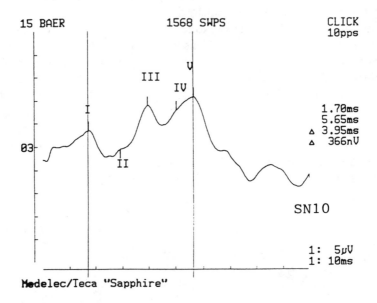

Figure 1.27 A typical ABR waveform

Test procedure

Step 1

This varies slightly from centre to centre, but usually three EEG-type recording electrodes are attached to the mastoid of the test ear, to the forehead or vertex (top of the head) and to the mastoid of the opposite ear.

Step 2

Infants need to be settled in a quiet darkened room with the parent and a feed if necessary. The audiologist needs to be prepared to begin the test when the baby falls asleep, as time is limited if the test is to be completed. Although sedation is unnecessary in younger infants, in older children it may be helpful. However, in such children, testing under a short term general anaesthetic often yields more satisfactory results.

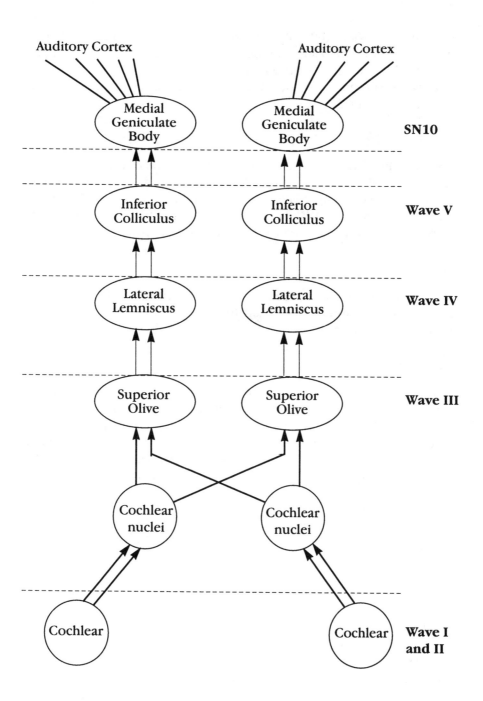

Figure 1.28 The anatomical origin of the auditory brainstem response

Step 3

During sleep, 1000–2000 clicks are presented at a rate of 20 to 40 clicks per second through a headphone. The background EEG is monitored and should be quiet. Testing when the EEG is active, i.e. when the child is awake or restless, can seriously affect interpretation of the results and should be avoided.

Step 4

The stimulus should be presented at suprathreshold level, but not at a level which will wake a sleeping infant. Observation of the child's behavioural response during the test can be informative, i.e. when the child is disturbed by the sound. The intensity level should be decreased in 20 dB steps, if a clear waveform is observed, until it disappears.

Step 5

If there is a difference between the ears of more than 50 dB, then broadband masking should be applied to the opposite (contralateral) ear (Reid and Thornton, 1983).

ABR results

The outcome of the ABR examination will be a threshold reported in dBnHL. This is a decibel scale for the click stimulus in which 0 dBnHL is the quietest audible sound for a group of normally hearing adults, biologically calibrated for the equipment in use. A threshold of 30 dBnHL or better is considered to be consistent with normal hearing on this decibel scale. An example of a normal waveform can be seen in Figure 1.29.

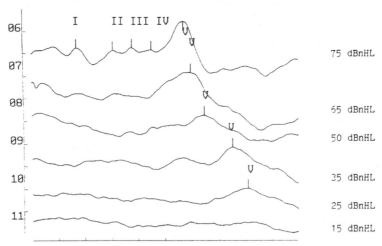

Figure 1.29 An example of a normal ABR waveform recorded down to 25 dBnHL

The latency of wave V lengthens as the intensity decreases and the amplitude of the waveform decreases. In threshold estimation, wave V or the largest wave is traced down until it disappears. In this example, Wave V is present at 25 dBnHL and has disappeared at 15 dBnHL. Wave III is usually the largest wave in neonatal ABRs and is used in threshold estimation. The SN10 is often used instead of wave V, but a longer analysis window of 20 ms is needed to keep the waveform within the window near to threshold.

The audiologist has to make a subjective decision about the presence of the waveform. This judgement can be helped by repeating the run and comparing or superimposing the two waves, which should be identical if the waveform is a genuine response. At threshold, two waveforms should always be recorded and compared. Figure 1.30 is an example of an abnormal ABR with no recordable waveform at 100 dBnHL.

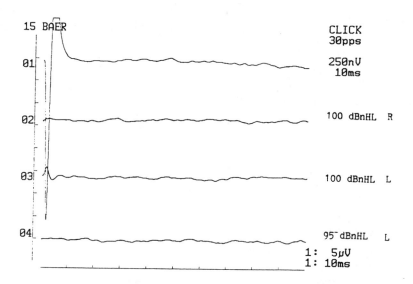

Figure 1.30 An example of an abnormal ABR waveform with no recordable response at 100 dBnHL

Interpretation of ABR results

Frequency specificity of ABR

The stimulus used in ABR is a click, which is broad-band. The stimulus needs to have a sharp rise time to enable a large number of auditory nerve fibres to fire synchronously. If frequency specific tone bursts or pips are used, synchronisation of the firing of the nerve fibres is reduced and the waveform is degraded. Interpretation of the waveform close to threshold is therefore very difficult (Hawes and Greenberg,1981).

However, a click-evoked ABR correlates with pure-tone audiometric findings between 2 kHz and 4 kHz, and in practice it gives a single point on the PTA (Davis et al., 1985; Gorga et al., 1985; Stappells et al., 1985; Keith and Grenville, 1987).

Information about low frequency hearing is therefore not available, and the same ABR threshold could be recorded for a child with severe high frequency hearing loss and a child with a profound loss across the frequency range. Both audiograms in Figure 1.31 would give the same ABR threshold.

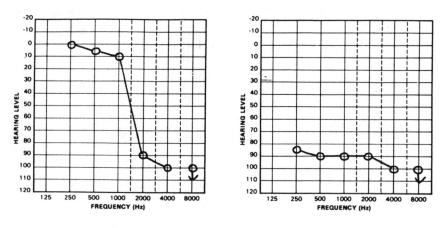

Figure 1.31 An example of two audiometric configurations in which the ABR threshold could be the same

Attempts have been made over the last two decades to improve the frequency specificity of the technique, but there are some difficulties that have not yet been overcome:

- The use of frequency specific stimuli such as tone bursts or filtered clicks (Picton et al., 1979; Kileny, 1981; Stappells and Picton, 1981; Gorga et al., 1988; Frattali et al., 1995).
- Masking frequency regions of the click stimulus with high-pass noise, noise with a notch at a specific frequency band, or with pure tones (Don and Eggermont, 1978; Picton et al., 1979; Mason, 1984a).
- Derived ABR responses obtained by subtracting the response to a click stimulus recorded in high-pass noise at one cut-off frequency (e.g., above 1 kHz) from another at a higher cut-off frequency (e.g., above 2 kHz) leaving a 'derived response' to the frequencies between the two cut-off settings (Parker and Thornton, 1978; Don et al., 1979).

The disadvantage of these techniques is that the recording efficiency of the ABR is reduced, making the response more difficult to interpret close to threshold. Validation of these techniques has proved difficult and there are discrepancies between the low frequency audiometric findings and the ABR thresholds of patients with low frequency hearing loss (Laukli, 1983; Sohmer and Kinarti, 1984). The procedures are often more time consuming and more uncomfortable for the patient, and the instrumentation is not commercially readily available.

Information about degree of hearing loss

The ABR correlates reasonably well with the degree of hearing loss between 2 kHz and 4 kHz when such recordings are undertaken in older children and adults. However ABR is now a well established method of measuring hearing loss in early infancy (Hyde et al., 1990; Durieux-Smith et al., 1991; Watkin et al., 1991).

The relationship between the ABR threshold at this age and subsequent behavioural thresholds is less predictable. If a raised ABR threshold is obtained early in infancy it may be difficult to exclude the presence of middle ear dysfunction overlying a sensorineural loss. The ABR also changes during infancy.

Fjermedal and Laukli (1989) compared ABR thresholds measured in infancy with the subsequently obtained pure-tone thresholds (averaged between 2 and 4 kHz) of 56 children. In 43 ears with different degrees of SNHL measured by PTA, the ABR threshold differed by as much as 40 dB in a positive or negative direction. However, children with an elevated ABR threshold of over 100 dBnHL always had some degree of SNHL, but this varied from 70 dB to more than 120 dB PTA average at 2–4 kHz. Children with ABR thresholds of 60 dBnHL and better often had normal hearing at PTA, but children with thresholds above 60 dBnHL all had some degree of SNHL.

These findings are in keeping with the authors' experience in which children with ABR thresholds above 60 dBnHL are carefully monitored. Such thresholds usually suggest that there is a SNHL or a sensorineural component to the hearing loss.

Interpretation of no response

No response in ABR, i.e. no recordable waveform at the limit of the audiometer, should be interpreted with caution. While this result is consistent with a profound SNHL it could also be consistent with a profound high frequency hearing loss. A 'no response' result should never be conveyed to the parent as 'no measurable hearing' as in the majority of children this is not the case.

There is also a little reported group of children with no response in ABR, whose eventual diagnosis has been normal hearing or a more moderate hearing loss than would be expected. Occasionally, hearing aids have been fitted and later removed. In some cases this is because of neurological illness affecting the brainstem and it has been reported in cases of hydrocephalus (Kraus et al., 1984) and hyperbilirubineamia, i.e., high levels of jaundice (Nakamura et al., 1985). It has also been reported in pre-term neonates, possibly because of a delay in maturation of the auditory pathway (Roberts et al., 1982).

Worthington and Peters (1980) reported four cases with no evidence of neurological illness whose ABRs were absent, but pure-tone audiometry demonstrated normal hearing to moderate hearing loss. They stress the importance of behavioural evaluation and follow-up in interpretation of ABR findings.

The ABR is often mistakenly viewed as the 'gold standard' audiological assessment, but interpretation of ABR findings must always be made in conjunction with ongoing behavioural assessment.

Information about type of hearing loss

Information about the type of loss is also available from the ABR. Information can be obtained from:

Bone conduction ABR

Bone conduction ABR is not used routinely by many centres in the UK, but it is reported to be feasible (Hooks and Weber, 1984; Stappells and Ruben, 1989; Yang and Stuart, 1990; Yang et al., 1993a). Yang et al. (1993b) found ABRs to bone conducted clicks to be as reliable and reproducible as conventionally recorded air conduction ABRs. The force with which the bone vibrator is applied to the skull affects the result and should be monitored (Yang et al., 1991). Bone conduction ABR can be successfully used to investigate the cochlear function of infants (Muchnik et al., 1995) and neonates (Webb and Stevens, 1991; Stuart et al., 1994), and comparison of air conduction and bone conduction ABR can be used in the diagnosis of conductive hearing loss. Currently the technique is under-utilised in the UK (Hall, 1992).

Latency/intensity curves

The latencies of the waveform can be plotted on the normal latency/intensity curve as in Figure 1.32. The latencies for conductive hearing loss are delayed but run parallel to the normal curve. In a cochlear recruiting hearing loss, latencies are delayed at the quieter levels but at louder levels they meet the normal curve.

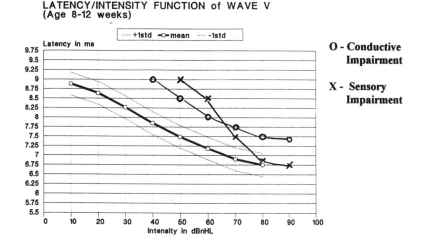

Figure 1.32 An example of a latency/intensity curve showing a conductive and a sensory hearing loss

Screening ABR

ABR is being increasingly used as a neonatal screening test and is most applicable to 'at risk' groups of neonates or the residents of special care baby units (SCBU or NICU) (Stevens et al., 1987, 1989; Durieux-Smith et al., 1991).

The screening test is shortened by the use of fixed intensities. In a study of 'at risk' neonates, ABR screening was carried out at 40 dBnHL and 60 dBnHL with two waveforms being recorded and compared at each level. The presence of a superimposable waveform at the lower intensity level constituted a pass. This was found to be a sensitive and specific method of screening this population of children (Watkin and Baldwin, 1991). Other centres have employed different screening criteria, depending upon the infants targeted for identification by the screen.

Automated ABR machines have been developed incorporating machine scoring, in which pairs of waveforms are compared for similarities and a pass or refer decision is made by the machine at a specific intensity level. The Nottingham ABR screener (Mason, 1984b, 1988) and the Algotek 2 (Kileny, 1988) are both such machines. They are aimed specifically at neonatal screening applications, so that less experienced testers do not have to make a decision about the presence of a response. This method of neonatal hearing screening is undoubtedly possible for high risk groups, and in some States in the USA has been adopted as the methodology for a universal neonatal screen.

ABR is a clinically useful tool both in diagnostic and screening applications. It currently remains a measure of high frequency hearing and is usefully employed in the assessment of children whose behavioural responses to sound are difficult to interpret. Although a normal ABR threshold is a positive indicator of normal peripheral auditory function to brainstem level, the child could still have problems in interpreting the sound at a higher cortical level.

The ABR threshold should always be interpreted in conjunction with other evidence available to the audiologist and not taken in isolation. It is often regarded as the ultimate investigation by parents and probably seems the most impressive, requiring complex equipment and an audiologist with a higher level of training. In fact the information obtained is often more limited than that achieved by apparently much simpler behavioural tests.

Otoacoustic emissions

In 1978, Kemp described the presence in the external ear canal of very low intensity sound energy emitted from the cochlea. The development of commercially available equipment able to identify these emissions under clinical conditions (Bray and Kemp, 1987) has made available a new test of auditory function.

The inner ear increases hearing sensitivity by acting as a sound amplifier. This is achieved by contraction of the outer hair cells. Amplified vibrations are then transmitted to the inner hair cells for transduction into nerve impulses. This outer hair cell mechanism produces the emissions. Several types have been described. However they are all part of the same normally-occurring physiological response, and the different types actually describe different testing conditions.

Spontaneous otoacoustic emissions (SOAEs) are pure tones found in the unstimulated ear. Emissions can also be recorded when two pure tones of slightly different frequencies are continuously presented to the ear. The emerging sound is more complex and includes distortion product otoacoustic emissions (DPOAEs). The clinical application of SOAEs and DPOAEs continues to be researched. A useful summary is presented by DeVries and Decker (1992). However, the simplest way of recording emissions is by evoking them with a transient stimulus such as a click. Clicks present a broad band of frequencies simultaneously to the ear and emissions from different parts of the cochlea can be recorded from the same stimulus. These emissions are known as transient evoked otoacoustic emissions (TEOAEs). Because currently this is the commonly used recording method, it will be discussed in this section. Illustrations are from recordings made with the ILO88 (Otodynamics) equipment.

A readily understood description of TEOAE instrumentation is presented by Kemp and Ryan (1993). TEOAEs are recorded by acousti-

cally sealing a probe in the external ear. The probe contains two transducers. The first is a miniature speaker that delivers the click stimuli into
the external ear canal, and the other is a miniature microphone that
picks up the emission (Figure 1.33).

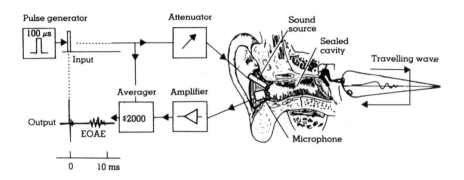

Figure 1.33 Basic method of recording TEOAEs (Published with permission of
D. Kemp)

Separation of the sound stimulus from the much quieter emission is
necessary, and this is achieved in several ways. Firstly, the emission is
recorded a short time (usually 2.5 ms) after the click, so much of the
stimulus is removed. A more ingenious method recognises that
emissions are physiological responses that grow non-linearly. Other
sounds in the external ear grow linearly, and this difference allows their
differentiation. To ensure that the emissions collected are not artefacts,
two waveforms are collected and correlated. Subtraction of one from
the other leaves the random components caused by contaminating
noise. The reproducible parts of the waveforms represent the true
emission signal, and this can be related to the noise as a signal to noise
ratio spectrographically displayed across the frequencies. The signal to
noise spectrogram derived from the two waveforms is illustrated in
Figure 1.34.

The waveforms consist of TEOAEs emitted from the different parts of
the cochlea. Thus the high frequency basal turn emits a high frequency
emission with the low frequency waveform being emitted from the apex.
Logically the high frequency emission will emerge first. The emission
latency (i.e. the time delay following stimulation) thus reveals its place of
origin within the cochlea. The latency of the 5 kHz emission is around
4 ms, with that from the 500Hz region being delayed to around 20 ms.
Because low frequency noise is often present in clinical conditions,
recording is undertaken from 2.5 to 12.5 ms, with loss of part of the low
frequency emission.

The use of a strong stimulus of around 80 dBSPL to elicit the response is recommended because a wide range of TEOAE frequencies can be obtained (Kemp et al., 1990). An emission threshold measurement is not useful because TEOAEs are an on-off phenomenon, being absent if there is cochlear hair cell dysfunction. The absence of an emission from a particular area of the cochlea thus relates well to the presence of a mild or worse degree of hearing loss at that frequency, even though the stimulation has been at high intensity.

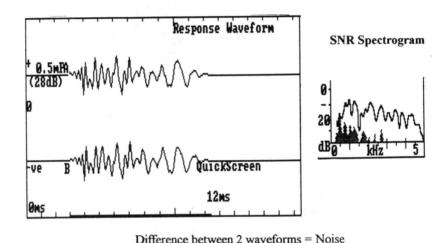

Difference between 2 waveforms = Noise
Cross Power Spectrum of 2 waveforms = Emission

Figure 1.34 Frequency analysis of the TEOAE waveform

The emission has to travel from the cochlea through the middle ear before it can be recorded in the external ear canal. Thus middle ear problems such as OME prevent a recording. Even eustachian tube dysfunction attenuates much of the response (Kemp et al., 1990). However, the recording of TEOAEs has allowed a window into the functioning of the hair cells in the inner ear, and this is its main use. If the outer hair cells are not functioning, an emission is absent. In Figure 1.35, example 'a' demonstrates a normal TEOAE with 'b' demonstrating the absence of an emission. The absence of the TEOAE could have been obtained with any degree of hearing loss present across the frequencies. If an area of the cochlea is physiologically normal, an emission should be obtainable from these functioning outer hair cells. This is illustrated for a child with a high frequency hearing impairment in Figure 1.36, example 'c'. The exact relationship between audiometry and emission spectrographic patterns in children is still being investigated.

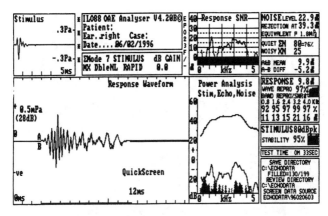

Example 'a' - A normal TEOAE

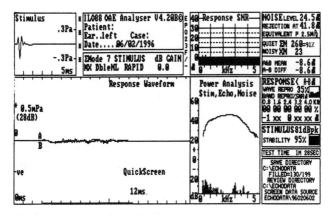

Example 'b' - An absent TEOAE

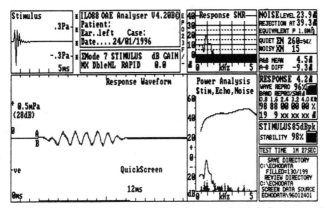

Example 'c' - An abnormal TEOAE - seen in high frequency hearing loss.

Figure 1.35 Examples of TEOAEs

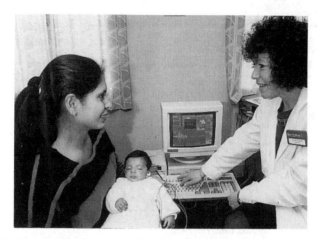

Figure 1.36 Photograph of a neonate being tested with TEOAEs

The instrumentation for recording TEOAEs is sophisticated. The test is objective, simple and quick to use, non-invasive and acceptable to most children (Figure 1.36). The greatest potential for use is as a method of neonatal hearing screening. Neonatal programmes have been successfully implemented (White and Behrens, 1993; Watkin, 1996). In fact the potential is such that the National Institutes of Health in the USA have recommended that every neonate has such a test (NIH, 1993).

TEOAE recording as an assessment of cochlear function within a diagnostic clinic also adds an extra dimension to the existing paediatric test battery. Many children are referred for diagnostic audiology specifically to exclude a hearing loss. Such requests are made especially by speech therapists and teachers. For such children, defining the presence of normal peripheral auditory function is as important as identifying the disability present in those with impaired hearing. TEOAE testing is useful in any situation where an element of uncertainty remains about the validity of the subjective results. Clearly it is essential to consider the results within the context of the other tests, and TEOAE recording is not always a simple procedure in the older infant or unco-operative toddler. Although test time averages 3 minutes, it may take considerably longer if the child is unsettled and the conditions noisy. Often techniques similar to those familiar in behavioural localisation tests are appropriate, with one tester holding the child's attention and another recording the emission.

Several paediatric applications afford significant advantage within a diagnostic clinic (Baldwin and Watkin, 1992):

- Children with functional or non-organic hearing losses present a common dilemma in diagnostic clinics. Baldwin and Watkin reported that out of 157 school children aged 7 years and older, newly referred to a diagnostic clinic, 28 (18%) had a functional hearing loss. Although the test battery approach was required, the recording of TEOAEs was the quickest and simplest way of establishing normal peripheral auditory function.

- Developmentally young children with learning difficulties may also be difficult to test to threshold. Baldwin and Watkin reported in a single school 44 children with severe learning difficulties who could not be tested accurately by the traditional behavioural tests. None of these children had been admitted for ABR under anaesthetic. Using TEOAE recording it was possible to test satisfactorily over two thirds of the ears without the use of sedation.
- More uncommonly, children with neurological damage require diagnostic audiological assessment and yet often such children have abnormal ABRs. The effect on their hearing is unclear. The ability of TEOAE testing to demonstrate the normality of peripheral auditory function in these children is of enormous benefit for their management. Others have successfully used TEOAE testing to routinely check the cochlear function of children who have suffered from meningitis (Richardson et al., 1995).

Whilst TEOAE recording has become an important component of the diagnostic assessment of children, it is important to emphasise that, like most other routine diagnostic tests, it assesses only part of the hearing mechanism. It examines the integrity of the outer hair cells, and of the middle ear. Although isolated inner hair cell dysfunction has not been reported in either adults or children (Patuzzi, 1993), central organic auditory disorders are of considerable educational importance, and are discussed in detail elsewhere. These will be undetected if there is indiscriminate reliance on a test that measures only cochlear hair cell function. However this may eventually be recognised as an advantage of TEOAE testing, allowing for clearer definition of the site of lesion in children with impaired hearing.

Case studies

The following case studies demonstrate the inter-relationship of the different procedures employed in diagnostic assessment.

Case 1: Anne

Anne was born prematurely at 28 weeks gestation, and required ventilation for 4 weeks. She had hydrocephalus and, fulfilling several 'at risk' criteria, was assessed by ABR screening prior to her discharge from the SCBU. At intensity levels of 40 dBnHL and 60 dBnHL, no repeatable waveforms were measured. A diagnostic ABR was therefore completed and no repeatable waveforms were present at 100 dBnHL.

Anne was seen again as an out-patient for further testing. The results can be seen in Figure 1.37. The ABR thresholds were now recorded at 70 dBnHL but were absent at 60 dBnHL. TEOAEs were recorded at the low frequencies with no recordable emission above 2 kHz. Tests of middle ear function were equivocal. Within the home the parents had noticed a definite reaction to loud sounds such as the dog barking and a door slamming. BOA showed eye-widening to a low frequency voice at 60 dBA with no change in her behaviour being noticed in response to the Manchester rattle or warble tones at 4 kHz. She startled to the drum at 90 dBA. These results were consistent with a high frequency hearing loss. The peripatetic teacher for the hearing-impaired was introduced to the family, but the parents decided against hearing aid fitting at this stage.

Anne made good developmental progress, and when she was sitting without support she was assessed using the infant distraction test. She turned consistently to low frequency stimuli at minimal levels, but required a raised level of 70 dBA at 2 kHz and 90 dBA at 4 kHz with no response to the Manchester rattle. Tests of middle ear function and auroscopic examination were normal. Although Anne had a high frequency sensorineural hearing loss typically seen as a result of perinatal illness, the parents could see no evidence of hearing loss at home. She continued to respond appropriately to environmental sounds and was vocalising with open vowel sounds. However they agreed to hearing aid fitting at this stage.

Anne's PTA can be seen in Figure 1.37. She has a severe high frequency sensorineural hearing loss. Her hearing is much better than would have been predicted from the first neonatal ABR. ABR in children with hydrocephalus can be difficult to interpret because of the effect of raised intracranial pressure. Her hydrocephalus had been treated with a shunt before the second diagnostic ABR and ongoing assessment was necessary to determine fully the degree and type of her hearing loss.

Case 2: Ben

Ben was born normally at full term and there were no risk factors for deafness. However he was born in a district which screens the hearing of all neonates. Otoacoustic emissions could not be recorded in either ear at 2 days old, but this is a common finding and repeat emissions were arranged and undertaken at 4 weeks. Once again emissions were not present and ABR testing was carried out. No waveforms were measured at 100 dBnHL in either ear. There was no APR at 90 dBA and no other behavioural response. The mother was shocked that a problem had been detected and reported no problems at home.

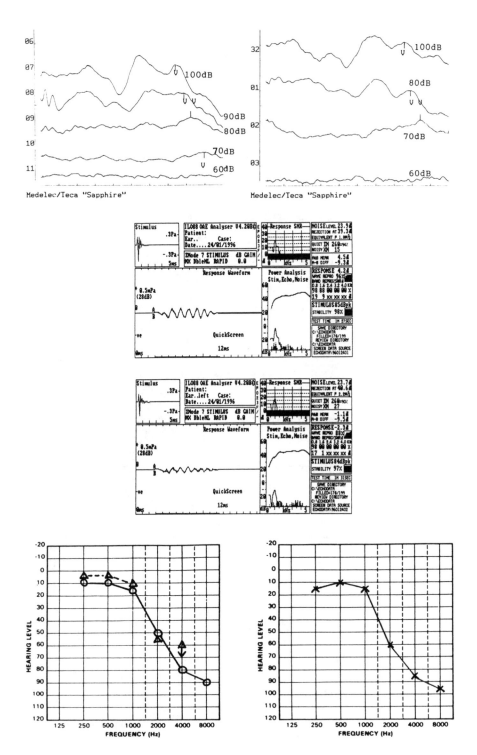

Figure 1.37 Case study 1

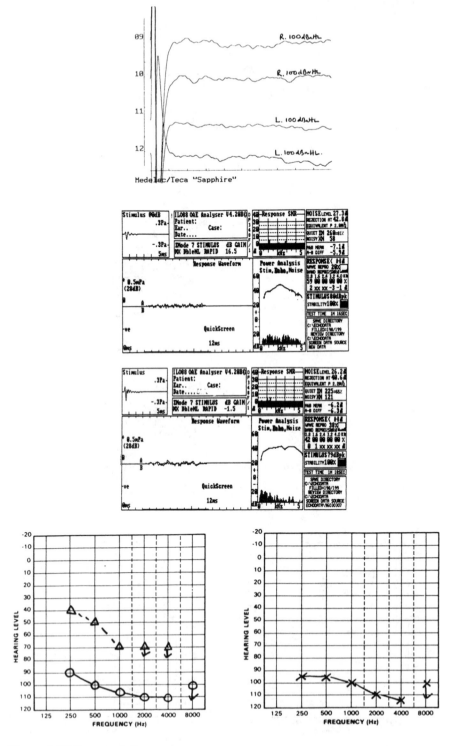

Figure 1.38 Case study 2

ABR testing was repeated and repeatable waveforms were once again absent at 100 dBnHL. The peripatetic teacher was involved with the family and early hearing aid fitting was possible.

As ABR can only give information about the 2–4 kHz region, BOA was used to assess his low frequency hearing. No behavioural changes were observed for loud low frequency stimuli such as the drum at 100 dBA. There was no APR. With his hearing aids in situ fleeting eye movements were noticed in reaction to broad-band stimuli and voice at 70 dBA.

At 7 months, Ben was noticeably more vocal with his hearing aids in. He was sitting without support but infant distraction testing proved difficult, as he had difficulty localising the stimuli. He quietened to low frequency stimuli such as the 500Hz warble tone and the C chime at 70 dBA. Visual reinforcement audiometry was more useful and at 12 months his aided thresholds using VRA were encouraging, with responses across the frequency range 500 Hz to 2 kHz at 60–65 dBSPL. Unaided, Ben responded only at 90 dBSPL at 500 Hz, confirming a profound hearing loss. Impedance testing was normal in both ears and the loss was entirely sensorineural.

Ben has now completed pure-tone audiometry and the audiogram can be seen in Figure 1.38. He has a profound sensorineural hearing loss.

Case 3: Sarah

Sarah was referred by the health visitor for diagnostic audiological assessment following the IDT hearing screen. There was no neonatal 'at risk' screen implemented in this particular district at this time, so referral had not been made earlier despite the fact that Sarah had been born at 24 weeks gestation.

The screening IDT was initially undertaken by the health visitor at a corrected age of 7 months, and this resulted in Sarah not being seen at the hearing assessment centre until just after her first birthday. She had quadriplegic cerebral palsy and blindness. Infant distraction testing was not appropriate as her localisation responses were affected by her motor and visual problems. Her lack of response to sounds using this method of testing could not be interpreted as a lack of hearing.

BOA was used to assess her responsiveness to sounds. She quietened to the sound of the Manchester rattle at 60 dBA, and eye-widened to low frequency voice sounds at 50–60 dBA. Behavioural responses to quieter stimuli could not be elicited. She had a clear APR at 80 dBA in both ears.

Tests of middle ear function were normal and an attempt was made to record otoacoustic emissions when she was relaxed and quiet. The recording was difficult, but possible, and the results from one ear can be seen in Figure 1.39. This shows a normal TEOAE from the left ear. The mother had not been worried about her hearing as Sarah was comforted by voice at quiet levels. This was witnessed in the clinic. The TEOAE recording demonstrating no peripheral cochlear hearing loss confirmed this behavioural observation.

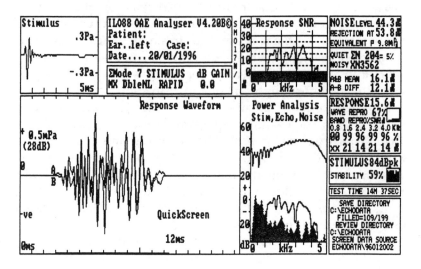

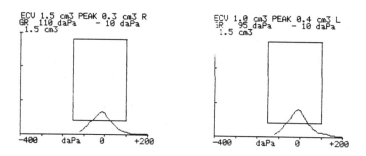

Figure 1.39 Case study 3

Case 4: Samantha

Samantha was referred for diagnostic audiological assessment by the paediatrician when she was seen at the child development centre at the age of 3 years. There were concerns about her general development and about her language development which was limited to a few single words. She was noted to have a dysmorphic right pinna and had seen a plastic surgeon since birth because of this. No 'at risk' referral had been made regarding her hearing and the family had not attended for IDT screening.

Samantha conditioned to warble tone audiometry in the free-field and she then co-operated with pure-tone audiometry. Initially a limited three-point audiogram was achieved as seen in Figure 1.40. Bone conduction thresholds were normal. Tympanometry demonstrated normal middle ear pressures and compliance. Her tympanic membranes appeared normal. Acoustic reflexes were absent in both ears.

At subsequent appointments a full pure-tone audiogram was obtained as in Figure 1.40. The loss appears to be bilateral and conductive, but until Samantha is testable with masking it is not possible to determine the degree of impairment in each ear. There is a masking dilemma however, and pure-tone audiometry requires the use of masking with insert earphones to isolate the ears.

Samantha has congenital stapes fixation. Her hearing loss is permanent and she was fitted with hearing aids. Aided thresholds undertaken in each ear separately confirmed the absence of a dead ear and allowed a binaural fitting.

Case 5: Rani

Rani was screened at school entry by the school nurse using sweep audiometry. She failed the screen in both ears and an appointment was arranged in the second tier audiology clinic for pure-tone audiometry. There were also educational concerns, but her teacher was uncertain whether this was because she was learning English as a second language.

Pure-tone audiometry in the second tier clinic was undertaken again by the school nurse without masking or bone conduction. The audiogram can be seen in Figure 1.41. It shows a mild loss in the right ear and a moderate loss on the left. There is no information about the type of hearing loss from this PTA. A full pure-tone audiogram was undertaken at the hearing assessment centre as part of a battery of tests. This can also be seen in Figure 1.41. Unmasked bone conduction was normal and masking was necessary to determine the true thresholds in the left ear. The unmasked air conduction thresholds were in fact a shadow of the normal bone conduction in the right ear, and when the right ear was masked, a profound loss was revealed on the left. The mild loss on the right was conductive and was due to otitis media with effusion (OME). Tympanometry revealed a flat trace in the right ear, and auroscopic examination confirmed the presence of a middle ear effusion. In the poorer hearing left ear middle ear function was normal and the loss was entirely sensorineural.

Case 6: Debbie

Debbie was 8 years old and having difficulties reading. She had had middle ear problems as a young child and had undergone surgical middle ear ventilation with insertion of grommets. She complained to her mother that she could not hear the teacher, and at the mother's request the GP referred her back to the hospital.

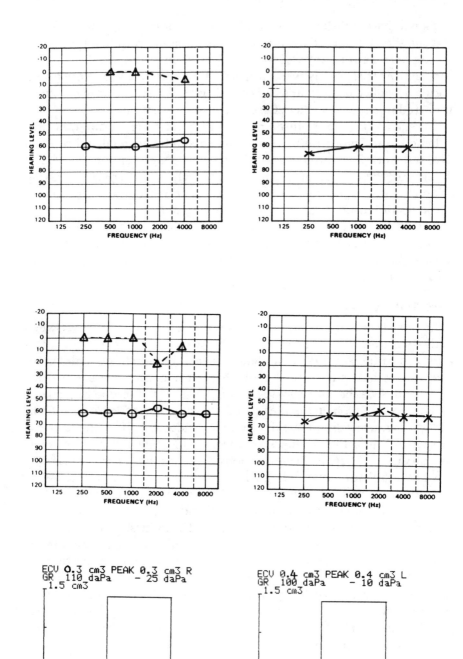

ECV 0.3 cm3 PEAK 0.3 cm3 R
GR 110 daPa   - 25 daPa
1.5 cm3

ECV 0.4 cm3 PEAK 0.4 cm3 L
GR 100 daPa   - 10 daPa
1.5 cm3

Figure 1.40 Case study 4

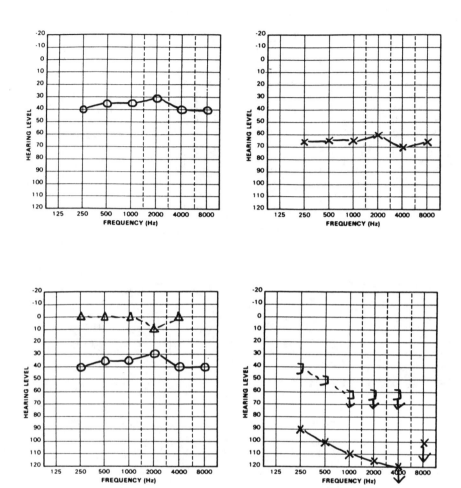

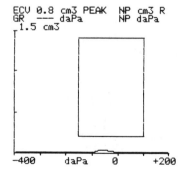

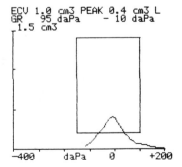

Figure 1.41 Case study 5

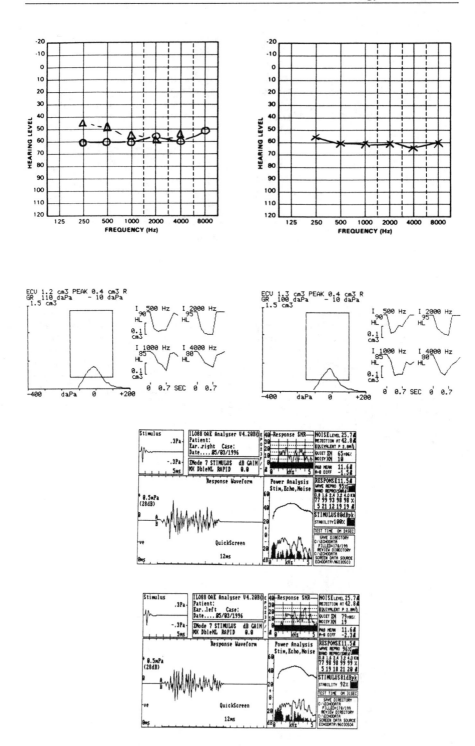

Figure 1.42 Case study 6

She was seen in a busy ENT outpatient clinic and assessed by pure-tone audiometry and otoadmittance testing. The audiogram obtained is illustrated in Figure 1.42. It shows a flat bilateral sensorineural hearing loss. The otoadmittance test was normal in both ears. It was concluded that she had a sensorineural hearing loss and she was referred to the hearing assessment centre for hearing aid fitting.

On meeting Debbie it was apparent that she had no difficulty hearing quiet conversational voice without lip reading. Her thresholds on pure-tone audiometry were a little unreliable and the audiologist suspected that the hearing loss was non-organic. Pure-tone audiometry with attention-raising revealed improved hearing thresholds. Debbie was asked to say "yes" when she heard the tone clearly, and "no" when she was unsure. She responded consistently down to normal levels. Other attention raising techniques include 'ear pointing' and counting the number of tones presented. AB words were presented through headphones. She made errors such as hearing "boat" for "ship", and "mat" for "rug". Nevertheless, the half peak level elevation was better than the pure-tone average in both ears. Auroscopy confirmed normal tympanic membranes, and tympanometry was normal with acoustic reflexes present in both ears. Otoacoustic emissions were recorded successfully from both ears.

Debbie had a non-organic hearing loss. It was not possible with subjective tests to ascertain the exact level of her hearing, but objective testing using otoacoustic emissions confirmed normal cochlear function.

Conclusion

The case studies demonstrate some of the difficulties encountered in achieving correct audiological diagnosis. They have a common end point: the measurement of hearing impairment. Audiological diagnostic procedures can never be an end in themselves. Such a point is artificially imposed and is only one step in a continuum of care. However, following identification, accurate measurement of the child's impairment is an essential precursor to the assessment of disability and provision of appropriate educational assistance. Whilst it may be unnecessary for test procedures to be known in detail by teachers of the deaf who are not implementing them, understanding the results, their limitations and their implications is an essential foundation upon which educational provision for the hearing-impaired is built.

References

"A Word in Your Ear" (1991) A TVF Medical Production for Nicholas Laboratories Limited (Video).

American Speech-Language-Hearing Association (1991) Guidelines for the audiological assessment of children from birth through 36 months of age. ASHA 33: 37-43.

Aplin DY, Kane JM (1985) Variables affecting pure tone and speech audiometry in experimentally simulated hearing loss. British Journal of Audiology 19: 219-228.

Baguley DM, Moffat DA, Nigam A (1988) Disposable electrodes in auditory brainstem response audiometry. British Journal of Audiology 22: 219-221.

Baldwin M, Watkin PM (1992) The clinical application of otoacoustic emissions in paediatric audiological assessment. Journal of Laryngology and Otology 106: 301-306.

Bamford J, McSporran E (1993) Visual reinforcement audiometry. In McCormick B (Ed) Paediatric Audiology 0-5 Years (2nd Edition). London: Whurr. pp 124-154.

Barr B (1960) Non-organic hearing problems in school children. Functional deafness. Acta Otolaryngology 52: 337.

Bellman S, Marcuson M (1991) A new toy test to investigate the hearing status of young children who have English as a second language: a preliminary report. British Journal of Audiology 25: 317-322.

Bench J, Collyer Y, Mentz L, Wilson I (1976) Studies in infant behavioural audiometry III ; Six month old infants. Audiology 15: 384-394.

Bench J, Kowal A, Bamford JM (1979) The BKB (Bamford-Kowal-Bench) sentence lists for partially hearing children. British Journal of Audiology 13: 108-112.

Bennett M, Mowat L (1981) Validity of impedance measurements and referral criteria in school hearing screening programmes. British Journal of Audiology 15: 147-150.

Berlin CI, Cullen JK (1980) The physical basis of impedance measurement. In Jerger J, Northern J (Eds) Clinical Impedance Audiometry (2nd Edition). New York: Georg Thieme Verlag.

Bonny IC (1989) Impedance and audiometric screening. Public Health 103: 427-431.

Boothroyd A (1968) Developments in Speech Audiometry. Sound 2: 3-10.

Boothroyd A (1986) A three-interval, forced-choice test of speech pattern contrast perception. New York: City University of New York and Lexington Centre.

Boothroyd A (1991) Assessment of speech perception capacity in profoundly deaf children. The American Journal of Otology 12: 67S-72S.

Boothroyd A, Cawkwell S (1970) Vibrotactile thresholds in pure tone audiometry. Acta Oto-Laryngologica 69: 381-387.

Borton TE, Nolen BL, Luks SB, Meline NC (1989) Clinical applicability of insert ear-phones for audiometry. Audiology 28: 61-70.

Brasier VJ (1974) Pitfalls in audiometry. Public Health 89: 31.

Bray P, Kemp DT (1987) An advanced cochlear echo technique suitable for infant screening. British Journal of Audiology 21: 191-204.

British Society of Audiology (1981a) Speech audiometric terminology. British Journal of Audiology 15: 143.

British Society of Audiology (1981b) Recommended procedures for pure tone audiometry using a manually operated instrument. British Journal of Audiology 15: 213-216.

British Society of Audiology (1985) Recommended procedure for pure-tone bone conduction audiometry without masking using a manually operated instrument. British Journal of Audiology 19: 281-282.

British Society of Audiology (1986) Recommended procedure for masking in pure tone threshold audiometry. British Journal of Audiology 20: 307-314.

British Society of Audiology (1988) Recommendation: descriptors for pure-tone audiograms. British Journal of Audiology 22: 123.

British Society of Audiology (1989) Recommended format for audiogram forms. British Journal of Audiology 23: 265-266.

British Society of Audiology (1992) Recommended procedure for tympanometry. British Journal of Audiology 26: 255-257.

Brooks DN (1968) An objective method of detecting fluid in the middle ear. International Audiology 7: 280-286.

Brooks DN, Geoghegan PM (1992) Non-organic hearing loss in young persons: Transient episode or indicator of deep-seated difficulty. British Journal of Audiology 26: 347-350.

Brown J, Watson E, Alberman E (1989) Screening infants for hearing loss. Archives of Disease in Childhood 64: 1488-1495.

Carhart R, Jerger J (1959) Preferred method for clinical determination of pure tone thresholds. Journal of Speech and Hearing Disorders 24: 330-345.

Chiveralls K (1974) What is a decibel? Journal of the British Association of Teachers of the Deaf 2(2): 48-49.

Cutting JA, Pisoni DB (1978) In Kavanagh JF, Strange W (Eds) Speech and Language in the Laboratory, School and Clinic. Cambridge: MIT Press.

Davis H, Hirsh SK, Turpin LL, Peacock ME (1985) Threshold sensitivity and frequency specificity in auditory brainstem response audiometry. Audiology 24:54-70.

DeVries SM, Decker TN (1992) Otoacoustic emissions: Overview of measurement methodologies. Seminar on Hearing 13(1): 15-23.

Don M, Eggermont JJ (1978) Analysis of the click evoked brainstem potentials in man using high-pass noise masking. Journal of the Acoustical Society of America 63: 1084-1092.

Don M, Eggermont JJ, Brackman DE (1979) Reconstruction of the audiogram using brainstem responses and high-pass noise masking. Annals of Otolaryngology, Rhinolaryngology and Laryngology 57: 1S-20S.

Durieux-Smith A, Picton TW, Bernard P, MacMurray B, Goodman JT (1991) Prognostic validity of brainstem electric response audiometry in infants of a neonatal intensive care unit. Audiology 30: 249-265.

Eisenberg RB (1983) Development of hearing in children. In Romand R (Ed) Development of Auditory and Vestibular Systems. New York: Academic Press.

Evans PIP (1987) Speech audiometry for differential diagnosis. In Martin M (Ed) Speech Audiometry. London: Taylor and Francis.

Ewing I, Ewing A (1944) The ascertainment of deafness in infancy and early childhood. Journal of Laryngology 59: 309-333.

Fjermedal O, Laukli E (1989) Paediatric auditory brainstem response and pure tone audiometry: threshold comparisons: A study of 142 difficult to test children. Scandinavian Audiology 18(2): 105-111.

Foster JR, Haggard M (1987) The Four-Alternative Auditory Feature test (FAAF) - Linguistic and psychometric properties of the material with normative data in noise. British Journal of Audiology 21(3): 165-174.

Frank T, Vavrek MJ (1992) Reference threshold levels for an ER-3A insert earphone. Journal of the American Academy of Audiology 3: 51-59.

Frattali MA, Sataloff RT, Hirshout D, Sokolow C, Hills J, Spiegel JR (1995) Audiogram reconstruction using frequency-specific auditory brainstem response (ABR) thresholds. Ear, Nose and Throat Journal 74(10): 691-700.

Froding CA (1960) Acoustic investigation of newborn infants. Acta Otolaryngology (Stockholm) 52: 31.

Froeschels E, Beebe H (1946) Testing hearing of newborn infants. Archives of Otolaryngology 44: 710-714.

Fry DB (1961) Word and sentence tests for use in speech audiometry. Lancet 2: 197-199.

Gans DP (1987) Improving behavioural observation audiometry testing and scoring procedures. Ear and Hearing 8: 92-100.

Gans DP, Flexer C (1982) Observer bias in the hearing testing of profoundly involved multi-handicapped children. Ear and Hearing 3: 309-313.

Gans DP, Gans KD (1993) Development of a hearing test protocol for profoundly involved multi-handicapped children. Ear and Hearing 14(2): 128–140.

Gorga MP, Kaminski JR, Beauchaine KA, Jesteadt W (1988) Auditory brainstem responses to tone bursts in normally hearing subjects. Journal of Speech and Hearing Research 31: 87-97.

Gorga MP, Worthington DW, Reiland JK, Beauchaine KA, Goldgar DE (1985) Some comparisons between auditory brainstem response thresholds, latencies, and pure tone audiogram. Ear and Hearing 6: 105-112.

Green R (1987) The uses and misuses of speech audiometry in rehabilitation. In Martin M (Ed) Speech Audiometry. London:Taylor and Francis.

Grimaldi P (1976) The value of impedance testing in the diagnosis of middle ear effusion. Journal of Laryngology and Otology 90: 141-152.

Haggard M, Hughes E (1991) Screening Children's Hearing. London: HMSO.

Haggard MP, Wood EJ, Carroll S (1984) Speech, admittance and tone tests in school screening. British Journal of Audiology 18: 133-153.

Hall DMB (Ed) (1996). Health for all Children: A Programme for Child Health Surveillance; The Report of the Joint Working Party on Child Health Surveillance (3rd Edition). Oxford: Oxford University Press.

Hall JW (1980) Predicting hearing loss from the acoustic reflex. In Jerger J, Northern JL (Eds) Clinical Impedance Audiometry (2nd Edition). New York: Georg Thieme Verlag.

Hall JW (1992) Handbook of Auditory Evoked Responses. Needham Heights, Allyn and Bacon .

Hallett CP (1982) The screening and epidemiology of middle ear disease in a population of primary school entrants. Journal of Laryngology and Otology 96: 899-914.

Hashimoto I (1992) Auditory evoked potentials from the human midbrain: Slow brainstem responses. Electroencephalography and Clinical Neurophysiology 53: 652-657.

Hawes MD, Greenberg H J (1981) Slow brain stem responses (SN10) to tone pips in normally hearing newborns and adults. Audiology 20: 113-122.

Hinchcliffe R (1981) Clinical tests of auditory function in the adult and the school-child. In Beagley HA (Ed) Audiology and Audiological Medicine. Volume 1. New York: Oxford University Press.

Hooks RG, Weber B A (1984) Auditory brainstem responses of premature infants to bone-conducted stimuli: A feasibility study. Ear and Hearing 5: 42-46.

Hughson W, Westlake H (1944) Manual program outline for rehabilitation of aural casualties both military and civilians. Transcription of the American Acadamy of Ophthalmology and Otolanyngology (Supplement 48): 1-15.

Hyde ML, Riko K, Malizia K (1990). Audiometric accuracy of the click ABR in infants at risk for hearing loss. Journal of the Academy of Audiology 1:59-74.

Jerger J (1970) Clinical experience with impedance audiometry. Archives of Otolaryngology 92: 311.

Jerger J, Northern JL (1980) (Eds.) Clinical Impedance Audiometry. Stuttgart: Thieme.

Jerger J, Tillman T (1960) A new method for the clinical determination of sensorineural acuity level (SAL). Archives of Otolaryngology 71: 948-953.

Jewett DL, Williston JS (1971) Auditory evoked far fields averaged from the scalp of humans. Brain 4: 681-696.

Jonathan DA, Chalmers P, Wong K (1986) Comparison of sonotubometry with tympanometry to assess Eustachian tube function in adults. British Journal of Audiology 20: 231-235.

Keith WJ, Grenville KA (1987) Effects of audiometric configuration on the auditory brainstem response. Ear and Hearing 8: 49-55.

Kemp DT (1978) Stimulated acoustic emissions within the human auditory system. Journal of the Acoustical Society of America 64: 1386-1391.

Kemp DT, Ryan S (1993) The use of transient evoked otoacoustic emissions in neonatal hearing screening programmes. Seminar on Hearing 14(1): 30-44.

Kemp DT, Ryan S, Bray P (1990) A guide to the effective use of otoacoustic emissions. Ear and Hearing 11: 93-105.

Kileny PR (1981) The frequency specificity of tone-pips evoked auditory brainstem responses. Ear and Hearing 2: 217-221.

Kileny PR (1982) Auditory brainstem responses as indicators of hearing aid performance. Annals of Otology 91: 61-64.

Kileny PR (1988) New insights on infant ABR hearing screening. Scandinavian Audiology 30: 81S-88S.

Killion M, Wilber L, Gudmundsen G (1985) Insert earphones for more interaural attenuation. Hearing Inst. 36: 34-36.

Kraus N, Ozdamar O, Heydemann P T, Stein L, Reed N L (1984). Auditory brainstem responses in hydrocephalic patients. Electroencephalography and Clinical Neurophysiology 59: 310-331.

Kryter KD, Ades HW (1943) Studies on the function of the higher acoustic nervous centres in the cat. American Journal of Psychology 56: 501-536.

Laukli E (1983) High-pass and notch noise masking in suprathreshold brainstem response audiometry. Scandinavian Audiology 12: 109-115.

Liden G, Kankkunen A (1969) Visual reinforcement audiometry. Acta Otolaryngology 67: 281-292.

Lutman ME (1987) Diagnostic Audiometry. In Kerr A (Ed) Scott-Brown's Otolaryngology (5th edition). London: Butterworth.

Lutman ME, Clark J (1986) Speech identification under simulated hearing aid frequency response characteristics in relation to sensitivity frequency resolution and temporal resolution. Journal of the Acoustical Society of America 80: 1030-1040.

Lutman ME, McCormick B (1987) Converting free field A-weighted sound levels to hearing levels. Journal of the British Association of Teachers of the Deaf 11(4): 127.

Lyregaard P (1987) Towards a theory of speech audiometry tests. In Martin M (Ed) Speech Audiometry. London: Taylor and Francis.

Marchbanks RJ, Martin AM (1984). Theoretical and experimental evaluation of the diagnostic potential of the TMD measuring system. Memorandum of the Institute of Sound and Vibration Research No. 652.

Markides A (1978) Speech discrimination functions for normal hearing subjects with AB isophonemic word lists. Scandinavian Audiology 7: 239-245.

Markides A (1980) The relationship between hearing loss for pure tones and hearing loss for speech among hearing impaired children. British Journal of Audiology 14: 115-121.

Martin JAM, Bentzen O, Colley JRT, et al. (1981) Childhood deafness in the European Community, Scandinavian Audiology 10: 165-174.

Mason SM (1984a) Effects of high-pass filtering on the detection of the auditory brainstem response. British Journal of Audiology 18: 155-161.

Mason SM (1984b) On-line computer scoring of the auditory brainstem response for estimation of hearing threshold. Audiology 23: 277-296.

Mason SM (1988) Automated system for screening hearing using the auditory brainstem response. British Journal of Audiology 22: 211-213.

McCormick B (1988) Screening for Hearing Impairment in Young Children. London: Croom Helm.

McCormick B (1993) Behavioural hearing tests 6 months to 3;6 years. In McCormick B (Ed) Practical Aspects of Paediatric Audiology 0-5 years (2nd Edition). London: Whurr. pp 102-123.

McCormick B (1996) Chapter 6: Screening and surveillance for hearing. In Kerr A (Ed) Scott-Brown's Otolaryngology (6th Edition). Oxford: Butterworth-Heinenmann.

McCormick B, Wood S A, Cope Y, Spavins F M (1984) Analysis of records from an open access audiology service. British Journal of Audiology, 18, 127-132.

Mendel MI (1968) Infant responses to recorded sounds. Journal of Speech and Hearing Research 11: 811-816.

Metz O (1946) The acoustic impedance measured on normal and pathological ears. Acta Otolaryngology 63: 1S.

Moore JM, Thompson G, Folsom RC (1992) Auditory responsiveness of premature infants utilizing visual reinforcement audiometry (VRA). Ear and Hearing 13(3): 187-194.

Moore JM, Thompson G, Thompson M (1975) Auditory localization of infants as a function of reinforcement conditions. Journal of Speech and Hearing Disorders 40: 29-34.

Moore JM, Wilson WR, Thompson G (1977) Visual reinforcement of head turn responses in infants under 12 months of age. Journal of Speech and Hearing Disorders 42: 328-334.

Morgan DE, Dirks DD, Bower DR (1979) Suggested theshold sound pressure levels for frequency-modulated (warble) tones in the sound field. Journal of Speech and Hearing Disorders 44: 37-54.

Muchnik G, Neeman R K, Hildesheimer M (1995) Auditory brainstem response to bone-conducted clicks in adults and infants with normal hearing and conductive hearing loss. Scandinavian Audiology 24(3): 185-191.

Nakamura H, Takada S, Shimabuku R, Matsuo MM, Matsuo T, Negishi H (1985) Auditory nerve and brainstem responses in newborn infants with hyperbilirubinemia. Pediatrics 75(4): 703-708.

National Deaf Children's Society (1983) Discovering Deafness. London: NDCS.

National Institutes of Health (1993) Early identification of hearing impairment in infants and young children. NIH Consensus Statement 11(1): 1-24.

Nolan M (1978) Guidance on the interpretation of information from a sound level meter. Journal of the British Association of Teachers of the Deaf 2: 328-334.

Northern JL, Downs MP (1984) Hearing in Children (3rd Edition). Baltimore MA: Williams and Wilkins.

Northern JL, Downs MP (1991) Hearing in Children (4th Edition). Baltimore: Williams and Wilkins.

Orchik DJ, Rintelmann WF (1978). Comparison of pure tone, warble tone and narrow band noise thresholds of young normal hearing children. Journal of the American Audiology Society 3: 214-220.

Palmer AR, Sheppard S, Marshall DM (1991) Prediction of hearing thresholds in children using an automated toy discrimination test. British Journal of Audiology 25: 351-356.

Parker DJ, Thornton ARD (1978) Derived cochlear nerve and brainstem evoked responses of the human auditory system. Scandinavian Audiology 7: 73-80.

Patuzzi R (1993) Otoacoustic emissions and the categorisation of cochlear and retro-cochlear lesions. British Journal of Audiology 27: 91-95.

Picton TW, Ouelette K, Hamel G, Smith AD (1979) Brainstem evoked potential to tone pips in notched noise. Journal of Otolaryngology 8: 289-314.

Priede VM, Coles RRA (1976) Speech discrimination tests in investigation of sensori-neural hearing loss. British Journal of Audiology 90: 1081-1092.

Rainville MJ (1959) New method of masking for the determination of bone conduction curves. Trans. Beltone Institute Hearing Institute: 11.

Redel RC, Calvert DR (1969) Factors in screening hearing of the newborn. The Journal of Auditory Research 3: 278-289.

Reid A, Thornton ARD (1983) The effects of contralateral masking upon brainstem electric responses. British Journal of Audiology 17: 155-162.

Richardson MP, Williamson TJ, Lenton SW, Tarlow MJ, Rudd PT (1995) Otoacoustic emissions as a screening test for hearing impairment in children. Archives of Disease in Childhood 72: 294-297.

Roberts JL, Davis GL, Phon TJ, Reichert EM, Sturtevant EM, Marshall RE (1982) Auditory brainstem responses in preterm neonates: maturation and follow-up. Journal of Pediatrics 101: 257-263.

Robertson C, Aldridge S, Jarman F, Saunders K, Poulakis Z, Oberklaid F (1995) Late diagnosis of congenital sensorineural hearing impairment: why are detection methods failing? Archives of Disease in Childhood 72: 11-15.

Robinson K (1987) Children of Silence - The Story of Sarah and Joanne. London: Victor Gollancz.

Rosen S, Corcoran T (1982) A video-recorded test of lip-reading for British English. British Journal of Audiology 16(4): 245-254.

Rudmin FW (1984) Brief clinical report on visual reinforcement audiometry with deaf infants. Journal of Otolaryngology 13(6): 367-369.

Seewald RC (1992) The desired sensation level method for fitting children: version 3.0. The Hearing Journal 45: 36-41.

Smith BL, Markides A (1981) Interaural attenuation for pure tones and speech. British Journal of Audiology 15: 49-54.

Sohmer H, Kinarti R (1984) Survey of attempts to use auditory evoked potentials to obtain an audiogram (review article). British Journal of Audiology 18: 237-244.

Stappells DR, Picton TW (1981) Technical aspects of brainstem evoked potential audiometry using tones. Ear and Hearing 2: 20-29.

Stappells DR, Ruben RJ (1989) Auditory brainstem responses to bone-conducted tones in infants. Annals of Otology, Rhinolaryngology and Laryngology 98: 941-949.

Stappells DR, Picton TW, Perez-Abalo M, Read D, Smith A (1985) Frequency specificity in evoked potential audiometry. In Jacobson JT (Ed) The Auditory Brainstem Response, London:Taylor and Francis. pp 147-180.

Stevens JC, Webb HD, Hutchinson J, Connell J, Smith MF, Buffin JT (1989) Click-evoked oto-acoustic emissions compared with brainstem electric response. Archives of Disease in Childhood 64: 1105-1111.

Stevens JC, Webb HD, Smith MF, Buffin JT, Ruddy H (1987) A comparison of oto-acoustic emissions and brainstem electric response audiometry in the normal newborn and babies admitted to the special care baby unit. Clinical Physics and Physiological Measurement 8: 95-104.

Stuart A, Yang EY, Green WB (1994) Neonatal auditory brainstem response thresholds to air and bone-conducted clicks: 0 to 96 hours postpartum. Journal of the American Academy of Audiology 5(3): 163-172.

Summerfield Q, Foster JR (1983) Audiovisual speech perception, lipreading and arti-ficial stimulation. In Lutman ME, Haggard MP (Eds) Hearing Science and Hearing Disorders. London: Academic Press. pp 132-182.

Suzuki T, Ogiba Y (1961) Conditioned orientation reflex audiometry. Archives of Otolaryngology 74: 84-90.

Talbott CB (1987) A longitudinal study comparing responses of hearing-impaired infants to pure tones using visual reinforcement and play audiometry. Ear and Hearing 8(3): 175-179.

Teele DW, Teele J (1984) Detection of middle ear effusion by acoustic reflectometry. In Lim DJ, Bluestone CD, Klein JO, Nelson JD (Eds) Recent Advances in Otitis Media with Effusion. Philadelphia: BC Decker. pp 237-238.

Thompson M, Thompson G (1972) Responses of infants and young children as a function of auditory stimuli and test methods. Speech and Hearing Research 15: 699-707.

Thompson M, Weber BA (1974) Responses of infants and young children to behav-iour observation audiometry (BOA). Journal of Speech and Hearing Disorder 39: 140-147.

Tucker I, Nolan M (1984) Educational Audiology. London: Croom Helm.

Tucker SM, Battacharya J (1992) Screening of hearing impairment in the newborn using the auditory response cradle. Archives of Disease in Childhood 67: pp. 911–919.

Walker G, Dillon H, Byrne D (1984) Sound field audiometry: Recommended stimuli and procedures. Ear and Hearing 5: 13-21.

Watkin PM (1991) The age of identification of childhood deafness - improvements since the 1970s. Public Health 105: 303-312.

Watkin PM (1996) Neonatal otoacoustic emission screening and the identification of deafness. Archives of Disease in Childhood 74: F16-F25.

Watkin PM, Baldwin M, Laoide S (1990) Parental suspicion and identification of hear-ing impairment. Archives of Disease in Childhood 65: 846-850.

Watkin PM, Baldwin M, McEnery G (1991) Neonatal at risk screening and the identifi-cation of deafness. Archives of Disease in Childhood 66: 1130-1135.

Watson TJ (1957) Speech Audiometry in Children. In Ewing AWG (Ed) Educational Guidance and the Deaf Child. Manchester: Manchester University Press.

Webb HD, Stevens JC (1991) Auditory screening in high risk neonates: selection of a test protocol. Clinical Physics and Physiological Measurement 12(1): 75-86.

White KR, Behrens TR (1993) The Rhode Island Hearing Assessment Project: Implications for universal newborn hearing screening. Seminars in Hearing 14(1): 1-105.

Worthington DW, Peters JF (1980) Quantifiable hearing and no ABR: Paradox or error? Ear and Hearing 1: 281-285.

Yang EY, Stuart A (1990) A Method of auditory brainstem response to bone-conduct-ed clicks in testing infants. Journal of Speech Language Pathology and Audiology 14(4), 69-76.

Yang EY, Stuart A, Mencher GT, Mencher LS, Vincer MJ (1993a) Auditory brainstem responses to air and bone-conducted clicks in the audiological assessment of at-risk infants. Ear and Hearing 14: 175-182.

Yang EY, Stuart A, Stenstrom R, Green W B (1993b) Test-retest variability of the audi-tory brainstem response to bone-conducted clicks in newborn infants. Audiology 32: 89-94.

Yang EY, Stuart A, Stenstrom R, Hollett S (1991) Effect of vibrator to head coupling force on the auditory brainstem response to bone-conducted clicks in newborn infants. Ear and Hearing 12(1): 55-60.

Chapter 2
Deafness: Its Implications

L STEWART and D ADAMS

Introduction

Deafness is multifaceted. Some children develop a form of communication based on sign language, but for the vast majority of children who have a permanent hearing loss, this is not the case. The implications of deafness vary along a number of dimensions and the impact on any individual and their family is unique.

One of the primary implications is the potential effect deafness has on the development of communication skills. Communication is central to the development of any individual. In order to effectively support the development of communication skills and the growth of learning, it is essential that the professionals involved understand the nature and causes of deafness, the implications of the type of hearing loss in relation to auditory perception and the knock-on effect this can have on the development of spoken language. In understanding these processes, professionals can help to ensure that the potential of individual children to benefit from high quality audiological management is realised.

The causes of hearing loss in children can be classified in a number of ways; congenital or acquired, genetic (dominant inheritance or recessive inheritance), conductive or sensorineural. Fraser (1976) pointed out that the search for a cause is not of purely academic interest, but does have considerable practical implications. Parents and siblings, as well as well as other relatives of the deaf child, need as much information as possible regarding the likelihood of deafness occurring elsewhere within a particular family.

There are three types of deafness: conductive, sensorineural and mixed. There are two other conditions that may present where there is no impairment to the peripheral hearing system: psychogenic deafness and central auditory processing disorder. It is essential to bear in mind that any description of deafness used here describes one small part of a whole child. Any form of intervention will only be effective if viewed holistically – the central point is always a child. Each child is unique, as are a family's hopes and aspirations.

Physiology

It is important for the understanding of deafness that the reader has a knowledge of the structure and functions of the ear.

The ear is divided into three principal parts; the outer ear, the middle ear and the inner ear. The eustachian tube connects the middle ear to the nasal cavity.

The outer ear

The outer ear is composed of the pinna and the external auditory meatus (canal) and is separated from the middle ear by the tympanic membrane (eardrum) (Figure 2.1).

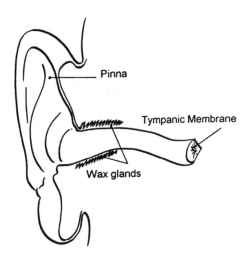

Figure 2.1 Structure of the outer ear

The pinna consists of a framework of flexible elastic cartilage covered by skin. It is claimed that the function of the pinna is to collect sound and direct it into the ear. There is a debate about how efficient this mechanism is in humans.

The external auditory meatus is about 2.5cm in length and serves to protect the inner ear to some degree. Wax glands are found only in the outer one-third of the canal, and it is important to remember that the ear has a very good self-cleansing mechanism (Figure 2.2). This self-cleansing mechanism is interfered with when parents use cotton buds in an attempt to remove ear wax, and their use should be strongly discouraged. There is also obviously a potential problem when children wear earmoulds for most of the day, because the moulds obstruct the outward movement of the wax.

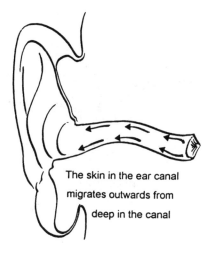

The skin in the ear canal
migrates outwards from
deep in the canal

Figure 2.2 The self-cleansing mechanism of the outer ear

The middle ear

The middle ear is an air conditioning cavity connected to the back of the nose (naso-pharynx) and to the mastoid air cells (Figure 2.3).

It is separated from the outer ear by the tympanic membrane, and contains three ossicles (Figure 2.4). The malleus is attached to the inner surface of the tympanic membrane, and the stapes is positioned in the oval window of the inner ear. Two small muscles (stapedius and tensor tympani) are attached to the stapes and the malleus respectively. These contract in response to loud sounds and may have some function in protecting the inner ear from damage caused by further or continued loud sounds. The stapedius reflex test makes use of this phenomenon (see Chapter 1).

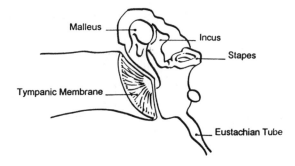

Figure 2.3 The middle ear

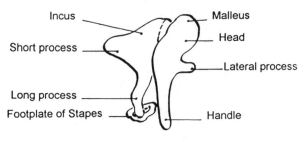

Right Ossicular Chain

Figure 2.4 The ossicles

Sound waves travelling along the ear canal cause the tympanic membrane to vibrate, and this vibration is transmitted via the ossicles to the oval window of the inner ear. The middle ear functions as an impedance matching device or transformer. Sound waves travel much more easily in fluid than in air, and in a situation where two such differing media interface, there is an impedance mismatch (Figure 2.5). Two mechanisms are involved in overcoming this mismatch and ensuring that the maximum sound energy reaches the inner ear fluids. The effective surface area of the tympanic membrane relative to that of the oval window is 14:1, and the leverage ratio of the malleus/incus is 1.3:1 (Figure 2.6). Overall, these mechanisms increase the sound energy transferred by a factor of about 18.

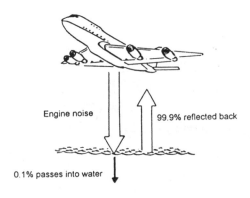

Figure 2.5 An example of impedance mismatch

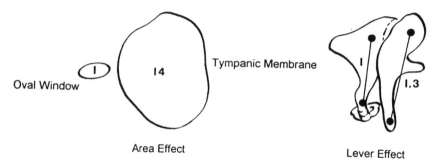

Figure 2.6 The mechanisms by which the middle ear acts as an impedance matcher

Eustachian tube

This is a bony and cartilaginous tube that connects the middle ear to the naso-pharynx (nasal cavity). Its function is to maintain air pressure in the middle ear at atmospheric level so that the tympanic membrane is able to move freely in response to sound. The eustachian tube is normally closed but is opened periodically by yawning or swallowing.

The inner ear

The inner ear has two functional parts, the cochlea (hearing) and the vestibular system (balance). The cochlea is a tube coiled into a snail-shell shape with 2.75 turns. A cross-section of the tube shows it to be divided into three compartments (Figure 2.7). The important functional compartment is the scala media (cochlea duct). In the scala media there are two rows of hair cells, outer and inner, which sit on the basilar membrane. Mechanical vibration of the stapes is transmitted to the inner hair cells through the oval window. This causes a wave to travel along the basilar membrane. The maximum amplitude of the wave is at a position

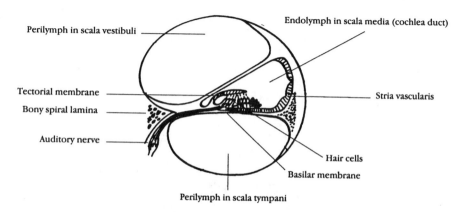

Figure 2.7 A cross-section of the cochlea

on the basilar membrane that is related to the frequency of the incoming vibration. High frequency sounds cause maximum deflection of the basilar membrane at the bottom of the cochlea (near the oval window), whereas low frequency sounds produce maximum amplitude of deflection towards the apex of the cochlea (Figure 2.8). This tuning of the basilar membrane so that different positions along it respond maximally to particular frequencies is known as tonopicity.

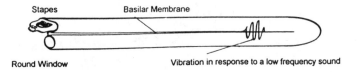

Figure 2.8 The travelling wave

The deflection of the basilar membrane causes bending of the hairs, and this in turn activates the hair cells to produce electrical impulses which are transmitted through the auditory pathway to the temporal lobe of the cerebral cortex (Figure 2.9). The nerve impulses arising from activity in the hair cells travel along the cochlear nerve to the cochlear nucleus in the brain stem. The brainstem nuclei can be compared to

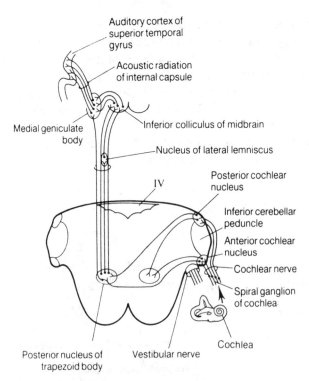

Figure 2.9 The nerve pathway

electrical junction boxes. From the cochlear nucleus, some nerve fibres pass upward on the same side (ipsilateral) in a bundle of fibres known as the lateral lemniscus to an area in the base of the brain (inferior colliculus and medical geniculate bodies). From there, new fibres radiate outwards to the temporal lobe of the cerebral cortex. Other fibres pass across the brainstem to the opposite side within the superior olivary bundle and ascend (contralaterally) eventually to reach the temporal lobe.

There has been considerable interest in the function of the outer hair cells for some time. They act as amplifiers or fine tuning devices and are the source of the otoacoustic emissions which have been described by Kemp (1978), and which are used as a screening device when testing hearing (see Chapter 1).

Conductive hearing loss

Conductive hearing loss results from an abnormality before the cochlea (Pickles, 1988). Any obstruction or malformation which impedes the transfer of sound from the environment through the outer and middle ear, thus attenuating it, will result in conductive deafness. This type of loss is within the mild to moderate range in audiological terms, characteristically ranging from 20 dBHL to a maximum of 60 dBHL. The primary effect of a conductive hearing loss is a loss of intensity, not impaired frequency selectivity. Conductive deafness is a feature of the conditions described in the following paragraphs.

Treacher Collins syndrome (mandibulofacial dysostosis)

This is a dominantly inherited syndrome. It is characterised by an under-development of the cheek bones usually associated with a similar disorder of the mandible (Figure 2.10). There may be deformities of the pinna, with stenosis (narrowing) of the external auditory canal. The tympanic membrane itself may be replaced by a bony plate. The ossicular chain has a variety of malformations and in some cases the middle ear cleft is absent. Occasionally there are also inner ear abnormalities. These children may be suitable for a bone-anchored hearing aid when the skull bones are sufficiently thick to accept the implanted prosthesis.

Pierre Robin syndrome

This is another dominantly inherited syndrome. The child will have a cleft palate, a small mandible, a large tongue, and often abnormalities of the lower limbs. The external ears may be cup shaped and appear to be very low set because of the small mandible. The middle ear may be absent or there may be abnormalities of the stapes footplate. There are occasionally abnormalities of the inner ear.

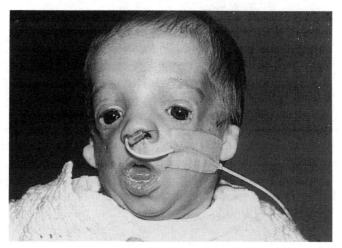

Figure 2.10 Treacher Collins syndrome (courtesy of Dr W Reardon)

Osteogenesis imperfecta

This is genetically inherited and results in the abnormal development of bone. In the ear, new soft bone is laid down in the region of the oval window (Schuknecht, 1993). Stewart and O'Reilly (1990) described their findings from a group of such patients and showed that the hearing loss first appeared in the first and second decades of life.

Cystic fibrosis

This is recessively inherited and occurs in approximately 1 in 2000 births. The nasal airway, eustachian tube and middle ear are blocked by thick mucus. There is also involvement of the salivary glands, bile duct and intestine which causes impaired digestion. Children with cystic fibrosis are susceptible to glue ear and middle ear infections. As cystic fibrosis is frequently treated with potentially ototoxic antibiotics in high dosage, children are at risk of developing a sensorineural deafness.

Cleft palate

The incidence of cleft lip/palate is one in 500-750 live births (Rood and Stool, 1981). Otitis media, especially with effusion is common. Paradise, Bluestone and Felder (1969) found that virtually all children with cleft palates under the age of 20 months had otitis media, usually with effusion. The problem may be due to a number of factors including regurgitation of irritant fluids and foods around the eustachian tube through the cleft. This causes swelling of the lower part of the eustachian tube. There is also failure of the eustachian tube to open properly when swallowing.

Down's syndrome

This is not an uncommon syndrome. It occurs in 1 in 600 of all live births. Three types of chromosomal anomaly have been distinguished in Down's syndrome:

1 Standard trisomy 21; this accounts for 95% of cases.
2 Translocations; these account for 4% of cases.
3 Mosaicism; this occurs in only 1% of cases (Rondall, 1994).

It is important to bear in mind that there is a huge diversity amongst children who have Down's syndrome. Each child will carry individual characteristics inherited from the parents, just as with any other child. The concept of a typical child who has Down's syndrome is just as unhelpful as imagining a typical deaf child.

Down's syndrome is associated with narrow external auditory canals, making it difficult to examine the tympanic membranes on occasions. It is also more difficult to insert ventilator tubes or grommets when treating glue ear (otitis media with effusion) in these children. The incidence of glue ear and ear infections is high in children with Down's syndrome (Schwartz and Schwartz, 1978). In addition there may be ossicular chain abnormalities, usually of the stapes. There can be an underlying sensorineural hearing loss, the commonest finding being that of a short cochlea. It is therefore very important to reassess hearing thresholds after insertion of ventilator tubes in children found to have glue ear, as residual hearing loss is an additional handicap in these children (Cunningham and McArthur, 1981). Pappas (1985) was of the opinion that the early detection and treatment of otological problems in children with Down's syndrome could result in the development of better communication skills and possibly a higher level of academic achievement. It is very important to note that whilst this syndrome is commonly associated with a conductive hearing loss, Buchanan (1990) reported a high incidence of acquired sensorineural loss within the first decade for this group. This is as a result of presbyacusis which is usually associated with early ageing.

Middle ear infection

Middle ear infections are very common in children. Infection is thought to get to the middle ear either via the eustachian tube, from the blood stream or through a pre-existing perforation. Perforations of the tympanic membrane are caused either by a trauma which may be as a direct result of a foreign body pushed through the membrane, or indirectly as a result of an explosion or slap in the ear. Perforations may also be caused by infection. Middle ear infections usually present with severe earache (otalgia) and hearing loss. If the infection progresses, the tympanic membrane may burst and blood-stained pus will run from the ear. The general practitioner will generally now prescribe an antibiotic, and this discharge will be prevented. Most middle ear infections have a short course and have no long term damaging effects on the ear.

Otitis media with effusion (glue ear)

There is enormous interest in this disorder, which may affect up to 50% of children under the age of 10 years at one time or another. The cause of the disorder is not yet properly understood. It may be related to dysfunction of the eustachian tube, caused for example by a large pad of adenoid, or by repeated upper respiratory tract infections. It may follow a partially resolved acute otitis media. Antibiotics, often given by the general practitioner, will sterilise the middle ear contents, but these are unable to escape down the eustachian tube. It is claimed that there is an association between the development of this disorder and parental smoking, bottle feeding and attendance at nursery school or playgroups (Paradise, Bluestone and Felder, 1969). It can be associated with speech and language delay as well as behavioural disorders. Children are often inappropriately labelled as disruptive or inattentive. Conductive hearing loss is asymptomatic and only detected when the child fails a screening test carried out by a health visitor at 7 months or by the school nurse during the first year at school. If however the child does have a hearing loss, it classically fluctuates.

It is generally agreed that there is no useful medical drug treatment for this condition. A variety of antihistamines, antibiotics and decongestants have been tried without much benefit. It is hoped that the multi-centre Medical Research Council target trial that is currently under way in the United Kingdom will provide some answers as to the best treatment options for these children. There is no doubt that many children with glue ear will get better spontaneously if they are left alone, and it is the authors' policy routinely to leave such children for 3 months before deciding whether or not to put ventilators (grommets) into their ears. The choice of surgery is also controversial. Some surgeons prefer to do only myringotomies and remove the fluid, while others take the opportunity to insert ventilator tubes while the child is under anaesthetic. Others also remove the adenoids in an attempt to improve eustachian tube function.

Trauma

Conductive deafness can be caused by either direct or indirect trauma to the ear. Direct trauma from a foreign body can perforate the tympanic membrane, as can a fracture of the bone in which the ear is housed.

Indirect trauma can result from a slap on the ear, an explosion or other cause of extreme sudden pressure change. Children are more likely than adults to have a dysfunction of the eustachian tube, and may experience problems when flying, usually during descent.

Language development: conductive hearing loss

The effect of conductive hearing loss on language development is a controversial area with many uncertainties. Research results are inconclusive (Klein and Rapin, 1988). If the 'critical period' for language learning exists, it will be affected by the reduced and inconsistent auditory input of a child with a conductive hearing loss. It is necessary to consider the inter-relationship between the age of onset, the degree, duration, and persistence of conductive hearing loss in assessing its effect on language acquisition. In general, children with a partial hearing loss should therefore not be classified as a homogeneous group for language learning.

Inconsistent auditory input

Inconsistent auditory input can start in infancy and persist until the early school years, i.e. the language learning years. Thresholds may vary from a negligible hearing loss up to a loss of 60 dBHL. For example, thresholds may vary as follows:

* normal hearing for 6 months,
* 30 dBHL loss for 2 months,
* normal hearing for 6 weeks,
* 20 dBHL loss for 3 months etc.

Northern and Downs (1984) outline the language deficit related to the acoustics of speech. The child cannot hear and process subtle information to make use of auditory strategies in order to predict or to compensate for missing information.

Prediction

Young children do not have the linguistic or auditory experience to predict the content of what is being said to them, and so they cannot compensate for the distorted stimuli they receive with a conductive hearing loss. They therefore make inaccurate decisions which impede language coding, because they do not have the strategies to cope with the same input in different acoustic formats; e.g., "cats" could be heard as "ca-", "-at" or "-a". The child may not realise that they are the same. This has a cumulative and an interactive effect. The lack of compensation means that the child suffers a communication breakdown which makes him unresponsive to further efforts at communication. The negative spiral may result in the child being understimulated, and this domino effect may exist because the input is either non-existent, fragmented, distorted or frustrating.

Receptive language development with a conductive hearing loss

Children with only 30-35 dBHL hearing loss can have a language delay of approximately 1 year on recognised tests of language skills (e.g., TROG test, Bishop,1982). Alterations in early auditory input affect speech discrimination of such high frequency sounds as voiceless fricatives s, sh, f, t, d. This means they miss the consonants that mark tense, possession and number. These consonants occur also in important function words, (Dobie and Berlin, 1979; Downs, 1985). Researchers suggest that pre-school children are still learning to discriminate voiceless fricatives (Prateate and Umano, 1981; Wardrip-Fruin and Peach, 1984). In spoken language, turn taking is dependent on the detection of the prosodic features of speech. Children with middle ear effusions may misunderstand both speech sounds and the prosodic message of language because the hearing loss affects all speech frequencies (Northern and Downs, 1984; Klein and Rapin, 1988).

The effects of a conductive hearing loss on auditory discrimination

It is essential for the teacher of the deaf to determine exactly what a child can discriminate, as this is the basis of any child's communication system. Whole word discrimination tests are more sensitive than sentences because the redundant stimuli make the sentence tests less sensitive to the auditory processing difficulties common to secretory otitis media (SOM). Problems for whole word discrimination may persist after the SOM has been resolved. Auditory discrimination tests such as Wepman (1958) or Morgan Barry (1988), or minimal pair picture pointing, would detect subtle discrepancies. In a noisy classroom the child may have difficulties in locating a sound quickly and this will prevent him from listening to the appropriate speaker (Bamford and Saunders, 1991).

The development of semantics and conductive hearing loss

Semantics means the linking of words to accepted meanings. This may not necessarily be a long standing problem for children with conductive hearing loss; poor scores may improve with time. However, the problem increases as the hearing loss increases. The initial vocabulary development may be slower, but should follow normal patterns, given appropriate stimulation. There may be some auditory confusions, such as between "mouth" and "mouse" (Bamford and Saunders, 1991).

Expressive language in children with a conductive hearing loss

Children with secretory otitis media use more simple syntax in sentences than children with normal hearing, i.e., more co-ordinate sentences joined by "and", with decreased use of more complete syntax such as prepositional phrases (e.g., "on the table"). They present with problems with morphological markers at the end of words (-s, -ed, n't, s, -est) which reflect their comprehension difficulties caused by the hearing loss. They also have errors of agreement between subject and verb, and verb tenses. Northern and Downs (1984) pointed out that a conductive hearing loss often affects the whole frequency range from 125 Hz to 8 kHz; therefore the child may have problems with phonology (segmental) and to a lesser degree with prosody (suprasegmental).

Typical segmental problems are open syllable speech (the final consonant in words is omitted), voiced/voiceless confusion (e.g., t/d confusion), and cluster reduction (e.g., "sk" becomes "k", and "sky" becomes "ky"). These all result from discrimination problems caused by inconsistent auditory input.

Controversial points to consider

Hasenstabb (1987) argues that children with conductive hearing loss may have additional disadvantages relative to children with sensorineural hearing loss, because of the following factors:

1 They do not have a stable level of acuity and therefore consistent auditory input.
2 Their environment (school or home) has not been adapted to suit their needs.
3 They are often not recognised as being hearing-impaired and are therefore not given what are perhaps much needed visual or raised intensity cues in communication.
4 They may not receive amplification and regular aural habilitation from the teacher of the deaf.

Conclusion

Conductive hearing loss affects cognitive and social development as well as linguistic development. Some authors would argue that it has a transient effect (Zinkus et al., 1978; Zinkus and Gottlieb, 1980; Brandes and Ehinger, 1981) and that in the long term they remain unaffected (Lous, Fiellau-Nikolajsen, 1984). The child needs consistent auditory input for optimum development. The effect of even a slight loss cannot be underestimated. It particularly affects children who may already face challenges in the learning process:

- Children with reading difficulties.
- Children who are already underachieving.
- Children who have behaviour problems.
- Children who are suffering from social and emotional problems.
- Children who already have poor attention skills.
- Children who do not have a rich language base.
- Children who already have underlying speech difficulties.
- Children who are frequently absent from school.

Sensorineural hearing loss

A sensorineural hearing loss is one which occurs as a result of damage to both the sensory and neural systems. Pathology or disease affecting the inner ear or neural pathways is irreversible. This type of hearing loss affects not only the ear's ability to hear sounds of varying intensity, but also its ability to discriminate between sounds of different frequencies. It makes it difficult for a child to cope in noisy situations, because loud sounds can appear to be much louder than they actually are. The difference between the level at which a child can just hear and the level at which a sound causes him pain (i.e., the dynamic range) can be very small.

Sensorineural deafness in children may be present at birth (congenital) or may appear at some time afterwards (acquired). This classification is not entirely satisfactory because there are a number of congenital conditions in which a child is born with normal hearing but develops a hearing loss during the first decade of life, such as Alport's Syndrome. Sensorineural deafness is a feature of the following:

Usher's syndrome

Usher's syndrome is a recessively inherited syndrome which affects both hearing and vision. Visual impairment is caused by retinitis pigmentosa which leads to loss of peripheral vision, in turn leading to tunnel vision and possible eventual blindness. This process begins in the early teens or twenties. There are three types of Usher's syndrome. Type I and Type II are by far the most common. In Type I, there is severe to profound deafness, absence of balance and the onset of retinitis pigmentosa before puberty. In Type II on the other hand, there is moderate to severe hearing loss, no balance problems and later onset of visual impairment. Usher's syndrome accounts for 3-6% of children who are congenitally deaf (Chan, 1994). Children with this syndrome present challenges for the teacher of the deaf, who must be aware of the implications for a child who potentially will have a dual sensory impairment.

Waardenburg syndrome

This is dominantly inherited and accounts for 2% of all children who have a congenital hearing loss (Chan, 1994). There are two types. In Type I the inner fold of the eye is displaced laterally, giving the bridge of the nose a broad appearance. In Type II the inner fold of the eye is not displaced, 20% of affected children have a white forelock, and 45% have different colours in one iris (heterochromia iridis) or have irides of different colours. Chan (1994) was of the opinion that Type II was 20 times more common than Type I. Newton, Liu and Read (1994) found that a profound sensorineural hearing loss associated with small blue irides was more common in children with Type I, whereas children with Type II usually have different coloured irides and asymmetrical audiograms. The unusual eye signs do not appear to cause any visual disturbance.

Alport's syndrome

This is principally a renal (kidney) disorder. Males tend to be more severely affected than females. The hearing loss is usually bilateral and at high frequencies. Children present with blood and protein in the urine in the first 10 years. In about 50% of patients the high frequency sensorineural hearing loss develops at 10 years of age. This progresses to become much more severe.

Rubella

The number of children affected by rubella has declined (Newton, 1985; Davis, 1993). In Newton's series 75% of the children who were deaf as a result of rubella were born to mothers who were not immunised. Deafness occurs in about one-third of rubella children, who may also have microcephaly and mental retardation with eye lesions and abnormalities of the cardiovascular system. Hemenway, Sando and McChesney (1969) described the abnormal findings in the ear. There may be abnormalities of the stapes including fixation of the stapes footplate. The cochlea and saccule of the inner ear are abnormal. As a result of these problems the sensorineural hearing loss is usually severe to profound.

Cytomegalovirus

There is controversy as to the importance of cytomegalovirus in the causation of congenital sensorineural deafness. It may well be of more importance than has been previously estimated (Pappas, 1983). Cytomegalovirus can be congenital, can occur during the perinatal period, or can be acquired. Newton (1985) felt that perinatal incidence was commoner than congenital, but caused less damage to hearing. The hearing loss is usually severe to profound and bilateral, but may in a few cases be unilateral (Strauss, 1990). There is some evidence that the hearing loss in these children is progressive (Hickson and Alcock, 1991). There is also concern that some of these children who have apparently normal hearing thresholds may in fact have a higher centre dysfunction (Connolly et al., 1992). The important clinical application of this finding relates to auditory processing by these children in noisy classroom situations.

Toxoplasmosis

This is much less common than either rubella or cytomegalovirus infection. It is usually not obvious at birth, but eventually manifests itself with progressive blindness, liver disease, epilepsy or hydrocephalus. It would appear that the hearing loss develops in only 10-15% of children with congenital toxoplasmosis, and even in these, does not become obvious until much later.

Perinatal disorders causing sensorineural hearing loss

There is no doubt that children who are pre-term with a low birth weight are much more at risk of having a hearing loss than a baby delivered at term (Newton, 1985; Davis Razi and Das, 1994). In this group there is more than one risk factor present and this makes the contribution of each difficult to ascertain. The three main risk factors are hypoxia (shortage of oxygen), hyperbilirubinaemia (jaundice) and pre-term delivery/low birth weight. Rhesus incompatibility used to be the commonest cause of hyperbilirubinaemia in the United Kingdom, but with modern methods of management and prevention, neonatal jaundice has virtually disappeared as a cause of congenital deafness. Low birth weight/ pre-term children are more at risk than mature children for many reasons; they may have suffered episodes of hypoxia, or have immature metabolic functions and spend some time in intensive care units in noisy incubators. In summary, it is often difficult to ascertain the causative agent in these children because of the number of potential risk factors. It is possible that these factors exert a synergistic effect on the auditory system.

Other childhood viral illnesses

Mumps is thought to be the commonest cause of unilateral sensorineural hearing loss in children. Measles may also rarely cause hearing loss which tends to be bilateral and moderate to severe.

Meningitis

The most frequent cause of acquired sensorineural hearing loss in childhood is meningitis (David and Wood, 1992). A useful review of literature was provided by Fortnum (1992). The incidence of post-meningitic hearing impairment is reported as varying from 3.5% to as high as 37.2%. It is likely however that the true incidence is somewhere in the region of 10%. The deafness is usually bilateral and profound, although it can be less severe in cases and unilateral. There have been reports of improvements in hearing after meningitis although these improvements are more often reported in cases with less severe problems. Fortnum (1992) described recent advances in both prevention and treatment of bacterial meningitis. Immunisation against one of the organisms, haemophilus influenzae, is now available. There is also considerable interest in the use of steroids in the early treatment of meningitis. There have been only a few documented cases of hearing impairment after viral meningitis. The author has not seen any to date.

Ototoxic drugs

The potential of many drugs to damage the inner ear is well recognised. The most important are aminoglycoside antibiotics. These are powerful antibiotics such as streptomycin and gentamycin which are normally used only in life threatening infections. In a study of Albanian children Kastanioudakis et al. (1993) found a significant number of children with hearing loss and vestibular damage due to the administration of streptomycin sulphate. Gray (1989) described a similar problem in India. The antibiotics would appear to damage the hair cells of the cochlea.

Trauma

Fractures of the bone in which the inner ear is housed can damage the cochlea. It is also important to remember that ear operations, even in minor procedures such as myringotomy, may very occasionally cause inner ear damage. Amplified music is a potential source of noise in our environment. Portable stereo cassette players with headphones can generate noise intensity levels that are potentially hazardous to human ears (Catalano and Levin, 1985). Concern has been expressed about the potential hearing loss caused by high powered hearing aids. Many authors have studied the problem, but found no evidence of deterioration of hearing caused by hearing aids (Fradis and Feighlin, 1984; Newton and Rowson, 1988).

Language acquisition: sensorineural hearing loss

The effects upon receptive and expressive language skills, both spoken and written, vary enormously from child to child and usually present as a range of difficulties rather than as one dimension. Bench and Bamford (1979) state that there are dangers in treating children with hearing loss as a homogeneous group, as it is not necessarily possible to predict the outcome from the degree of hearing loss. Mild or moderate hearing loss can cause subtle problems with reading, spelling and conceptual skills in an educational context. Children with a unilateral hearing loss may have language related problems caused by discrimination difficulties in noisy environments (Davis, 1986). Averaging the hearing loss across the frequencies belies the difficulties children with high frequency ski-slope losses will experience in discriminating high frequency consonants (Mogford, 1988).

For the deaf child, as soon as development diverges from the norm, language learning processes change, becoming more visual as the child attempts to utilise any available information to assist in communication. It is important that a mother is able to gauge the level of her child's language and to pitch her own language level appropriately. This may not be the case with hearing mothers of hearing-impaired children. Gross (1970) found that hearing mothers of deaf children spoke to them less, tended not to use normal intonation patterns and were less likely to use verbal praise than mothers of hearing children. Wedell-Monig and Lumley (1980) found that hearing parents of deaf children used more utterances to control and direct behaviour, and frequently 'flooded' the children with language. Researchers have found that the communication climate of deaf mothers with deaf children was similar to that of hearing mothers with hearing children, i.e., elaborating, extending, contingent, child initiated, encouraging enjoyment of communication.

The pre-verbal stage

Babbling is not altered in the first months of life for the deaf child, with normal crying and cooing sounds. After this, babbling decreases gradually with age due to lack of environmental stimulation and auditory feedback. The babble of children with sensorineural loss differs qualitatively and quantitatively, having fewer multi-syllabic utterances incorporating with consonants. Mothers tended to ignore these vocalisations, as they were less speech-like (Mogford, 1988).

Vocal imitation relates directly to speech development and emerges from a mother's imitation of her child's vocalisations. When babble incorporates speech-like qualities, these vocalisations are incorporated into the mother's dialogue (Mogford and Gregory, 1982). Failure to produce speech-like sounds at this early stage can have a 'knock-on' effect. Late diagnosis of hearing loss and consequently late fitting of hearing aids further compounds this problem. Early mother–child inter- actions are characterised by a high level of synchrony (Schaffer, 1977). Turn-taking as a particular feature of mother–baby vocalisations. In addition, early looking behaviour is usually baby-led, with the mother following the infant's line of gaze. When an infant has a severe or profound hearing loss, this close synchrony is under threat. Verbal inter- changes are likely to be quantitatively reduced, and infants will miss comments relating to the immediate visual environment. By the age of seven months, mother and baby (and often father and baby) have a well worked-out routine for communicating with each other non-verbally (Harris et al., 1986).

In the case of a deaf infant with hearing parents this is not the case. Hearing impairment disrupts the process. Labelling of objects, people, and pictures needs shared visual attention through pointing and mutual gaze monitoring. Some vocal play usually follows. Without skilled inter- vention the child is likely to have great difficulty in co-ordinating vocal and visual input from his mother, delaying labelling.

Structure of language

It is useful to look in detail at the four levels of language, using an analogy of a house to explain how each level functions:

Foundations (= pragmatics)

"Pragmatics is the study of how utterances are used to convey meaning in different social and environmental contexts" (Bishop and Mogford, 1994). This involves the desire to communicate and the knowledge of how and when to communicate. This level is essential and without this any other level of language is meaningless (the house will not be built). There is no reason for the different use of language or intentions expressed by a deaf child, but problems occur in recognising the inten- tions of others and acquiring linguistic devices to mark pragmatic functions. When language structure is delayed, intentions are marked by less sophisticated devices. Initially using non-verbal means or single words, the child will indicate a wide range of pragmatic intentions. Syntactic problems may eventually be pragmatic because the child may not know how or when to use pragmatic devices.

Conversations

In order to allow the deaf child to (1) respond appropriately, (2) partner, (3) initiate and (4) sustain conversation, his conversational partner (for example his mother) must provide him with a great number and variety of appropriate opportunities in which he can engage with her. Mother/child or teacher/child interaction will vary with the age and the maturity of the child. In children who are 2 years old for example, mothers initiate interaction and dominate the conversation, and the child has minimal verbal abilities. With 5 year olds, mothers adapt their language to the child's language levels rather than to his cognitive levels. When a child is unable to respond appropriately to a pause in the conversation, the conversational partner will respond by reducing the linguistic demands being made. Thus the cognitive level of a child may be masked by the child's ability to engage in dialogue. The flow of dialogue may be limited because of fewer 'responses' from the child. This suggests that dialogue develops along with linguistic ability.

In the case of children who are 5–11 years old, a teacher may exhibit a high level of control of conversation by, for example, frequent use of questions. This results in a decrease in the length of the child's contribution and in the number of opportunities given to the child to initiate conversations. With reduced teacher control, there is an opportunity for the child to develop more conversational initiative and thus make longer contributions. In this way he can demonstrate awareness of conversational structure, for instance, that a question must be followed by an answer, or that a comment is followed by a free contribution (Wood and Wood, 1992). Younger children exhibit problems initiating and developing conversations, as well as problems in establishing mutually relevant themes. They often give short ambiguous contributions, and teachers have problems dealing with misunderstandings without interrupting the conversational flow. There needs to be much more research into the difficulties that children with hearing impairment have in understanding and in making themselves understood with adults in conversation.

Walls (= semantics)

"This involves the study of meaning" (Bishop and Mogford, 1994). This aspect of language is fundamental to the functioning of the remaining levels. It is at this level that meaning is attached to a sound or a sign system that enables the deaf child to interpret what is being said and to convey meaning. Without the walls we can have no windows, door or roof. Early research (Templin, 1950) on children with sensorineural hearing loss looked at vocabulary and found it to be restricted or delayed. It contains fewer abstract and more concrete nouns. Standardised tests used by Davis (1986) on basic concepts found that 75% were below the 10th percentile of norms (with a moderate to severe hearing loss). Here children with milder losses did significantly better. The most difficult concepts for them were time and quantity, while the spatial concepts were the most accessible. There was a patchiness of response and no difference in performance with age. Location is one of the earliest developing semantic functions due to the dominance of visual/spatial aspects. Early language labelling shows greater cognitive maturity (due to a longer pre-verbal stage) in using more abstract qualities of size, colour and number. Other studies looked at understanding of the temporal order of events (i.e., before, after, first, last). These resembled a younger child's performance, where they responded to complex sentences as though they occurred in the order mentioned. In adulthood those semantic fields occurring or acquired late were not always used by the hearing-impaired, although a coherent and systematic picture has not yet been developed.

Windows/Doors (= syntax)

"Syntax – a system of rules which accounts for the ways in which different parts of speech may be legitimately combined to form sentences in a language" (Bishop and Mogford, 1994). Syntax involves using grammatical rules of language to combine words. This is the useful part of language, i.e. how we make language work for us by combining words using the rules of our language. We use doors and windows as flexible and manoeuvrable parts of the house. Early studies by Templin in 1950 show the use of circumlocution with increased use of content words, i.e. nouns and verbs, and decreased use of 'function' words, i.e. conjunctions, verbal auxiliaries, prepositions and pronouns. It is therefore concluded that deaf children use telegraphic language and that they also have more errors in written language. Their expressive language may lack flexibility and appear to be stereotyped and repetitious, with overuse of Subject Verb Object (SVO) structures and infrequent conjoined and complex sentences. Taught phrases are used repeatedly, in which certain simple word orders are rigidly adhered to. Bench and Bamford (1979) used LARSP (Crystal et al., 1976) profiles and found a marked lack of use of word level and morphological markers, to a greater degree than that found with children who have a conductive hearing loss.

At phrase and clause level there is a decreased use of advanced level combinations, i.e. a shorter mean sentence length. In summary, there is a reduced use of complex sentences and sentence connectivity. Quigley (1984) used the test of syntactic abilities and found that, even when deaf children understood the vocabulary and concepts, they had problems in understanding the syntactic structures. They showed some differences in order of acquisition and treated all sentences as SVO patterns, missing, for example, the passive voice, e.g. "The boy was helped by the girl" read as "The boy helped the girl". A linear order of words dominated, with some aspects of language being deviant and delayed. Bishop feels that the development of understanding of grammatical contrasts is not simply delayed, but involves different processing strategies. Bishop (1983) found that these strategies are not exclusive to the

deaf, but are used by other groups with syntactic difficulties. This under-
mines the assumption that the language learning facility remains
unaffected when lip-reading and residual hearing are used to overcome
the perceptual barrier. This is another controversial area.

Roof (= phonology)

"Phonology – the study of how speech sounds function to signal
contrasts in meaning in a language" Bishop and Mogford (1994). The
differing sounds combining in a system of contrasts enables us to
identify objects, actions and thoughts. We also use intonation to communicate our feelings and opinions. To describe phonological development
it is easiest to break it into two parts:

1 segmental – phonemes, the smallest segment of sound that can be
   distinguished within a word
2 suprasegmental – prosody, the stress, length, tone and intonation.

Both parts are affected by difficulties with control of voice quality and
articulatory accuracy. Normally they are acquired primarily by auditory
means, with some complementary visual perception, i.e. visual clues
where auditory discrimination is difficult and vice versa.

Segmental

For the child with severe or profound sensorineural hearing loss, there
is a greater challenge; he/she has to rely on minimal auditory cues, and
this affects speech intelligibility. This does not indicate the absence of
meaningful contrasts, but unintelligibility may be due instead to
phonetic inaccuracy. Information about the vowels, together with
rhythm, intonation and stress, is mainly carried in the low frequencies. A
child may be able to make sufficient use of his/her low frequency
residual hearing to discriminate vowels with the use of a hearing aid.
However, depending on audiometric configuration of hearing loss,
he/she may gain little or nothing from the high frequencies. It is
primarily the high frequencies that the listener uses to distinguish
consonants. The importance of consonants is effectively demonstrated
when they are removed from the following simple sentence;

-a- e -ou -a--e- i- -ou- -o- e -o-- -e-?
(Have you handed in your homework yet?).

A child with very little hearing in the high frequencies may pick up
some secondary cues from the low frequencies (formants), which
explains why their speech may be much clearer than anticipated in spite
of their difficulties in discriminating consonants. This underlines the
critical importance of ensuring a high quality of audiological manage-

ment, enabling a child with a profound hearing loss to have access to minimal auditory cues. Lack of this is often reflected in the speech of deaf children, when consonants are omitted or mispronounced. With a severe hearing loss, the phonology may well resemble that of a younger child and may exhibit a range of immature processes:

- Cluster reduction, e.g., spoon becomes -poon.
- Final consonant deletion, e.g., bag becomes -ba.
- Voicing avoidance, e.g., boy becomes -poy.
- Velar plosive avoidance, e.g., car becomes -tar.
- Fronting, e.g., good becomes -dood.
- Stopping, e.g., ship becomes -dip.

Most of these children have an adequate vowel system. For children with profound losses the vowel system is also affected and this severely affects intelligibility. It is vital that the child develops a system of contrastive sounds that can enable him to convey changes in meaning.

Suprasegmental

If a child has a severe/profound hearing loss, the quality of the voice may be hypernasal and there will be additional difficulties controlling vocal cord vibration. There will also be problems of varying degrees with volume control, rhythm, stress, and pitch, with abnormal or reduced intonation. The rate of speech may be slow and laboured. In some cases the air stream may be ingressive, and the use of injectives rather than the normal use of egressive pulmonic air stream will be noted. Effective early intervention can ensure that these difficulties are minimised.

The factors governing the effect of hearing loss on speech and language development can be summarised as follows:

1 The type of hearing loss (as discussed above).
2 The age of onset. The effect of hearing loss will vary greatly dependent on when the hearing loss has occurred, i.e. on whether the child is pre-lingually or post-lingually deaf.
3 The age of diagnosis. Early identification is vital. Early diagnosis and early and appropriate intervention give the deaf child the maximum opportunity to achieve his potential.
4 Amplification. Immediate and accurate hearing aid fitting is essential as soon as the hearing loss has been diagnosed.
5 Acceptance of hearing aids. The teacher of the deaf may have to work hard to achieve this goal on behalf of the parents and family of the deaf child and on behalf of the child himself. Only when this happens will vital listening opportunities be made available routinely to the child. The aid must be working efficiently, and the earmould must be a good fit if this end is to be achieved.

6   Effectiveness of parent guidance. Counselling is of paramount impor-
    tance. The teacher of the deaf must focus on creating positive
    attitudes to the hearing aids and to the deaf child. Parent guidance
    must focus on promoting the use of a stimulating language environ-
    ment for the child. It is vital for all professionals involved in the team
    working with the family to have a holistic approach, avoiding any
    conflict of advice to the family which could cause them confusion and
    distress.
7   The presence of additional challenges. Hearing impairment may also
    be accompanied by the following:
    •   learning disabilities of varying degrees, e.g., Tay-sachs, Hurler's
        syndrome,
    •   visual impairment, e.g., Usher's syndrome,
    •   physical disability, e.g., cerebral palsy.
        More hidden problems which are easily overlooked and should
        be assessed separately by the appropriate professionals include:
    •   language disorder,
    •   speech problems which can also occur in normally hearing
        children and which may also present in deaf children's speech,
    •   central auditory processing,
    •   dyspraxia,
    •   dysarthria,
    •   dyslexia.
8   The individual child's personality, intelligence and emotional
    development.
9   The educational input which he/she receives. This will be influenced
    by the type of school, size of class, quality of teaching as well as the
    language policies of the school.
10 If there is a difference between the language used at home and at
    school, this can delay the child's acquisition of language initially. As
    soon as a first language is acquired this plays a much smaller role. The
    types of language input include: BSL, English, another spoken
    language and signed English.

Non-organic deafness (psychogenic deafness)

There are three types of non-organic hearing loss; functional deafness,
malingering, and organic deafness with psychogenic overlay. In
functional or hysterical deafness the hearing loss is generated by the
subconscious. It may be a reaction to stress, especially when the child is
not doing as well at school as the parents would like. In some cases it is a
means of identifying with another member of the family who has a
hearing problem. Clinically, the child's hearing is usually better than the
audiogram would suggest, and the audiograms are not repeatable.
Malingering is rare in children because they are not usually sophisticated

enough to maintain the pretence for long and there is rarely the motivation for financial gain as is sometimes seen in adults.

Central auditory processing disorders (CAPD)

It is impossible to know how many children have CAPD because no standard definition of terminology is used (Keith, 1995). The disorder should be suspected when children with normal audiograms show the following features:

- Inconsistent response to auditory stimuli.
- Short attention span.
- Distraction by both auditory and visual stimuli.
- Difficulty with location.
- Requests for information to be repeated.
- Problems with short and long term memory.
- Difficulty relating what is heard to words on paper.
- Possible difficulties with spelling.
- Possible difficulties in monitoring own voice level.
- Possible difficulty in rapidly processing auditory information.
- Possible difficulty retrieving appropriate words when speaking (English and Adkins, 1996).

The disorder may be caused by a number of problems, including delayed maturation of the central nervous system and injury of the brain from trauma or infection. There is also a suggestion that persistent glue ear may result in auditory learning difficulties (Keith, 1995). The management of this condition presents a number of challenges, involving auditory training or a language development approach (Keith, 1995).

Conclusion

Deafness in various types and degrees has far-reaching implications for the development of language, and therefore presents enormous challenges to teachers of the deaf. The house analogy in this chapter is a simplified attempt to clarify a complicated process involving four inter-related and interdependent levels of language. There are many overlaps; however, the fundamental principle of considering the language development of children by looking firstly at the pragmatic and semantic levels and then considering syntax and phonology, reflects normal developmental patterns. Teachers of the deaf, speech and language therapists and other professionals must therefore have an informed and mutually supportive approach to empower families so that their child can achieve the most effective communication system possible. Early identification of hearing loss is vital to allow the fast, efficient and appropriate provision of intervention. This will enable maximum use of residual hearing. It is essential that all involved understand the need for effective audiological management to promote good quality listening to aid language development.

References

Bamford JM, Saunders E (1991) Hearing Impairment, auditory perception and language disability. Whurr: London.

Bench J, Bamford JM (1979) Speech tests and the spoken language of hearing impaired children. Academic Press, London.

Bishop D (1982) TROG–Test for the Reception of Grammar. Medical Research Council.

Bishop D (1983) Comprehension of English syntax by profoundly deaf children. Journal of Child Psychology and Psychiatry 24: 415–434.

Bishop D, Mogford K (1994), Language in Exceptional Circumstances. Hove: Laurence Erlbaum.

Brandes PJ, Ehinger DM (1981) The effects of early middle ear pathology on auditory perception and academic achievement. Journal of Speech and Hearing Disorders, 46: 301–307.

Buchanan LH (1990) Early onset of presbycusis in Down's Syndrome. Scandinavian Audiology 19: 103–110.

Catalano PJ, Levin SM (1985) Noise induced hearing loss and portable radio with headphones. International Journal of Paediatric Otorhinolaryngology 9, 59–67.

Chan KH (1994) Sensorineural hearing loss in children - classification and evaluation. Paediatric Otology, Otolaryngologic Clinics of North America 27: 473–486.

Connolly PK, Jerger S, Williamson WD, Smith RJH, Denmler G (1992) Evaluation of higher level auditory function in children with asymptomatic congenital cytomegalovirus infection. American Journal of Otology 13: 185–192.

Crystal D, Fletcher P, Gamian M (1976) The Grammatical Analysis of Language Disability. A procedure for assessment and remediation. London: Edward Arnold.

Cunningham CC, McArthur K (1981) Hearing loss and treatment in young Down's syndrome children. Child Care Health and Development 7: 357–374.

David A, Wood S (1992) The epidemiology of childhood hearing impairment: factors relevant to planning of services. British Journal of Audiology 26: 77–90.

Davis A (1993) The prevalance of deafness. In: Ballantyne J, Martin MC, Martin A (Eds) Deafness (5th Edition). London: Whurr.

Davis J (1974) Performance of young hearing impaired children on a test of basic concepts. Journal of Speech and Hearing Disorders 17: 342–357.

Davis J (1986) Effects of mild and moderate hearing impairments in language, education and psychosocial behaviour in children. Journal of Speech and Hearing Disorders, 51: 530–562.

Davis J, Razi MS, Das VK (1994) Effects of adverse perinatal events on hearing. International Journal of Paediatric Otorhinolaryngology. 30: 29–40.

Dobie RA, Berlin C (1979) Influence of otitis media on hearing and development. Annals of Otology, Rhinology and Laryngology, suppl. 60: 45–53.

Downs MP (1985) Effect of mild hearing loss on auditory processing. Otolaryngologic Clinics of North America 18: 337–344.

English K, Adkins T (Eds) (1996) CAPD, the basics. In: Educational Audiology Association newsletter, Spring,: 6.

Fortnum HM (1992) Hearing impairment after bacterial meningitis. Archives of Disease in Childhood 67: 1128–1133.

Fradis M, Feighlin H (1984) Effects of hearing aids on hearing. Laryngoscope 94: 113–117.

Fraser GR (1976) The cause of profound deafness in childhood. London: Ballière Tindall.

Gray RJ (1989) Causes of deafness in schools for the deaf in Madras. International Journal of Pediatric Otorhinolaryngology 18: 97–106.

Gross RN (1970) Language used by mothers of deaf children and mothers of hearing children. American Annals of the Deaf 115: 93–96.

Harris M, Jones D, Brookes S, Grant J (1986) Relations between the non-verbal context of maternal speech and the rate of language development. British Journal of Deveolpmental Psychology 4: 261–268.

Hasenstabb S (1987) Language Learning and Otitis Media. Taylor and Francis.

Hemenway W, Sando I, McChesney D (1969) Temptoral bone pathology following maternal rubella. Archive fur Klinische und Experimentelle Ohren–Nasen and Kehlkopfheilkunde 193: 287–300.

Hickson LM, Alcock D (1991) Progressive hearing loss in children with congenital hearing cytomegalovirus. Journal of Paediatrics and Child Health 27: 105–107.

Kanstanioudakis J, Skevas A, Asimakopoulous D, Anastassopoulos D (1993) Hearing loss and vestibular dysfunction in childhood from use of streptomycin in Albania. International Journal of Pediatric Otorhinolaryngology 26: 109–115.

Keith RW (1995) Test of central auditory processing. In: Roeser R, Downs M (Eds) Auditory disorders in children. (3rd edition) New York: Thieme Medical Publishers.

Kemp DT (1978) Stimulated acoustic emissions within the human auditory system. Journal of the Acoustical Society of America 64: 1386–1391.

Klein SK, Rapin I (1988) Intermittent conductive hearing loss and language development. In: Bishop D, Mogford K (Eds) Language in Exceptional Circumstances. Hove: Lawrence Erlbaum.

Lous J, Fiellau-Nikolajsen M (1984) A five year prospective case control study of the influence of early otitis media with effusion on reading achievement. International Journal of Pediatric Otorhinlaryngology 8: 19–30.

Mogford K (1988) Oral language in the prelingually deaf. In: Bishop D, Mogford K (Eds) Language in Exceptional Circumstances. Hove: Lawrence Erlbaum.

Mogford K, Gregory S (1982) The development of communication skills in young deaf children: picture book reading with mother; cited in Bishop D, Mogford K, Language in Exceptional Circumstances, Hove: Lawrence Erlbaum.

Morgan Barry R (1988) The Auditory Discrimination and Attention Test. Windsor: NFER/Nelson.

Newton V (1985) Aetiology of bilateral sensori-neural hearing loss in young children. Journal of Laryngology and Otology Suppl. 10.

Newton VE, Rowson VJ (1988) Progressive sensorineural hearing loss in young children. Journal of Laryngology and Otology. Suppl 10. 1–57.

Newton VE, Liu X - Z, Read A (1994) The association of sensorineural hearing loss and pigmentation abnormalities in Waardenburg syndrome. Journal of Audiological Medicine. 3: 69–78.

Northern JL, Downs MP (1984) Hearing in Children. Baltimore: Williams and Wilkins.

Pappas DG (1983) Hearing Impairment and vestibular abnormalities among children with subclinical cytomegalovirus. Annals of Otology, Rhinology and Laryngology 92: 552–557.

Pappas DG (1985) Diagnosis and Treatment of Hearing Impairment in Children. London: Taylor and Francis.

Paradise JL, Bluestone CD, Felder H (1969) The Universality of otitis media in 50 infants with cleft palate. Paediatrics 44: 35–42.

Pickles JO (1988) An introduction to the physiology of hearing. London and New York: Academic Press.

Prateate DD, Umano H (1981) Auditory discrimination of voiceless fricatives in children. Journal of Speech and Hearing Research. 24: 162–168.

Quigley SP, Power DJ, Steinkamp MW (1977) The Language Structure of Deaf Children. Volta Review. 79: 73–84.

Quigley SP (1984) Language and Deafness. San Diego: College Hill, London: Croom Helm.

Rondall JA (1994) Down's syndrome. In Bishop D, Mogford K (Eds) Language in Exceptional Circumstances. Hove: Lawrence Erlbaum.

Rood SR, Stool SE (1981) Current concepts of aetiology, diagnosis and management of cleft palate related otopathologic disease. Otolaryngology Clinics in North America 14: 865–884.

Schaffer HR (1977) Studies in Mother Child Interaction. New York: Academic Press.

Schuknecht HF (1993) Pathology of the Ear. (2nd edition) Philadelphia: Lea and Febiger.

Schwartz DM, Schwartz RM (1978) Acoustic impedance and otosopic findings in young children with Down's syndrome. Archives of Otolaryngology 100: 258–260.

Stewart EJ, O'Reilly BF (1990) A clinical and audiological investigation of osteogenesis imperfecta in Scottish patients. Clinical Otolaryngology 15: 93 (abstract).

Strauss M (1990) Human Cytomegalovirus labyrinithitis. American Journal of Otolaryngology 11: 292–298.

Templin MC (1950) The development of reasoning in children with normal and defective hearing. Minnesota: University of Minnesota.

Wardrip-Fruin C, Peach S (1984). Developmental aspects of the perception of acoustic cues in determining the voicing feature of final stop consonants. Language and Speech 27: 367–379.

Wedell-Monig J, Lumley JM (1980) Child deafness and mother interaction. Child Development 51: 766–774.

Wepman J (1958) Auditory Discrimination Test. Los Angeles: CA Western Psychological Services.

Wood D, Wood H (1992) Teaching and Talking with Deaf Children. Chichester: Wiley.

Zinkus PW, Gottlieb MI, Schapiro M (1978) Developmental and psycho-educational sequelae of chronic otitis media. American Journal of Diseases in Children 132: 1100–1104.

Zinkus PW, Gottlieb MI (1980) Patterns of perceptual and academic defecits related to early chronic otitis media. Paediatrics 66: 246–253.

Chapter 3
The Multiply Handicapped Deaf Child

F CONINX and J M MOORE

Illustrations by H. Rosier

Introduction

Although 'multiply disabled' has to be considered as the better termi-nology, throughout this chapter 'multiply handicapped' will be used, because it is more widely used and familiar. A person is referred to as 'multiply handicapped' when he/she has more than one (primary) disability, and where there is a complicating, negative interference between the various handicaps. In those cases, assessment and treat-ment is more complex than with the handicaps in isolated form.

The group of multiply handicapped deaf children is characterised by its high heterogeneity, representing a wide spectrum of sensory, physical, emotional, intellectual, social and educational needs. Some main classes and typical problems in hearing assessment and aural rehabilitation are:

- Deaf-blind children, who pose serious problems in hearing assess-ment because of the lack of visual functions (i.e. absent or insufficient visual control or reinforcement possibilities), or extremely delayed mental development (that is, difficulties in conditioning for assess-ment tasks). In working and playing situations, the parent or teacher is typically in close proximity to the child, so that gain requirements in hearing aids have to be lowered to prevent over-amplification.
- Deaf children with severe learning disability, with specific difficulties in conditioning for assessment tasks. Goals of aural rehabilitation may have to be adjusted for non-symbolic (non-verbal) hearing levels. Personal care of hearing aids is generally impossible.
- Down's syndrome, with a high incidence of hearing impairment; Downs (1980) reported an incidence of 78%. Narrow external ear canals and abnormal external ear configurations means earmould production and hearing aid use may be problematic. There is a dominance of conductive losses, and a high risk for recurring otitis media, implying

fluctuating or increasing hearing loss. Accelerated auditory ageing has been reported by Buchanan (1990), with presbyacusis symptoms within the first decade. This stresses the need for regular auditory check-ups.

- Cerebral palsy, characterised by uncontrollable motor spasms due to brain lesion, and resulting in poor head control (excluding the use of head-turn type responses, such as in VRA) and hand motor control (inability to perform regular play-audiometry tasks). Also, these children may show serious problems in handling their hearing aids, and increased risk for auditory feedback when seated in specially designed chairs with head restraints.

- Autism, characterised by an inability to attend to auditory stimuli or to respond consistently to them. There may be an over-sensitivity to background noises. Preoccupation with certain activities and stimuli, quite often in the visual domain, makes the child pervasively lacking in adequate responses. Hearing assessment with behavioural procedures is extremely difficult. The use of visual stimuli in trying to condition the child for audiometrical tests must be avoided, as the child will likely process them as the dominant stimulus, and fading to auditory stimuli might then be impossible.

The profession of audiology has the task of identifying these children, assessing their needs, initiating therapeutic programmes and supporting educational services. In this context, the role of the teacher of the deaf is indispensable. All hearing assessment and aural rehabilitative measures have to be strongly individualised and applied adaptively to the child's possibilities and restrictions in all areas of development. The teacher has the unique opportunity to complement and support the audiologist's task (McCracken, 1994).

Rationale and general consideration of aural rehabilitation for multiply handicapped children will be described below. Next, this chapter will concentrate on behavioural assessment procedures, as they are particularly different from the procedures that can be successfully applied in the non-multiply handicapped hearing-impaired child. Finally, issues related to the selection and fitting of hearing prostheses for multiply handicapped hearing-impaired children will be reviewed.

Rationale for aural rehabilitation

The goals of aural rehabilitation for hearing-impaired children without additional handicaps generally focus on the acquisition of spoken language. For multiply handicapped children, these goals may have to be adjusted to more appropriate and realistic levels. For this purpose, it seems helpful to distinguish between four different levels of hearing:

basic level, signal level, symbolic level and sensorimotor feedback level.

At the basic level, the child detects the environmental sounds with various effects. These effects concern the state of arousal, the awareness of the acoustical environment, social involvement, the emotional responses to sound and music, and sensing space by perceiving invisible parts of the world. At the signal level, the child processes alerting acoustic signals and recognises environmental and referential sounds that are relevant to his/her daily life. At the symbolic level, the child has to process speech sounds in a linguistic context. Listening skills at this level represent the recognition of an acoustically based code consisting of abstract and conventional elements (phonemes) which are being combined into meaningful sets (words). At the sensorimotor feedback level, hearing is used to control (gross and fine) motor activities, to manage speech production, with special reference to phonation and articulation.

The first three levels are receptive in nature and have been described by Ramsdell (1977). The fourth level relates to the feedback loop integrating productive and receptive skills.

Aural rehabilitation at the symbolic level

Generally, children with profound learning disability and hearing-impairment will face the greatest challenge in achieving skills at the symbolic level. However, the possibility of developing receptive and productive skills in the spoken language should not be neglected or ruled out. Instead, the aural rehabilitation goals at the symbolic level should be carefully considered on an individual basis.

Several cases have been reported in the literature that provide evidence that spoken language skills can be mastered by multiply handicapped hearing-impaired children, even when the aural rehabilitation programme starts at a later age and/or with profound hearing loss (for instance, van Hedel-van Grinsven, 1980).

Some evidence of success at the symbolic level is also available from a study on 15 deaf-blind subjects (Coninx, 1995). The chronological ages varied from 6 to 20 years. Everyday listening performance and benefit from the hearing aid were assessed using the Meaningful Auditory Integration Scale inventory, MAIS (Robbins et al., 1991). The MAIS inventory includes 10 questions, addressing three major aspects of children's ability to make meaningful use of sound in everyday situations: bonding to the device, alerting to sound, and the ability to derive meaning from auditory phenomena (Robbins et al., 1991, p.145). These three aspects closely match the aforementioned first three levels of hearing, that is, basic, signal and symbolic levels. As a consequence, scores below eight indicate basic level skills only, scores between 8 and 28 indicate skills at the basic and symbolic levels, whereas scores above 28 must imply at least some level of symbolic hearing.

The MAIS scores for the 15 deaf-blind subjects have been plotted in Figure 3.1, as a function of average hearing loss. As expected, average hearing loss is an important factor that determines the student's level of auditory functioning. Almost all children seem to benefit from amplification. Some reach the symbolic level, as long as hearing loss does not exceed 100–110 dB. Others benefit from hearing aids only at the basic and signal levels. The importance of sound perception for these children will be described below.

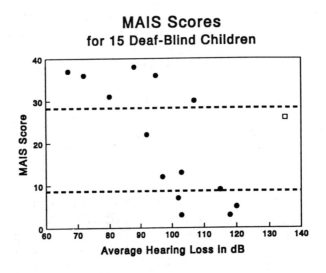

**MAIS Scores
for 15 Deaf-Blind Children**

Figure 3.1 Scores on the MAIS (Meaningful Auditory Integration Scale) for 15 deaf-blind subjects as a function of average hearing loss (at 500, 1000 and 2000 Hz) Closed circles correspond to hearing aid users; the open square corresponds to a cochlear implant user (with 135 dB pre-operative hearing loss)

Aural rehabilitation at the basic, signal and sensorimotor feedback levels

Many hearing-impaired children with additional handicaps are unable to acquire spoken language. Modified goals restricted to the basic, signal and sensorimotor levels of hearing (see above) make it still worthwhile and valid to offer these children an aural rehabilitation programme. Goals must be defined that are realistic and appropriate in terms of a child's developmental as well as auditory status. A number of goals have been listed below, which can be related to the aforementioned hearing levels:

- To reduce children's isolation and to improve their involvement with the environment (basic level).

- To enlarge and enrich the very limited 'within-reaching-distance' world of deaf-blind children (basic level).
- To increase the activity level, i.e., state of arousal, of passive or even apathetic children (basic level).
- To calm and reassure restless or hyperactive children, or to reduce counter-productive visual self-stimulation (basic level).
- To allow experience and enjoyment of the sounds of music; its rhythm, melody and spectral colours (basic level).
- To prevent deaf-blind children from having frightening experiences resulting from sudden tactile encounters without auditory anticipation (basic and signal level).
- To develop an alerting and warning function of sound, increasing the child's state of arousal (signal level).
- To support the perception and recognition of objects and persons in the child's environment and thus develop a better space orientation and mobility for deaf-blind children in particular (signal level).
- To use non-verbal sounds as referential objects, and a limited number of (onomatopoeic) verbal sounds as well (signal level).
- To stimulate and reinforce the functional use of voicing in an expressive communicative sense, i.e., asking for attention (sensory motor feedback level).
- To reduce and extinguish annoying and uncontrolled voicing, i.e., unwanted, socially unacceptable phonations without a communicative function, by making the children aware of the sound they produce (sensory motor feedback level).
- To facilitate cognitive development, i.e., stimulating the child in sensorimotor learning stages (Piaget, sensory motor feedback level).

In order to achieve the goals mentioned above, one needs to apply more structured approaches as compared with children who are only hearing-impaired. A few of these approaches are described below.

Pollack (1985) presents modifications for her 'acoupedic approach', making it applicable for multiply handicapped children. In particular for the low-functioning multiply handicapped children, Pollack suggests that "only a rigorous program of stimulus and reinforcement presentation – or operant conditioning – seems to work" (Pollack, 1985, p.334). In this approach, specific task-learning receives, temporarily or permanently, more attention than generic learning processes within the child. Pollack proposes to use onomatopoeic words as a bridge between the signal and symbolic levels of hearing.

Robbins (1964) published an auditory training programme for deaf-blind children. Robbins considers structured activities or formal training to be an important component of an aural rehabilitation programme, like Pollack, but also stresses the importance of exploiting natural opportunities. Training should proceed along three parallel lines of content: environmental sounds, music, and speech. Early exposure to this range of sounds is an important aspect of effective auditory training. Robbins (1964) distinguishes between structuring the acoustical environment of the deaf-blind child, and filling that environment with as much sound as possible (saturated approach). For multiply handicapped children, Robbins advocates the structured approach, especially in the first stages of auditory development, i.e., immediately after fitting hearing aids. Although Robbins' publication goes back to the early days of hearing aids, it contains a number of useful concepts and practical suggestions.

McInnes and Treffry (1982) published a developmental guide for deaf-blind infants and children. In contrast the frequent denial of amplification for deaf-blind children because of blindness, severity of hearing impairment and/or learning disability, McInnes and Treffry advocate the use of amplification for almost all deaf-blind children. They emphasise the need for a stepwise introduction of hearing aids. "Most deaf-blind children do not take to amplification like 'ducks to water'. They need a carefully designed program to teach them to tolerate, accept, and use an aid." (McInnes and Treffry, 1982, p.189). Many deaf-blind children acquire the habit of disregarding sounds (Van Dijk, 1995). It is necessary to guide them in learning to recognise and integrate auditory input.

Franklin (1987) reports results from a field trial experiment aimed at comparing the values of two types of tactile prostheses used by six deaf-blind children aged 2–18 years. Instead of defining holistic training goals, Franklin implemented well-defined and structured task- and function-specific target behaviours, such as the reduction of self-stimulatory behaviour and self-abuse, the production of purposeful vocalisations and improvement of on-task behaviour. At the level of these specific tasks and functions, Franklin was able to demonstrate effective use of tactile prostheses.

Hearing assessment procedures

General procedures and considerations

Electro-physiological (objective) test procedures for the assessment of auditory sensitivity are being used on a large scale in clinical practice. The specific potentials and limitations of tests such as brainstem electric response audiometry, otoacoustic emissions, impedance audiometry (including stapedius reflex measurements and tympanometry), and others, have been reviewed by several authors (Gorga et al., 1995; Maurizi et al., 1995; Stein, 1995). The availability of these objective test procedures will expand and help to speed up the process of obtaining a clear picture of the child's auditory detection abilities.

Although the electro-physiological procedures are widely used, there is a general consensus that hearing assessment in persons with severe developmental disabilities and multiply handicaps requires a more extended approach, that is, one that also includes behavioural procedures (Northern and Downs, 1991). With regard to the behavioural procedures, the literature has been somewhat ambivalent. On the one hand, there has been a serious call for their implementation. On the other hand, it has been repeatedly underlined that they are rather complex, and at risk of being unreliable with the same (difficult-to-test) persons for which they are mostly invoked.

In the complex field of multiply handicapped hearing-impaired children where no two children will display the same degree and combination of problems, it is impossible to be highly prescriptive as to how the audiological assessment should be undertaken, and all that can be offered are general guidelines. The success of the assessment will be largely determined by the skill and ingenuity of the testers (McCormick, 1995).

Flexer and Gans (1985) investigated responses to sound in two groups of children with the same developmental ages of 2–4 months. One group was developmentally normal, whereas the other was profoundly multiply handicapped (with chronological ages of 3–9 years). Speech and noise stimuli were used at levels of 40, 60, and 80 dBHL. The responsiveness of children within the two groups was not significantly different. These results provide support for the 'development theory' (Zigler, 1969), i.e., the principle of evaluating multiply handicapped children on the basis of developmental level.

It is common practice to evaluate children's hearing on the basis of their developmental ages (Bench et al., 1976; Eisenberg, 1976). Results are being related to normal infants of similar developmental ages (Cox and Lloyd, 1976; Gerber et al., 1977; Northern and Downs, 1991). The person running the hearing assessment has to make a judgement of the child's capabilities for the task, and creatively adapt the test protocols accordingly. Factors like the child's physical response capabilities and social and emotional behaviour have to be taken into consideration. The absence of a response to a sound may be due to a hearing impairment, but may also be the consequence of a motoric or cognitive disability.

Behavioural observation audiometry (BOA)

One of the most commonly applied behavioural procedures is behavioural observation audiometry, which consists of the observation of the child's behaviour in relation to sound stimuli (Northern and Downs, 1991). The observer's task is to recognise those aspects of the child's behaviour that occur or change in concomitance with the perception of the sound stimuli presented by the audiologist. Drawbacks of this procedure are: (a) reactions may not be very obvious and can vary according to different situations or child's status and attention, and (b) the interest in, and reaction to, sound stimuli may be reliable only when the stimuli are quite intense (well above the child's thresholds).

The teacher of the deaf may play an important role in a modified version of clinical BOA, as described below (see "Suggestions for the teacher's role in assessment procedures").

The distraction test

The work of Ewing and Ewing (1944) provided a first behavioural test technique for young children. The distraction test provides a procedure for assessing auditory responsiveness in infants with developmental ages of about 6 months and above, and is based on the principle that babies naturally turn their head to locate sounds when their attention is suitably controlled. The procedure uses powerful human reinforcers such as smiles, vocal responses and tactile based contacts. For children with mental ages above 30 months, the distraction test becomes less feasible because of the child's increased social awareness and self-control.

The performance test

This procedure, also often referred to as 'play audiometry', provides another method of auditory testing, and can be used effectively with multiply handicapped children once they have reached a mental age of 2–3 years. In the performance test the child is conditioned to wait for a (sound) signal and then to respond with some play activity as soon as the signal is detected. The procedure offers flexibility, as the use of materials and response activity can be adapted to the child's capabilities, and is useful when the child is multiply handicapped (see Figure 3.2).

Tangible reinforcement operant conditioning audiometry (TROCA)

Lloyd et al. (1979) exploited the use of sweets and small toys to reinforce play audiometry responses with older children who could be trained to press a button or pull a lever in response to a sound. This test technique is known as tangible reinforcement operant conditioning audiometry (TROCA) and similar techniques have been reported by Bricker and Bricker (1969) and Spradlin et al. (1969).

Yarnall (1983) assessed the benefits of utilising various reinforcers (for example, food, sounds, and vibrators) in an operant conditioning audiometry task with the deaf-blind. Lancioni et al. (1989) report the successful application of TROCA as an alternative to visual reinforcement audiometry (see below) for deaf-blind children.

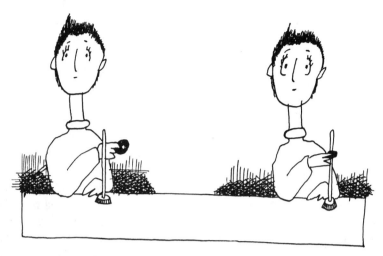

Figure 3.2 Play audiometry
Left: the child is waiting for a sound stimulus. Right: the ring can be put away

Suggestions for the teacher's role in assessment procedures

The preparation of multiply handicapped children for hearing assessment sessions may be of crucial importance. On the one hand, Hill and Birtles (1986) suggest that preparation or training for behavioural hearing assessment procedures in deaf-blind children should preferably be done in a familiar context (environment, persons, stimuli and materials); on the other hand the child also needs to get familiar with the test room and its typical characteristics. The taking of a full history will help to collect indicators of the most appropriate test technique. For that purpose, the parents/caregivers are to be questioned in some detail about their expectations of response patterns, their observations of spontaneous reactions to sound in the home, and their suspicions of hearing problems.

A practical procedure to elicit and collect responses to sound in a structured way has been worked out by Kershman and Napier (1982). The procedure can be used by teachers and parents, and provides an opportunity to work co-operatively on a shared problem. It includes observation methods and registration forms which build on behavioural definitions of response features (such as response intensity: no-low-medium-high; response type: cessation of activity, quieting, increased activity, vocalisation, jerk/startle, crying, laughing, etc.) and the classification and description of various sound stimuli (high frequency, low frequency, etc.). These procedures supply clinicians with reliable information and may draw parents' and teachers' attention to the acoustic environment of the home, and provide information about the child's responsiveness to sound. This behavioural observation procedure for non-clinical environments can be a solid basis or valuable extension of BOA, i.e., tests which utilise observations of general behavioural changes to sounds. A literature review is given by Fulton and Lloyd (1975) and Wilson and Thompson (1984). For infants with developmental ages below 6 months, BOA may be the only applicable technique other than objective testing.

Autistic children are by far the most difficult to test with behavioural observation procedures. Bizarre patterns of behaviour are frequently exhibited, and eye contact may be absent. It is only possible to observe reliable auditory responses to sound with patience and perseverance. The choice of sound type and response pattern have to be selected carefully on an individual basis. It seems helpful in many cases that the testing room is free of distracting materials, and that audiometers and other testing equipment are moved out of the room. Many autistic children will be fascinated with reflections and lights. Therefore, it might also be helpful to switch off most of the lights.

Behavioural procedures: visual reinforcement audiometry (VRA)

While there are many choices regarding the most appropriate hearing assessment procedure (Fulton and Lloyd, 1975; Wilson and Thompson, 1984; Worthington and Peters, 1984; Lancioni et al., 1990; Folsom, 1990; Moore, 1990), the use of a localisation-type response to sound has been widely reported in the literature, and is one of the most frequently evoked responses in the auditory assessment of infants and young children. The response is reliable, easy to observe and often within the repertoire of young and low-functioning children.

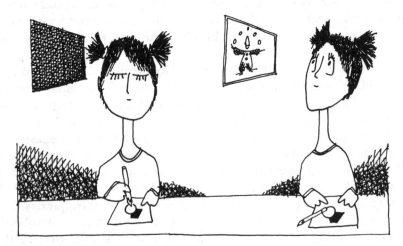

Figure 3.3 Visual reinforcement audiometry (VRA)
Left: the child's attention is directed to the table top because of drawing activity.
Right: after correctly detecting the sound stimulus, the child turns to the activated visual reinforcer (e.g. a slide, etc)

Half a century ago, Dix and Hallpike (1947) described a method of enhancing response patterns by means of a peepshow which illuminated when the child responded correctly in a performance/audiometry type test situation. Suzuki and Ogiba (1961) described a subsequent modification of this principle for the very young and they named it conditioned orientation reflex (COR) testing. In this test, sounds are presented by loudspeakers, and illuminated dolls on top of them act as reinforcers. The COR test has been applied with children with severe learning disability (Fulton and Graham, 1966; Thompson et al., 1979) and has later become known as visual reinforcement audiometry (VRA), a term first used by Liden and Kankkunen (1969) (see Figure 3.4). Thompson et al. (1992) investigated strategies for increasing the maximum number of responses that could be obtained from very young children (1–2 years of age) when using VRA methods. They found that 2 year olds habituated more rapidly than 1 year olds, and the use of two reinforcers led to more responses before habituation than the use of a single reinforcer.

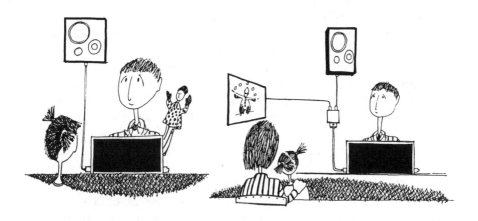

Figure 3.4 Visual reinforcement audiometry (VRA) in free-field condition
The examiner controls the sound generating system and the visual reinforcer, either by hand-held animals/dolls (left) or by electronically switched slides or illuminated toys (right)

The VRA testing procedure requires that the infant sits in a chair, or on the parent's lap, behind a small table in the centre of a sound-treated room. An examiner is seated to the infant's left side and attempts to maintain the infant's attention focused to the midline with soft colourful toys. Auditory stimuli are presented only when the infant is in a ready state (i.e., quietly facing forward, not vocalising or being fretful).

A visual reinforcer is located at eye level next to the loudspeaker to the right (or left) of the child's midline of vision. The visual reinforcer consists of a colourful animated toy animal that moves when electrically activated. The toy animal is contained in a smoked Plexiglas box and can only be observed when illuminated. Primus and Thompson (1985) found that responsiveness was substantially increased using novel reinforcement. According to this finding, Wilson and Thompson (1984) suggested that using several animated toy animals will maintain responsiveness longer than using one visual reinforcer. The visual reinforcers (toy animals) should be wired so that they may easily be interchanged or stacked in the smoked containers.

Prior to the collection of data, the children must be conditioned to the VRA task. It has been demonstrated through research and clinical VRA experience that most normal-functioning infants learn the task in four training trials (Primus and Thompson, 1985; Thompson and Folsom, 1985; Thompson et al., 1989). For multiply handicapped hearing-impaired children an average number of 16 trials has been reported by Lancioni, Coninx and Smeets (1989). During these training trials, the auditory stimulus is presented and the visual reinforcer is activated and paired with the auditory stimulus. If a child does not demonstrate a head-turn response after the addition of the visual reinforcer, the examiner in the test room shapes a head-turn response by assisting the infant in locating the source of the auditory stimulus/visual reinforcer. If the infant shows a natural orientation towards the sound source, the visual reinforcer is immediately activated.

A supra-threshold band-pass noise is recommended as the initial auditory stimulus because it can easily be calibrated in the sound field, and has been shown to be effective in eliciting responses from infants (Eisenberg, 1965; Hoversten and Moncur, 1969; Thompson and Thompson, 1972; Moore et al., 1975; Primus and Thompson, 1985).

Following the training trials, a series of stimulus and control trials begins. The stimulus trials consist of a presentation of auditory stimuli, with the initiation of visual reinforcement only if the infant demonstrates a head-turn response to the auditory signal within a 4 second hit window. This time window may be individualised and adapted to the child's response time. The visual reinforcer is only activated if the examiner (or possibly both of two examiners) votes positive during the hit window. If the infant does not respond, the visual reinforcer is not activated. Testing continues on a 100% reinforcement schedule until the required data are collected or the child habituates to the task. In addition to the stimulus trials, the infant receives one non-stimulus control trial randomly included in each set of three stimulus trials. Each control trial is identical to a stimulus presentation except that no stimulus is delivered. The purpose of the control trial is to check false-positive behaviour in order to insure valid results.

Normal developing infants from 6 to 18 months of age can perform the VRA task, but there is an increase in habituation rate between 12 and

24 months of age, indicating that the procedure begins to lose its effectiveness (Primus and Thompson, 1985). Clinical experience confirms the notion that VRA is very effective with infants between the age of approximately 6 months and 18–24 months, at which time a child may need a more active procedure such as play audiometry.

Greenberg et al. (1978) investigated VRA with children with Down's syndrome between the ages of 6 months and 6 years. Since chronological age is not expected to be a good predictor of success, the Bayley scale of infant development (Bayley, 1969) was used to provide an estimate of developmental age. Whereas previous studies with normally developing infants had shown a high response rate at approximately 6 months of age, substantial variability was observed with the children with Down's syndrome. Greenberg et al. found that the children with Down's syndrome did not achieve a high rate of success until a mental age equivalent of 10 to 12 months. The results revealed that the VRA test procedure yielded reliable audiometric thresholds in one visit for 76% of the children.

Decker and Wilson (1977) applied the VRA procedure to 28 institutionalised profoundly learning disabled children and adults who were unable to complete standard audiometric testing or play audiometry. Within one thirty minute session per child, 70% of the children and adults were found to respond correctly to auditory stimuli below 25 dBHL. This study demonstrated that VRA quickly separated 70% of the residents from a pool of 'untestables', and allowed the audiologist to follow-up with more time consuming techniques for those who did not respond.

Thompson et al. (1979) studied the use of VRA with a group of low-functioning children in a clinical setting. They found that VRA was effective for 71% of all children tested. If children who were found to be at a developmental age of 9 months or younger were excluded, the success rate was 88%. They concluded that a developmental age of approximately 10 months was needed for an expection of a high success rate.

While the research suggests that low-functioning children need a developmental age of approximately 10 months to succeed with VRA testing, clinical experience suggests that children who are more profoundly disabled may also respond to the VRA procedure. Goetz et al. (1982) developed a head-turn response programme used in the classroom for severely handicapped and deaf-blind children. They called their approach visual reinforcement localisation (VRL) and used noise-makers and lights to condition children for formal audiological testing. Folsom and Moore (1984), Moore (1987) and Coninx (1987) reported the use of the VRA paradigm with children who were labelled 'deaf-blind'. Despite this label, most of these children were rarely totally deaf or blind and were found to be hard-of-hearing with partial sight, reduced visual field and/or tunnel vision. These children with multiple disabilities (including dual sensory impairments) were often found to have enough sensory capability to be tested if a team approach was utilised. It was found essential to incorporate the assistance of the educational staff, the parents and/or the residential staff when planning for the comprehensive assessment of children who have been labelled 'difficult-to-test' and, unfortunately, in some cases mislabelled 'untestable'. The use of a team allows for maximum input from those who know the child (McInnes and Treffry, 1982). Information can be gathered to select the child's favourite activities or toys as reinforcers, and better understand the child's motor and cognitive abilities. The team members can also provide assistance in preparing the child for formal testing, which allows for broader ownership and support of the conditioning, assessment and follow-up process (Michael and Paul, 1990).

In order to maximise the potential for success, it is essential that a proper waiting posture, an adequate stimulus, a consistent response, an appropriate reinforcer, and the use of non-stimulus control trials be incorporated into the testing protocol. The waiting posture is defined as a position where the child indicates to the examiner that he or she is in a ready state to receive a stimulus. The waiting position also helps the child focus on the task. The child must be able to maintain the waiting posture long enough to allow the audiologist to vary the presentation rate and probe for threshold. It is important not to present the stimulus as soon as the waiting posture is achieved, so as not to teach the child that the waiting posture is the cue to respond immediately and receive reinforcement. The waiting posture for children with multiple disabilities is usually facing midline, but may be any position where the child's eyes and head are not facing the reinforcer.

The response, using VRA, is generally a head-turn towards some type of visual reinforcer. However, with children with severe learning disability who may not have good head control, it may be that eye movement is acceptable as long as the response is easily detectable and consistent. It is also possible that the visual reinforcer needs to be placed closer to the child (as opposed to being placed on or next to the loudspeaker) in order to accommodate reduced head-turn movement, if this is more appropriate for the child's abilities.

The desired stimulus is an auditory signal. However, with some low-functioning children, especially those with expected severe-to-profound hearing loss, it may be beneficial to start with a stimulus that creates both auditory and vibro-tactile sensations. For example, intense, low frequency signals presented through a loudspeaker may also carry tactile cues. Once the child has learned to respond to the conditioning stimulus, the vibro-tactile cue is eliminated and hearing testing is initiated. It is also enlightening to observe some children with dual sensory impairments, who only respond when tactile cues are presented, cease to respond to auditory stimuli only, and then respond again when the tactile cues are reintroduced. This behaviour pattern has been observed with deaf-blind children who are able to perform the task, but only receive stimulation when vibro-tactile cues are present.

In conclusion, the usefulness and effectiveness of the VRA procedure for developmentally impaired children can be summarised through the case reported by Folsom and Moore (1984). The case concerns a 5-year-old child with multiply disabilities who was in a residential setting, and according to past records was untestable. The young girl had a complex medical history of microcephaly, congenital toxiplasma, spastic quadriplegia, scoliosis, vision problems and possible hearing loss. Observations and discussions with the classroom staff revealed that she could slowly turn her head to the right (but not the left), had some vision and appeared occasionally to respond to voices. The child was accompanied by her teacher to the sound suite and immediately conditioned to VRA using a slow head-turn response to a visual reinforcer located close to her right side. She was tested for sound field and earphone thresholds in six 20-minute sessions.

Discrimination testing

The VRA paradigm has been modified to meet the needs of researchers interested in issues of developmental change in speech discrimination skills with infants and later applied to low-functioning children. Eilers et al. (1977) developed this modified VRA procedure called visually reinforced infant speech discrimination (VRISD). The primary difference between VRA and VRISD is that, rather than teaching the children to respond with a head-turn to the presence of a sound, they are now reinforced to a change from an ongoing background sound to a new sound. Essentially, the child is conditioned to respond with a head-turn when any change in a background auditory stimulus is detected, in order to receive visual reinforcement.

With 'normal infants', the VRISD procedure has been well utilised to test very difficult and subtle comparisons of infant speech perception, and more recently with a fully computerised testing programme (Eilers et al., 1979; Kuhl, 1979; Hillenbrand, 1984; Kuhl, 1986; Nozza et al., 1990; Nozza et al., 1991; Kuhl, 1993; Goodsitt et al., 1993).

The VRISD procedure has also been applied to a small sample of low-functioning, learning disabled children (Thompson et al., 1979). The children ranged in chronological age from 10 months to $6\frac{1}{2}$ years. Their developmental ages ranged from 1 month to 4 years, 9 months. They were medically diagnosed as having Down's syndrome or undifferentiated learning disability. Of those who were successfully tested for threshold assessment using VRA, slightly more than half of the children (56%) demonstrated successful performance on a discrimination task. Children who successfully demonstrated discrimination abilities ranged in developmental age between 12 and 30 months. Some children with developmental delays, however, could not complete the task without an intensity cue, and one child could not complete the task even with an intensity cue.

These results suggest that the discrimination task may be more difficult for children with severe learning disability than for normal infants at comparable mental ages. The VRISD procedure has potential for use with non-verbal children with severe learning disabilities where information regarding discrimination abilities is desired. For example, the decision to recommend one hearing aid rather than another, based on improved pure-tone and speech reception thresholds, might be supplemented with discrimination information using VRISD. While this procedure has been utilised and adapted for the study of infant speech development, the clinical utility has not yet been well demonstrated. The question remains as to whether there is a need for more sophisticated discrimination assessment with individuals with severe learning disabilities. If this need is established, it would be necessary to develop a standardised clinical VRISD protocol, collect normative data and demonstrate usefulness for populations with severe learning disability.

Conclusions

The use of VRA is a very powerful and robust procedure for children with severe learning disability who are conditionable. One primary advantage is the very short time frame in which children can be successfully tested (if they are conditionable) and the use of specific auditory stimuli to elicit an easy to observe behavioural response. Obviously, the benefit of VRA over BOA is the specificity of the auditory signal and the more precise threshold information, while the advantage over play audiometry may be the reduction of time required to condition and test. Some suggestions to improve VRA success with low-functioning children include: (1) the initial use of low frequency auditory stimuli with vibrotactile cues during conditioning, to be sure the child is being stimulated, (2) the use of multiple visual reinforcers to increase response rate, (3) the use of control trials to monitor for false-positive behaviour, and (4) the use of a team approach to share ownership in the process and assist with testing and follow-up. In addition, the creative attention to the key elements of testing (i.e., waiting posture, stimulus, response and reinforcement) will improve the success rate of VRA as a tool to gather audiological information on low-functioning children.

Behavioural procedures: air puff audiometry (APA)

Although the VRA procedure has proved to be very powerful, problems may still exist. For example, visual stimuli could prove only partially reinforcing, rapidly lead to saturation, or be totally inadequate (e.g., if the children are affected by severe visual handicaps), with the consequence that the procedure is inapplicable or ineffective in consolidating response. It may also be that the children have a severe learning disability, and are not capable of associating responses to sound and reinforcement. In a situation in which the child fails to learn, the audiologist would have to determine whether the failure is caused by the child's low motivation and limited performance, or by the child's inability to hear the sound used in the test.

A behavioural procedure based on classical conditioning may solve some of the problems related to VRA. For example, it might reduce problems of saturation and might more easily ensure that the unconditioned stimuli will be paired to the sound. Classical conditioning consists of the transfer of stimulus control from a stimulus that reliably elicits a response (unconditioned stimulus – UCS) to one that was previously neutral or irrelevant (conditioned stimulus – CS). The establishment of a CS–UCS contingency results in the so-called conditioned response (Rescorla, 1967).

Lancioni, Coninx and Smeets (1989) have evaluated a classical conditioning procedure used for hearing assessment, based on an air puff as the UCS. The air puff can be directed at the child's face, and elicits defensive responses such as eye-blinking and head-turning. Sound serves as the neutral stimulus that is to be paired to the UCS (thus to become a conditioned stimulus). Conditioning means that the children will show the same response that they have toward the air puff also in relation to the sound stimuli. The assessment procedure is called air puff audiometry (APA).

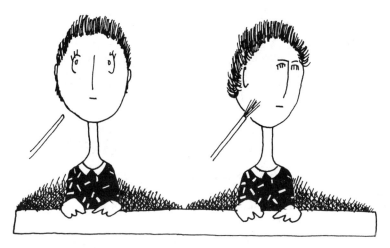

Figure 3.5 Air puff audiometry (APA)
Left: the child is waiting. Right: after detecting the sound stimulus, the child anticipates (with a defensive response) the air puff to come

Equipment for APA

The equipment consists of an audiometer, or some other sound generating system, a cylinder filled with filtered compressed air, a central
control unit, and the audiologist's hand-held control box. Since persons
with severe developmental disabilities and multiple handicaps may be
tactile defensive and so find headphones threatening, free-field presentation of the sound stimuli is a better, or even the only possible, alternative option. The cylinder filled with air is connected to an adjustable
pressure reducing ventile and an electrically controlled valve. This
enables the presentation of an air puff with well-defined duration and
intensity. The central control unit provides timing functions and inter-
faces the audiologist's control box with the sound generating system and
the electrical valve. More specifically, the central unit controls (a) the
audiologist's presentation of trials (e.g., it prevents too short or too
regular inter-trial intervals, (b) the timing of the stimuli, i.e., sound
signal and air puff, and (c) the inter-stimulus intervals (the time gap
between the onset of the sound signal and the onset of the air puff).

The audiologist's control box contains regulators of sound intensity
and frequency, a trial-type selector (test or control) and push buttons for
starting the trials and recording the responses. The air puffs are delivered through a flexible (plastic) tube of 2.5mm in diameter.

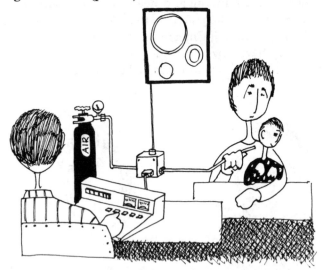

Figure 3.6 Air puff audiometry (APA) in free-field condition
The examiner controls the sound generating system; the air puff is delivered through
an electronic timing and switching device

Conditions for APA

Air puff audiometry includes three procedural phases: baseline, criterion conditioning and hearing assessment.

The baseline phase uses two sets of trials. The first set is used to verify that sound stimuli, to be applied in the assessment phase, are not followed by air puff specific defensive responses. Within the second set of trials the air puff is introduced and an optimal direction and intensity of the puff to obtain a strong defensive reaction (unconditioned response) is found. The response to the air puff may be a prolonged/repeated closure of the eyes and/or head-turning. The criterion conditioning phase is aimed at bringing the defensive response under the control of a 250 Hz sound signal.

The 3-second sound signals are paired with the air puff for a maximum of 90 trials (training trials). The puff occurs during the last 0.9 seconds of the sound. Signs of learning (association of sound and puff) are expected to be visible within the inter-stimulus intervals (i.e., as defensive responses following the onset of the sound and preceding the onset of the air puff). Test trials (omitting the air puff to check specifically for the presence of the aforementioned defensive responses during the sound) may not be strictly necessary and can be kept to a minimum. Criterion conditioning is reached when the children show the anticipatory defensive responses in training and test trials, and do not show the same responses in control trials (in which neither the sound nor the puff is presented).

The hearing assessment phase is aimed at testing the child's response to new sound stimuli. As in the previous phase, the procedure relies heavily on training trials and anticipatory defensive responses. It is recommended that a tracking method is used, starting with a 500 Hz signal. The level of this stimulus is decreased or increased in 10 dB steps depending upon whether the response is positive or negative. Whenever possible, 5 dB steps might be used.

Study

One of the experimental evaluations of the APA procedure was carried out in an institutional centre in the Netherlands (Lancioni, Coninx and Smeets, 1989). Twenty-three people were included in the study. Their chronological ages varied from 3.8 to 20.3 (M = 9.8) years. Their social ages (Vineland adaptive behaviour scales) were between 1.8 and 4.5 (M = 2.7) years. Severe learning disability was combined with learning and behavioural (neurological) problems and often with visual handicaps as well. Three children were totally blind. All of the subjects in the trial had a clinical diagnosis of hearing impairment. Most of them were provided with hearing aids, in spite of incomplete audiometric data.

All subjects were assessed with APA and VRA. Both procedures were used according to the three phases described above. Within the VRA procedure, several visual reinforcers (which could be changed within and across sessions) were used. The visual reinforcer was delivered when both the audiologist and a reliability observer pressed their response buttons within 4 seconds of the start of the sound stimulus, indicating head-turn response. For the blind participants, the VRA was modified into a TROCA-based procedure (see Northern and Downs, 1991). Edible reinforcers were used instead of the visual reinforcers, and a sideways reaching response replaced the head-turn response.

The results indicated that eight of the 23 subjects failed in the VRA (or modified version of it) while only two of the 23 failed in the APA procedure. Of importance is that none of the subjects failed in both procedures. The mean number of training trials required by the 13 subjects who completed both procedures was 81.1 for the VRA and 99.6 for the APA procedure. This difference in the number of training trials is not statistically significant.

With regard to the thresholds obtained for the 13 successful subjects in the two procedures, there were only two differences between procedures that reached 20 dB; in both cases, the APA procedure provided the lower threshold. All other differences were 10 dB or less. A display of these data is presented in Figure 3.7.

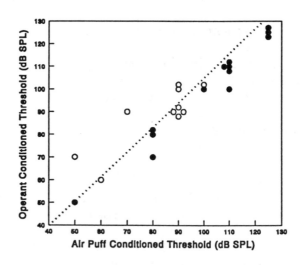

Figure 3.7 Thresholds at 500 Hz (open circles) and 2000 Hz (closed circles) for the 13 subjects who succeeded in both the air puff and the operant (VRA) procedures

In a second study with multiply handicapped persons, carried out in an institutional setting in Italy (Lancioni et al., 1990), the results of APA were compared with BERA outcomes. Twelve people with chronological ages from 9.6 to 32.4 (M = 17.5) years, participated. The age equivalents for their daily living skills (Vineland adaptive behaviour scales) ranged from about 0.3 to 3.4 years (M = 2 years). The results of the APA procedure indicated that 10 of the 12 subjects reached criterion conditioning (see above).

With regard to the thresholds obtained with the APA procedure and the BERA, there was overall agreement at 2 kHz for six subjects. For three of these, the BERA did not produce any response at the highest intensity level (95 dBHL) and the APA procedure showed reliable responding at 100 dBHL. In these cases, the results of APA seemed to add information that could be particularly valuable for deciding whether to use a hearing aid, and its fitting.

The difference between APA findings and BERA was quite large (and favoured the BERA) for two subjects. One of these had been observed to respond to intensities lower than those at which the threshold was found, but that responding could not be stabilised. For the other child, on the contrary, the performance with the APA procedure (supported by the child's history) had indicated profound deafness. One possible explanation for the discrepancy is that the BERA responses may be more peripheral and primitive than the behavioural (APA) responses which involve a level of sound awareness. If so, this would certainly emphasise the importance of combining diverse strategies in the hearing assessment of children with multiple handicaps (Northern and Downs, 1991).

Hearing prostheses

Introduction

Amplification for multiply handicapped hearing-impaired children is not a simple and straightforward response to the assessment of the hearing impairment. An appropriate form of amplification has to take into account variables such as the sensory, physical, emotional, intellectual, social and educational needs of the child (McCracken and Bamford, 1995). These needs will show a changing hierarchy over the years, and it is within this hierarchy that the place of aural rehabilitation and amplification has to be chosen.

Fitting issues

The adjustment of acoustical hearing aids, the mapping of cochlear implant sound processors and tactile aids is described extensively in Section B of this book. For multiply handicapped hearing-impaired children these procedures can be used only partially, or even not at all. One example has been worked out by McCracken and Bamford (1995) and relates to the desired sensation level (DSL) procedure (Seewald et al., 1985).

In brief, this procedure aims at amplifying the long term average speech spectrum (LTASS) to a level that is appropriately above threshold, without exceeding uncomfortable listening levels (ULLs). The audiologist can select real ear gain and maximum output values of the hearing aid, recommended by software and based on relevant thresholds of the child.

Having fitted the selected hearing aids, the actual real ear gain and real ear maximum output have to be measured in order to verify the required or recommended amplification. This can be directly by probe microphone measurements. Alternatively, functional gain can be measured, that is, the difference between the aided and unaided thresholds.

Following verification of the basic hearing aid fitting, the audiologist may want to evaluate the child's improvement in listening. Depending upon age, hearing loss, other handicaps, family circumstances, etc., various indicators of progress in hearing due to the hearing aid fitting should start to develop (see also Coninx, 1995) – for example, increased responsiveness to sound, more (appropriate) vocalisations, improved pre-verbal communication, willingness to wear the hearing aid all day, and so on. Such observations from caretakers, teachers and parents, using instruments as described above (Robbins MAIS and Kerhman's systematic procedures), will be an important contribution to ongoing monitoring and to supplying the audiologist with valuable feedback.

McCracken and Bamford (1995) summarise a number of points in the DSL procedure where implementation for children with multiple handicaps may be particularly difficult. Specifically, these are:

1 Threshold information may be lacking. For many multiply handicapped hearing-impaired children reliable and accurate (sound field) testing is not possible, and the DSL tables or software have to be entered with partial or unreliable threshold data.
2 In most multiply handicapped hearing-impaired children it will be impossible to assess uncomfortable listening levels with any accuracy.
3 For many multiply handicapped hearing-impaired children, probe-tube microphone measurements will not be possible because of excessive movement, tactile defensiveness, and so on. Therefore, average RECD values (real ear to coupler differences) will have to be used, with the disadvantage of ignoring significant individual variability. This is particularly the case for children with cranio-facial abnormality; for example, if the ear canals are unusually small, average RECDs will underestimate the actual RECD considerably. As a consequence, the selected aids will have greater real ear levels (gain and maximum output) than required. This is likely to happen in children with Down's syndrome (Balkany, 1980). In these cases, the initial use of the hearing aid should be monitored with extreme care, as an incorrect fitting may cause strong rejection due to uncomfortable loudness sensations.

4 Lack of co-operation, distress at (potentially) threatening situations or tactile defensiveness can make the insertion of earmoulds and placement of hearing aids impossible. Creative and incremental approaches, in a relaxed atmosphere and with the necessary patience, have to be used.

The problems in the hearing aid fitting procedure, as such, should never deter the team from providing the multiply handicapped hearing-impaired child with amplification. Small benefits from amplification may, in relative terms, be of great importance.

The fitting of hearing aids with multiply-handicapped hearing-impaired children is not only a challenging issue due to electro-acoustic aspects, but also because of ergonomic factors. McCracken and Bamford (1995) describe a number of illustrative examples, such as:

- The problems associated with cranio-facial abnormalities can make it impossible to 'attach' behind the ear (BTE) aids properly. The use of toupe tape, 'huckies' or a baby's sock pinned to a shirt (Condon, 1991) may present solutions in individual cases.
- Chairs that provide head restraint for physically handicapped children may give rise to considerable problems with acoustic feedback (whistling) of behind the ear (BTE) aids. The use of body-worn (BW) aids, contralateral routing of signal (CROS) systems or, when available, hearing aids with digital feedback suppression can offer solutions.
- Children with profound dual sensory impairments who may often spend much of their time in co-active situations, and thus in close proximity with the carer. This might result in over-amplification which has to be compensated for.
- For children wearing spectacles, the use of in the ear (ITE) aids should, whenever possible, be considered, as it eliminates interference between hearing aid and spectacles.
- Tactile aids may provide structured somatosensory stimulation to children who exhibit tactile defensive and self-injurious behaviour (Sears, 1981; Royeen, 1985; Royeen and Lane, 1991). Acoustical hearing aids may be of less use for this group, as they fail to establish a positive communication situation.
- For multiply handicapped hearing-impaired children, the effort required to perform any perceptive/cognitive task may be substantially higher than that of a normally hearing peer. Rabbitt (1966) and Downs and Crum (1978) showed that learning effort and mental load correlated positively with the presence of (disturbing) noise. For multiply handicapped hearing-impaired children, therefore, all measures that reduce the problems of listening in noise are more than usually important. Directional microphones, induction loop

and FM systems are highly recommended. The use of these systems has to be judged against the background of the daily living situation of the child, which might already be demanding.

- Multiply handicapped hearing-impaired children may inadvertently nudge a volume control, resulting in over-amplification and uncomfortable loudness sensations. With an output controlled by automatic gain control (AGC), tolerance levels may not be exceeded.

Alternatives to hearing aids: cochlear implant (CI)

Cochlear implant (CI), as an electrical sensory aid, is described in Chapter 6. As compared with deaf children without additional handicaps, the selection procedure for CI is more complicated and uncertain for multiply handicapped hearing-impaired children. The children's implant profile (ChIP) relates to 11 different areas that should be checked before a child is accepted into a CI programme (Hellman et al., 1991). These factors include speech and language abilities, family structure and support, cognitive/learning styles, educational environment and availability of support services. For children who are multiply handicapped and profoundly deaf, the assessment of the ChIP factor may pose a major challenge. Diagnostic tools to assess language, cognitive ability, emotional and psychological status for multiply handicapped hearing-impaired children are lacking to a large extent. It is, however, becoming evident that children who have multiple handicaps defy our clinical ability to predict likely benefit from cochlear implantation (McCracken and Bamford, 1995). One group which has been successfully implanted is children with a dual sensory handicap, such as occurs in Usher's syndrome. This syndrome is characterised by severe to profound sensorineural hearing loss and retinitis pigmentosa (Boughman et al., 1983). Experiences with CI in deaf children and adults with Usher's syndrome have been reported by Young et al. (1994) and Vermeulen et al. (1994).

Young reports on the early identification programme for Usher's syndrome used in the Children's Memorial Medical Centre in Chicago. The aim is an early implantation, before the full effects of retinitis pigmentosa become manifest. All implanted children are reported to have received significant benefit from their CI. The mean age of implantation was 4.6 years (range 2 years to 5.0 years), and the mean age of diagnosis of Usher's syndrome was 3.3 years (range 0.5 to 5.0 years).

Vermeulen et al. report on the results of four implanted deaf persons with Usher's syndrome (Type I), who received their CI at 13, 20, 20 and 28 years of age. Speech perception tests indicate an improvement (audio and audio-visual) in speech and environmental sound recognition. Even larger improvement was found in the clients' subjective evaluations. They feel less stressed in communication and orientation/mobility, and feel less dependent and more self-confident.

Alternatives for hearing aids: tactile aids

Cochlear implantation certainly offers considerable benefit to a range of profoundly deaf children, including multiply handicapped children. Nevertheless, the emotional and ethical issues involved should not be ignored. Against that background, tactile aids can offer a non-invasive sensory input (see Chapter 7). An example of an alternative specialised approach to using Tactaid II for deaf-blind children has been developed and evaluated by Franklin (1989).

Summary

The process of aural rehabilitation aims at helping the individual hearing-impaired child to improve its perceptive power, within a meaningful and functional context. As soon as the child has acquired a critical 'perceptive mass', it will be able spontaneously and naturally to develop further listening skills as part of, and serving, the learning of a wider range of skills and tasks.

For multiply handicapped hearing-impaired children this is basically the same. Goals may have to be adjusted to realistic and achievable levels of hearing, and training procedures may have to be more structured. However, the basic rationale for aural rehabilitation remains unchanged; the educator/teacher should offer effective challenges by creating an appropriately stimulating environment, so that the child can and will develop listening skills and integrate them in his/her personal living circumstances.

The task of the teacher of the deaf is to initiate, perform, manage and support this process. This includes the initial hearing assessment needed for diagnosis, hearing aid fitting and the selection of the initial goals of the child's individual educational programme. It also includes ongoing evaluative assessment, documenting the child's progress and determining possible modifications to the educational programme. Most of the generally applied hearing assessment procedures are of the behavioural type, and have been described in this chapter. The teacher of the deaf will have to play a significant role in these procedures.

References

Balkany JT (1980) Otological aspects of Down's syndrome. In Northern JL, Downs M (Eds) Seminars in Speech and Hearing, Vol I. New York: Thieme Stratton. pp 39-48.

Bayley N (1969) Bayley scales of infant development: birth to two years. Psychological Corporation.

Bench J, Watson T, Dowding T (1976) Children's use of hearing aids. Lancet 1: 1192.

Boughman J, Vernon M, Shaver K (1983) Usher syndrome: definition and estimate of prevalence from two high-risk populations. Journal of Chronic Diseases 36: 595-603.

Bricker D, Bricker W (1969) A programmed approach to operant audiometry for low-functioning children. Journal of Speech and Hearing Disorders 34: 312-320.

Buchanan LH (1990) Early onset of presbyacusis in Down Syndrome. Scandinavian Audiology 19: 103-110.

Condon M (1991) Unique challenges: children with multiple handicaps. In: Paediatric Amplification: Proceeding of National Conference, Boys Town Center, Omaha: 183-193.

Coninx F (1987) Air-puff audiometry for the hearing assessment of deaf-blind children. In Proceedings of the 9th IAEDB International Conference. Poitiers, France: pp 428-430.

Coninx F (1995) Aural rehabilitation issues with multiply handicapped hearing-impaired children. Scandinavian Audiology 24(41): 61-65.

Cox BP, Lloyd LL (1976) Audiologic considerations. In Lloyd LL (Ed) Communication Assessment and Intervention Strategies. Baltimore: University Park Press.

Decker TN, Wilson WR (1977) The use of visual reinforcement audiometry (VRA) with profoundly retarded residents. Mental Retardation 15: 40-41.

Dix MR, Hallpike CS (1947) The peepshow: A new technique for pure-tone audiometry in young children. British Medical Journal 2: 719-723.

Downs DW, Crum MA (1978) Processing demands during auditory learning under degraded listening conditions. Journal of Speech and Hearing Research 21: 702-714.

Downs MP (Ed) (1980) Communication disorders in Down's syndrome. Seminars in Speech, Language and Hearing 1.

Eilers RE, Gavin W, Wilson WR (1979) Linguistic experience and phonemic perception in infancy: a cross-linguistic study. Child Development 50: 14-18.

Eilers RE, Wilson WR, Moore JM (1977) Developmental changes in speech discrimination in infants. Journal of Speech and Hearing Research 20: 766-780.

Eisenberg R (1965) Auditory behaviour in the human neonate: methodologic problems and the logical design of research procedures. Journal of Audiological Research 5: 159-177.

Eisenberg RB (1976) Auditory Competence in Early Life. Baltimore: University Park Press.

Ewing IR, Ewing AWG (1944) The ascertainment of deafness in infancy and childhood. Journal of Laryngology and Otology 59: 309-338.

Flexer C, Gans DP (1985) Comparative evaluation of the auditory responsiveness of normal infants and profoundly multihandicapped children. Journal of Speech and Hearing Research 28: 163-168.

Folsom RC (1990) Identification of hearing loss in infants using auditory brainstem response: strategies and program choices. In Diefendorf A (Ed) Paediatric Audiology Seminars in Hearing. New York: Thieme Medical. pp 333-341.

Folsom RC, Moore JM (1984) An approach to the audiologic assessment of multihandicapped deaf-blind children: Insight in sight. In Proceedings of the 5th Canadian Interdisciplinary Conference on the Visually Impaired Child, Vancouver BC. pp 43-57.

Franklin B (1987) Effects of tactile aids on communication skills of deaf-blind children. In Proceedings of the 9th IAEDB International Conference. Poitiers, France: pp 327–337.

Franklin BA (1989) Tactaid II Training Program for Deaf Blind Children. San Francisco: San Francisco State University.

Fulton RT, Graham JD (1966) Conditioned orientation reflex audiometry with the mentally retarded. American Journal of Mental Deficiency 70: 703-708.

Fulton RT, Lloyd LL (1975) Auditory Assessment of the Difficult-to-Test. Baltimore: Williams and Wilkins.

Gerber SE, Jones BL, Costello JM (1977) Behavioural measures. In Gerber SE (Ed) Audiometry in Infancy. New York: Williams and Wilkins. pp 85-97.

Goetz L, Utley B, Gee K, Baldwin M, Sailor W (1982) Auditory assessment and programming for severely handicapped deaf-blind students. San Francisco State University: Bay area severely handicapped deaf-blind project, U.S. department of education contract 300-78-0338. Washington D.C.: U.S. Government Printing Office.

Goodsitt JV, Morgan JL, Kuhl PK (1993) Perceptual strategies in prelingual speech segmentation. Journal of Child Language 20: 229-252.

Gorga M, Beauchaine K, Bergman B, Kamenski J, Stover L (1995) The application of otoacoustic emissions in the assessment of hearing loss. Scandinavian Audiology 24(41): 8-17.

Greenberg DB, Wilson WR, Moore JM, Thompson G (1978) Visual reinforcement audiometry (VRA) with young Down's syndrome children. Journal of Speech and Hearing Disorders 43: 448-458.

Hellman SA, Chute PM, Kretschmer RE, Parisier SC, Thurston LC (1991) The development of a children's implant profile. American Annals of the Deaf 136(2): 77-81.

Hill AL, Birtles GJ (1986) A behavioural hearing assessment programme for multiply handicapped children. Australian Journal of Audiology 8: 31-34.

Hillenbrand J (1984) Speech perception by infants: categorization based on nasal consonants place of articulation. Journal of the Acoustical Society of America 75: 1613-1622.

Hoversten G, Moncur J (1969) Stimuli and intensity factors in testing infants. Journal of Speech and Hearing Research 12: 687-702.

Karchmer MA (1985) A demographic perspective. In Cherow E, Matkin ND, Trybus RJ, Hearing Impaired Children and Youth with Developmental Disabilities. Washington: Gallaudet College: 36-59.

Kershman SM, Napier D (1982) Systematic procedures for eliciting and recording responses to sound stimuli in deaf-blind multihandicapped children. The Volta Review 1982, May: 226-237.

Kuhl PK (1979) Speech perception in early infancy: perceptual constancy for spectrally dissimilar vowel categories. Journal of the Acoustical Society of America 66: 1679-1688.

Kuhl PK (1986) Infants' perception of speech: constraints on characterizations of the initial state. In Lindblom B, Zetterstrom R (Eds) Precursors of Early Speech. International Symposium Proceedings. Stockholm: Wenner-Gren Centre. pp 219-244.

Kuhl PK (1993) Developmental speech perception: implications for model of languages impairments. Annals of the New York Academy of Science 682: 248-263.

Lancioni GE, Coninx F (1995) A classical conditioning procedure for auditory testing: Air puff audiometry. Scandinavian Audiology 24(41): 43-48.

Lancioni GE, Coninx F, Brozzi G, Oliva D, Hoogeveen FR (1990) Air-puff conditioning audiometry: extending its applicability with multiply handicapped individuals. International Journal of Rehabilitation Research 13: 67-70.

Lancioni GE, Coninx F, Smeets PM (1989) A classical conditioning procedure for the hearing assessment of multiply handicapped persons. Journal of Speech and Hearing Disorders 54: 88-93.

Liden G, Kankkunen A (1969) Visual reinforcement audiometry. Acta Otolaryngology 67: 281-292.

Lloyd LL, Spradlin JE, Reid MJ (1979) An operant audiometric procedure for difficult-to-test patients. Journal of Speech and Hearing Disorders 33: 236-245.

Maurizi M, Ottaviani F, Paludetti G (1995) Overview of the field of objective auditory tests. Scandinavian Audiology 24(41): 5-7.

McCormick B (1994) Screening for Hearing Impairment in Young Children. London: Whurr.

McCormick B (1995) Assessment in low-functioning children. Scandinavian Audiology 24(41): 31-35.

McCracken W (1994) Deaf children with complex needs: a piece in the puzzle. Journal of the British Association of Teachers of the Deaf 18: 54-60.

McCracken W, Bamford JM (1995) Auditory prostheses for children with multiple handicaps. Scandinavian Audiology 24(41): 51-60.

McInnes JM, Treffry JA (1982) Deaf-blind Infants and Children: A Developmental Guide. Toronto: University of Toronto Press.

Michael MG, Paul PV (1990) Early intervention for infants with deaf-blindness. Except Child 57: 200-210.

Moore JM (1987) The hearing assessment of deaf-blind children. In Proceedings of the 9th IAEDB International Conference. Poitiers, France. pp 55-80.

Moore JM (1990) Hearing assessment of deaf-blind children using behavioral conditioning. Seminar on Hearing 11: 342-356.

Moore JM, Thompson G, Thompson M (1975) Auditory localization of infants as a function of reinforcement conditions. Journal of Speech and Hearing Disorders 40: 29-34.

Northern JL, Downs MP (1991) Hearing in Children (4th Edition). Baltimore: Williams and Wilkins.

Nozza RJ, Rossman RN, Bond LC (1991) Infant-adult differences in unmasked thresholds for the discrimination of consonant-vowel syllable pairs. Audiology 30: 102-112.

Nozza RJ, Rossman RN, Bond LC, Miller SL (1990) Infant speech-sound discrimination in noise. Journal of the Acoustical Society of America 87: 339-350.

Pollack D (1985) Educational Audiology for the Limited-Hearing Infant and Preschooler. Springfield, Ill.: Charles C Thomas.

Primus M, Thompson G (1985) Response strength of young children in operant audiometry. Journal of Speech and Hearing Research 28: 539-547.

Rabbitt PM (1966) Recognition memory for whole words correctly heard in noise. Psychonomic Science 6: 383-384.

Ramsdell D (1977) The psychology of the hard of hearing and the deafened adult. In Davis H, Silverman R (Eds) Hearing and Deafness. New York: Holt.

Rescorla RA (1967) Pavlovian conditioning and its proper control procedures. Psychological Review 74: 71-80.

Robbins AM, Renshaw JJ, Berry SW (1991) Evaluating meaningful auditory integration in profoundly hearing-impaired children. American Journal of Otology 12: 144S-150S.

Robbins N (1964) Auditory Training in the Perkins Deaf-Blind Department. Watertown (MA, USA): Perkins Publication No.23. pp 1-90.

Royeen CB (1985) Domain specifications of the construct tactile defensiveness. American Journal of Occupational Therapy 39: 596-599.

Royeen CB, Lane SJ (1991) Tactile processing and sensory defensiveness. In Fisher AG, Murray EA, Bundy AC (Eds) Sensory Integration Theory and Practise. Philadelphia: Davis. pp 108-136.

Sears C (1981) The tactilely defensive child. Academic Therapy 16: 565-569.

Seewald RC, Ross M, Spiro MK (1985) Selecting amplification characteristics for young hearing-impaired children. Ear and Hearing 6: 48-53.

Spradlin JE, Locke WJ, Fulton RT (1969) Conditioning and audiological assessment. In Fulton RT, Lloyd LL (Eds) Audiometry for the Retarded: With Implications for the Difficult-to-Test. Baltimore: Williams and Wilkins.

Stein L (1995) New developments: Clinical potentials of ERPs. Scandinavian Audiology 24(41) 18-30.

Suzuki T, Ogiba Y (1961) Conditioned orientation reflex audiometry. Archives of Otolaryngology 74: 192-198.

Thompson G, Folsom RC (1985) Reinforced and nonreinforced head turn responses of infants as a function of stimulus bandwidth. Ear and Hearing 6: 125-129.

Thompson G, Thompson M, McCall A (1992) Strategies for increasing response behaviour of 1- and 2-year-old children during visual reinforcement audiometry (VRA). Ear and Hearing 13: 236-240.

Thompson G, Wilson W, Moore J (1979) Application of visual reinforcement audiometry (VRA) in low functioning children. Journal of Speech and Hearing Disorders 44: 80-90.

Thompson M, Thompson G (1972) Responses of infants and young children as a function of auditory stimuli and test methods. Journal of Speech and Hearing Research 5: 7-19.

Thompson M, Thompson G, Vethivelu S (1989) A comparison of audiometric test methods for 2-year-old children. Journal of Speech and Hearing Disorders 54: 174-179.

Van Dijk J (1995) Hearing aid fitting and auditory training: A cautionary note. Scandinavian Audiology 24(41): 66-67.

Van Hedel-van Grinsven M (1980) Hoe een volledig doofblind kind tot verbale communicatie kwam. Logopedie & Foniatrie 52: 235-240.

Vermeulen L, van Dijk J, Hinderink H, van den Broek P (1994) Some results of cochlear implants in 4 persons with Usher's syndrome Type I. Low Vision: 419-422.

Wilson WR, Thompson G (1984) Behavioural audiometry. In Jerger J (Ed) Paediatric Audiology. London: Taylor and Francis. pp 1-44.

Worthington DW, Peters JF (1984) Electrophysiologic audiometry. In Jerger J (Ed) Paediatric Audiology. San Diego: College Hill. pp 95-124.

Yarnall GD (1983) Comparison of operant and conventional audiometric procedures with the multihandicappped (deaf-blind) children. The Volta Review 1983; Feb-Mar: 69-82.

Young NM, Mets MB, Johnson KC (1994) Cochlear Implants in Young Children with Usher Syndrome. In Clark GM, Cowan RSC (Eds.) Proceedings of the International Cochlear Implant Speech and Hearing Symposium, Melbourne 1994. pp 319.

Zigler E (1969) Development versus difference theories of mental retardation and the problem of motivation. American Journal of Mental Deficiency 73: 536-556.

Section B
Listening/learning devices

Introduction

Audiological assessments update the audiological needs of the child following diagnosis. The continually evolving options which are available for children present major challenges to the teacher of the deaf. This section considers acoustical aids, earmoulds, tactile and electrical aids and the environment in which they are used. In probing these options it gives a comprehensive description for the teacher of the deaf involved in the ongoing management of listening devices. It is essential that new technology, such as digital hearing aids, and old problems, for example acoustic feedback, are tackled with efficiency and confidence. The teacher of the deaf must be able to understand, identify and manage acoustic problems which will arise during all of the child's waking hours not just at home and in the classroom. An awareness of the many variables involved promotes effective management of situations which might otherwise inhibit or completely undermine effective learning.

Chapter 4
Hearing Aids

M SMITH

Introduction

Our aim in providing amplification for a hearing-impaired child is a simple one. Since the development of expressive speech and language skills is dependent on the quality of the received auditory signal, we have to ensure that we amplify sound to a level which provides the hearing-impaired child with access to as much of the speech signal as possible. The fitting of appropriate amplification for young children with mild, moderate and severe losses has been an achievable goal for some time. However, during the past 10 to 15 years the development of very high gain, low frequency aids has enabled more profoundly hearing-impaired children to benefit from amplification (Sung and Sung, 1982; Punch and Beck, 1986; Dyrlund, 1988; Franck, 1991). In addition, the introduction of sophisticated hybrid and digital aids has allowed a degree of flexibility and accuracy in fitting many losses which has not previously been attainable.

The simplified version of the Erber (1982) model (Figure 4.1) illustrates the overall aim in amplification for a hearing loss. Conversational speech is the desired input signal and is amplified to an optimum listening level in the dynamic range between the child's level of detection and the level of discomfort. The amount by which the hearing aid amplifies the signal is represented as the gain. The maximum output of the hearing aid is set to prevent the amplified signal exceeding the child's level of discomfort. The responsibility of the professional management team is to ensure that amplification is fitted early, is appropriate, is used consistently and is well maintained.

Hearing aids make sounds louder across a relatively narrow frequency range. Most hearing-impaired children do not require simple linear amplification, but need some form of signal processing, depending upon the nature of their loss. Many children would be assisted by output limiting, which may be dependent on the environment in which they are expected to function, and which may be related

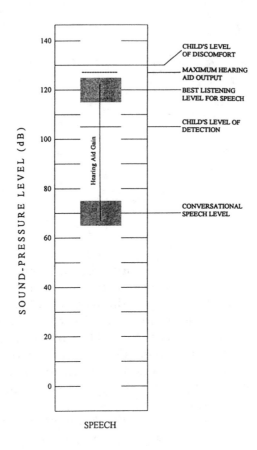

Figure 4.1 The aim of amplification. Schematic model based on that of Erber (1982)

to the reduction in dynamic range as the degree of hearing loss increases. Hearing aids can constitute the most effective habilitative tool we have for maximising the child's potential for acquiring speech and language. Correctly fitted, worn, managed and maintained, they will provide the child with access to the running speech signal, and so allow him to face the challenge of making sense of the world around him. Hearing aids are now smaller and more technically advanced than ever. Our knowledge of the development of language in hearing children has also improved, and our awareness of the facilitative features of interaction with hearing-impaired children continues to grow. All of these factors contribute to the provision of wider choice and opportunities for children with a hearing loss.

Despite the obvious benefits which effective amplification can bring, hearing aids are not an all-encompassing panacea for childhood deafness. They do not restore hearing to normal levels in the way that spectacles might correct visual problems. By their nature they can only amplify sound via an imperfect or damaged auditory pathway. Yet the provision and maintenance of effective amplification, combined with appropriate educational management, can lead to remarkable levels of achievement for hearing-impaired young people (Geers and Moog, 1989; Harrison, Simpson and Stuart, 1991; Lewis, 1994).

Basic hearing aid terminology

It is important that the professionals responsible for hearing aid management fully understand the basic terminology used in hearing aid specifications. The following definitions briefly summarise the most commonly used terms.

Gain

Gain can be defined as the amount in dB by which the sound pressure level developed by the hearing aid receiver in a coupler exceeds the sound pressure level in the sound field at the face of the hearing aid microphone. In simple terms, gain (dB) equals the output from the aid minus the input to the aid; e.g., output = 130 dBSPL, input = 60 dBSPL, therefore gain = 70 dB.

Frequency response

The frequency response of an aid is the graphical representation of the acoustic output against the frequency of the sound input for a constant input level. The usable range of the frequency response is often described as the frequency range with the low and high frequency limits being expressed in Hz.

Saturation sound pressure level

The saturation sound pressure level (SSPL) represents the maximum root mean square (rms) sound pressure level obtainable in a coupler, generated by the hearing aid. It therefore indicates what the hearing aid will do when working 'flat out'.

Harmonic distortion

Harmonic distortion reflects the presence of signals appearing at the output that were not present at the input. Distortion products may occur when part of the energy at the input stage is distributed in multiples (harmonics) of the fundamental frequency of the input signal. Harmonic distortion can be caused by overloading the hearing aid amplifier or receiver, and results when signals pass through a non-linear amplifier. If the non-linearity of the amplifier is significant, so too will be the amplitude of the distortion products. For example, a 250 Hz input signal passing via a non-linear amplifier would produce distortion products at 500 Hz, 750 Hz, 1 kHz and so on. The intentional use of peak clipping to limit output in a hearing aid inevitably produces harmonic and intermodulation distortion.

Intermodulation distortion

If two input signals of equal amplitude but with no harmonic relation-ship pass through a non-linear system, arithmetic sums and differences of the input signals will result, and can be measured as intermodulation distortion. This arises with complex input signals such as speech in noise.

Hearing aid microphones

The function of a microphone is to convert acoustic energy into mechan-ical energy and mechanical energy into electrical energy. Originally, carbon or crystal (piezoelectric) microphones were used in wearable hearing aids, with electromagnetic microphones being adopted by the 1950s. Early microphones of this type were poor performers in the low frequency range and were relatively sensitive to vibration, being easily damaged if dropped. Electret microphones are now almost universally used in hearing aid applications and have particular advantages. Their frequency response can be essentially constant (i.e., 'flat') or they can be tailored to produce specific response requirements. The construction of electret microphones can also result in very small diaphragm mass, which is less sensitive to damage if the hearing aid is knocked or dropped against hard surfaces. Since the mass is small, less acoustic energy is required to set it in motion, providing excellent sensitivity. The development of electret microphones has also allowed the microphone and the receiver to be housed in very close proximity without feedback problems. They are more reliable, with lower internal noise, and provide good sound quality.

Directional/omnidirectional microphones

Directional microphones are commonly used in hearing aids since they are more sensitive to sounds from preset angles of incidence than they are to those from other angles. A directional microphone would usually be more responsive to sounds from the front than to those from behind. This is obviously desirable in many conversational situations for the hearing-impaired listener, when an effective reduction in background noise is sought. Standard microphones without directional preference (omnidirectional microphones) are used in many hearing aids, and some aids have a switchable omnidirectional to directional facility. Omnidirectional microphones are usually referred to as pressure-type, as they respond to sound pressure fluctuations with similar sensitivity, regardless of azimuth. In practice, however, the mounting of an omnidirectional microphone in a forward facing position in a post-aural aid introduces some directionality, except at low frequencies where background noise may interfere with the signal. Directional microphones are also called gradient-type since their output depends on a pressure difference at two points of reference within the sound field (Figure 4.2). Two acoustic inlets are required (teachers will be familiar with these on some of the larger Type 1 FM systems used by children) with one opening on each side of the diaphragm. The requirement in separating the acoustic inlets either with tubing or an acoustic delay element is to create a sound delay between entering the front portal and entering the rear. The consequence is that sound entering the microphone from behind the hearing aid wearer is subject to a self cancelling effect resulting from internal delay. Sound entering the rear port from the front travels via the same time delayed route and then is further delayed by the equal internal and external delay to result in non-cancellation of the signal. In practice the microphone becomes around 15-20 dB more sensitive to sounds from the front than the back. Some studies have reported only limited benefit from the use of directional microphone technology, highlighting the fact that they are only advantageous under anechoic conditions, and that the benefits decrease as the reverberation time increases (Studebaker, Cox and Formby, 1980).

Hearing aids have been introduced recently which allow electronic switching, via a remote control unit, between directional and omnidirectional microphone characteristics, in an effort to improve the signal to noise ratio in different conditions. The improvements in speech recognition in noise using such systems are reported by Valente, Fabry and Potts (1995).

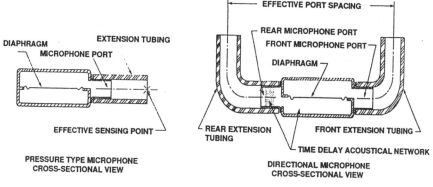

Figure 4.2 Omnidirectional and directional microphones (Knowles TB 21, 1989)

Hearing aid amplifiers

The amplifier's function is to increase the amplitude of weak electric voltages produced by the microphone and typically to process them through several stages of amplification. In development, amplifiers have been defined by classes of operation beginning with class A. These are known as single-ended output stage amplifiers and are used when low gain levels are required (not greater at peak than 50 dB). The power consumed by such an amplifier is constant, regardless of the signal level, and the low power application plus constant current drain of such a device has meant that class A amplifiers are rarely used in modern hearing aids.

With the development of class B amplifiers, higher power requirements were satisfied using push-pull technology in which there are at least two active transistors. If no signal is present, neither device draws a significant current, resulting in very low current drain. During amplification, power is drawn as the two devices alternate in their amplification of the negative and positive cycles of the input waveform. Thus, the efficiency of the amplifier is increased, whilst the energy consumed in terms of current drain is reduced whilst the device is active. In addition to the efficiency improvements over a class A amplifier, class B types allow greater output amplitude, particularly in the high frequency range. It is important, however, to obtain a smooth transition between the two devices in a push-pull amplifier to avoid cross-over distortion.

The introduction of class D amplifiers in hearing aid technology brought the advantages of class B in terms of efficiency, but with lower levels of distortion, improved broad-band performance with extended high frequency response and very low battery drain. Class D amplifiers can also be integrated into the receiver with the obvious advantages of saving space and also an extension in battery life of up to 50% (Figure 4.3). For a full description of the class D amplifier see Carlson, 1988.

A recent development within the class D family of amplifiers is the K-AMP (Killion, Etymotic Research Inc.) which can amplify a wide bandwidth with minimal distortion even at very high input levels (up to 115 dBSPL). The K-AMP circuit has a level-dependent frequency response, where the level of the input signal produces a change in the frequency response. The function of the circuit is to amplify quiet sounds with more high frequency emphasis whilst preventing loud sounds from being over-amplified to uncomfortable levels. K-AMP aids may be recommended for users with mild to moderate high frequency losses.

Receivers

Receivers in hearing aids perform the reverse function of microphones, by converting electrical energy into acoustic energy. The most frequently

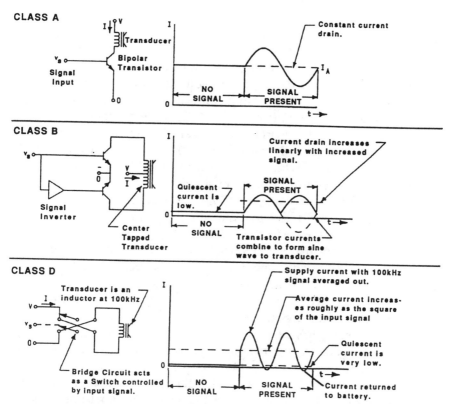

Figure 4.3 Circuits and waveforms of the three main classes of hearing aid amplifiers (Knowles EP Integrated Receiver Notes (1989). Report 10676-3, Knowles Electronics Inc)

used type of receiver in body worn aids is the moving iron magnetic earphone, which is designed to match the electrical impedance of the amplifier circuit, and can operate very efficiently from the output stage. In BTE, ITE, and in the canal (ITC) aids, internal receivers are used which are usually of the balanced armature magnetic type, and can provide good performance within a small space. Smaller receivers have a very wide frequency range amplifying up to and beyond 6 kHz. However, they are more prone to feedback and are less sensitive than the large type. The problem of improving fidelity in small receivers is constantly being addressed by hearing aid manufacturers.

In bone vibrator units the diaphragm is attached firmly to the plastic case and in turn has a magnetic system supporting it at the edge. As the electric current flows through the coil in response to the microphone function, the pull of the magnet varies. This variation results in the large mass of the magnet and case moving in relation to each other, giving rise to vibration.

Hearing aid controls

The microphone, earphone, amplifier, tone hook and mould can all be manipulated and designed to produce a given frequency response in a hearing aid. At the amplifier stage, the most commonly used control in conventional aids is the user operated volume control. A predetermined taper can be built into the volume control, allowing equal increases in loudness with proportionate rotation of the volume wheel.

Internally, the overall gain of the aid can be controlled by the adjustment of a trimmer (usually marked 'G'). This can be set to prevent the aid from overloading for wearers with tolerance or recruitment problems. The maximum output of the aid may be adjusted using an internal control (usually marked 'SSPL' or 'MPO'). Often the available adjustment is 15-25 dB, to allow the audiologist to set the SSPL control without exceeding the wearer's discomfort level.

Frequency response characteristics can be adjusted by electronic tone controls with potentiometer or switch adjustment. On hearing aids used by children, most teachers of the deaf and parents will be aware of the switch-operated external tone controls. A close eye needs to be kept on the position of these switches to ensure the child has not accidentally changed the frequency response of his aid to provide, for example, a marked high frequency cut. In some body worn aids, blanking plates are available to prevent this happening.

If the tone control is internally adjustable by potentiometer, the filter network uses low, high or sometimes band-pass filtering to produce the desired response. Thus the control allows for low cut-off, high cut-off or the suppression of a band of frequencies in a multi-channel aid. Some aids incorporate tone controls with L, N and H settings. N represents the normal or reference response for the aid whilst L can indicate high frequency cut-off (low-pass filter). The H setting can likewise represent a low frequency cut-off (high-pass filter). There is little uniformity in the labelling of tone controls, and what may appear to be a low frequency emphasis setting may actually be a low frequency cut-off. In such cases it is essential to refer to the manufacturer's data for guidance (Figure 4.4).

The required level at which an automatic gain control (AGC) becomes effective can be adjusted on some aids using an internal potentiometer. This level, known as the 'knee point' will be discussed in more detail under output limiting.

The introduction of digital technology in hearing aid programming has obviated the need for manually adjusted potentiometers. The parameters for output, gain, frequency response and other parameters can now be controlled and adjusted by a direct link from a computer to the aid whilst it is being worn. A visual indication on a monitor or LCD screen confirms the operation of the program and the resultant settings of the aid.

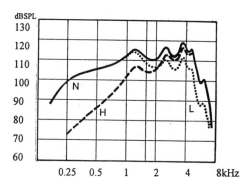

Figure 4.4 Typical effects of tone controls on the frequency response of a hearing aid

Output limiting

Output limiting is desirable in hearing aids to ensure that the amplified signal is accommodated within the listener's dynamic range of hearing, i.e., the window between threshold and uncomfortable listening level. The type of limiting used to keep the signal below the uncomfortable listening level will depend on the circuitry within the aid.

Output limiting can be achieved by simple 'peak clipping' where the amplifier affects the output signal above a given input level by clipping the peaks and troughs of the amplified waveform. In this situation, the input signal may steadily increase, but eventually the output will remain constant. The point at which the output becomes constant (and the waveform is clipped) can often be controlled using a potentiometer on the aid. Although a relatively simple and effective method of output limiting, peak clipping introduces levels of distortion which may be reflected in poorer sound quality.

Linear amplifiers produce an output directly proportional to the input up to the point where saturation is reached. It can be illustrated as in Figure 4.5 and is described in various terms: constant gain, 45 slope or 1:1 dB ratio over the available range. In practice most linear amplifiers approach saturation when the input signal level reaches 90 dBSPL. Fortune, Preves and Woodruff (1991) note that linear hearing aids with a higher maximum output (SSPL90) are less likely to exceed the user's aided uncomfortable listening levels than aids with a lower maximum output but higher levels of distortion. The gap between the combination of the peak input level plus the gain and the level when peak clipping is introduced is known as the 'headroom', and is illustrated in Figure 4.6. The work of Fortune et al. (1991) indicates that instruments with higher headroom and less distortion are more likely to be worn at gain settings which provide appropriate benefit.

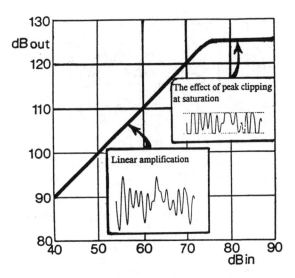

Figure 4.5 Linear amplification and the effect of peak clipping on a waveform

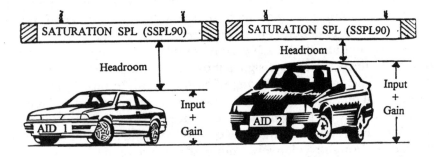

Figure 4.6 The concept of headroom
Research suggests that linear hearing aids with a higher headroom and less distortion are more likely to be worn at gain settings which provide most benefit. As such more effective use may be made of AID 1 than of AID 2

An alternative approach involves the use of compression amplification, often described as AGC (automatic gain control) or sometimes as AVC (automatic volume control) (Figure 4.7). Instead of clipping the peaks and troughs of the amplified signal, the waveform is compressed, with less resultant distortion than peak clipping introduces. Compression circuitry may be designed to be either input-dependent or output-dependent (Figure 4.8). Using input-dependent compression, an aid's gain depends on the signal level just before the volume control in the circuit. Using this technique with children, we need to remember that the child could alter the output level reaching the ear canal by adjusting the volume wheel. For an older child this may be acceptable and perhaps desirable, since it allows individual adjustment of the maximum output in different listening conditions. In the case of young children, input-dependent compression may be less appropriate.

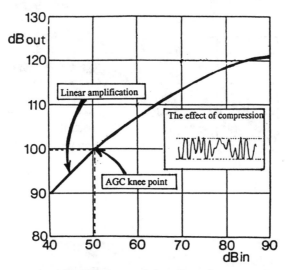

Figure 4.7 Compression amplification and the effect of compression on a waveform

The use of output-dependent compression, where the gain depends on the signal level after the volume control, may eliminate the potential risks of a child being exposed to amplification which exceeds their level of discomfort. As such, it may be desirable to use output-dependent compression for younger children. For a detailed review of the literature on compression and output limiting, see Walker and Dillon, 1982 and Staab and Lybarger, 1994.

Attack/release times

In output-dependent compression circuits, attack time refers to the length of time required for the controlling action to take effect after the loud signal is present at the earphone stage. In input-dependent compression circuits, it refers to the same time taken after the loud signal is present at the stage prior to the gain control. In other words, attack time defines the time taken for the compression circuit to react to loud input signals. Release time refers to the length of time required for the system to return to its normal amplification function after the loud signal has ceased. In technical specifications, hearing aid manufacturers usually define attack and release times in milliseconds, and these times can be critical in terms of sound experience for the hearing aid user (Figure 4.9).

There may be a loss of temporal resolution as the temporal pattern of masking is affected by sensorineural hearing loss. A weak sound may be inaudible if it is preceded by a loud sound, due to excessive masking such

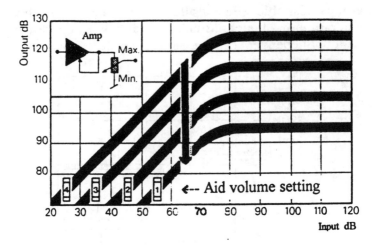

A

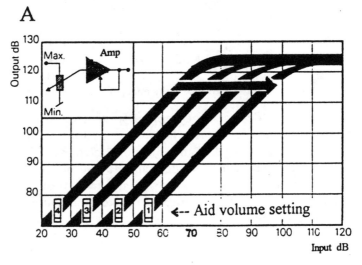

B

Figure 4.8 Input/output characteristics of hearing aids with (A) input-dependent compression and (B) output-dependent compression

as a vowel followed by a low energy consonant. Non-stationary noise might affect a hearing-impaired person disproportionately, since the moments of silence will be masked. Hearing aid manufacturers have attempted to overcome this problem with more sophisticated compression circuits to ameliorate the experience of the wearer in the presence of varying noise.

When a high-energy sound is processed by a hearing aid with AGC, the circuit may react too slowly and release too quickly, or vice versa, if the attack/release times are incorrectly set. This may cause discomfort and could result in poor speech discrimination – incorrect AGC function leaves hearing aid wearers describing a 'breathing', 'pumping' or

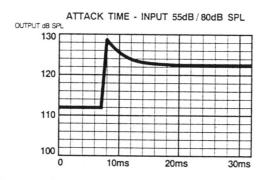

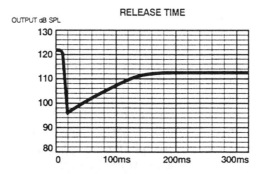

Figure 4.9 Graphical illustration of attack time and release time (note the difference in timescale)

'glugging' sound quality. It is important to ensure that the AGC circuit is not triggered unnecessarily to transient sounds. Walker and Dillon (1982) suggest an attack time of 0.5–20ms and a recovery time of 60–150ms.

The attack and release times of the compression circuit are the primary determinants of the dynamic behaviour of the compression system. It is important that the time between the onset of the loud signal prior to full activation of the system (known as undershoot), and the time taken to return to normal after signal cessation (overshoot), do not interfere with speech cues. The complexities of the application of compression are not fully documented in terms of auditory function much beyond pure-tone audiometry, and the recent arrival of multi-channel compression aids requires even more critical scrutiny (Dreschler, 1992).

Telecoil/loop

Most hearing aids accommodate an electromagnetic induction input mode known as a telephone coil or telecoil. The original purpose of this device was to allow hearing-impaired wearers to use their hearing aids to amplify signals from the telephone. In practice, telecoil technology has been used in many situations in which amplification for hearing aid wearers in group settings was required. It was particularly popular in schools for the deaf in the 1960s and 1970s prior to the advent of FM systems.

The principle of electromagnetic induction is that, when a conductor (a wire) carries a current, a magnetic field is set up around the wire. When a second conductor (the aid telecoil) is placed within this field, a current is induced into the telecoil in response to current fluctuations in the wire. The telecoil of the aid then passes on the current to the amplifier circuit.

When a hearing aid is set to 'T', it will usually receive telecoil signals only, and the microphone is often not active. Some aids have an 'MT' facility where both the microphone and the telecoil are simultaneously active, allowing the listener to monitor his/her own voice whilst listening to the telecoil-received signal. Telecoil or loop systems are commonly used in churches, theatres and auditoriums for group assemblies, but they have a number of disadvantages when used with hearing-impaired children.

The low frequency performance of telecoil circuitry is not particularly good, and for some children with limited residual hearing, loop systems are not an alternative to other remote microphone options. There can be weak or dead spots within the electromagnetic field in which the child may be placed. A naive listener may not be able to report when his/her hearing aid is not functioning as a result of this. The strength of the received signal will depend to some extent on the orientation of the telecoil within the magnetic field, giving rise to peaks and troughs in the signal as the child moves his/her head. Telecoils are additionally sensitive to interference from TV/computer monitors and fluorescent lighting systems. The commonest use for a loop system for children is in conjunction with a television at home via the audio output. In practice, however, a correctly fitted FM transmitter used with appropriate direct input from a TV/video will provide a far superior acoustic signal.

Hearing aid tone hooks

The tone hook (ear hook or acoustic elbow) can play a critical part in influencing the acoustic properties of the signal reaching the ear from a BTE aid. Several options in tone hook design are often available for the same aid, and particular care should be taken when fitting tone hooks appropriate for a child user. First, the size of the hook should be taken into account. Most hearing aids are designed primarily for adults and then adapted for the paediatric market. One effective way of making the aid a better fit in ergonomic terms is to use a tone hook that is smaller and is angled more sharply than the adult version. This has the effect of keeping the aid more firmly in place on the child's head, and ensuring that the top-mounted microphone remains forward facing (and not skyward-facing as is often the case when adult size hooks are used).

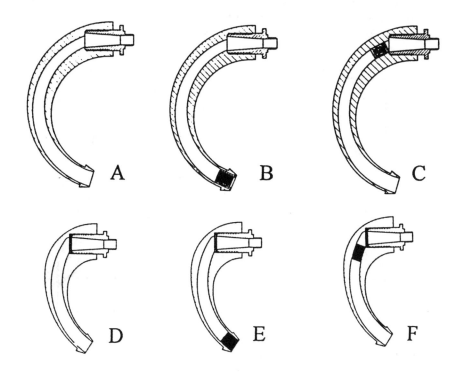

Figure 4.10 Examples of optional tone hooks
A–C illustrate adult size (regular) tone hooks whilst D–F illustrate mini hooks which may be more appropriate for children. A = regular tone hook, B = regular damped tone hook for moderate gain aids, C = regular damped tone hook for high gain aids, D = mini tone hook, E = mini damped tone hook for moderate gain aids, F = mini damped tone hook for high gain aids

Acoustic dampers may be fitted to the tone hook to shape the frequency response more closely to the child's requirements, often with the effect of reducing undesirable peaks in the signal. Alternatively, peak damping elements (sintered filters) can be inserted into the hook and can tailor the response of the output signal in a variety of predetermined ways (Figures 4.10 and 4.11). Highly specialised tone hooks are also available for use in cases of unusual audiogram configurations, particularly those with 'ski-slope' hearing losses. High-pass, low-pass and notch-filter tone hooks are available to accommodate a variety of audiogram shapes. Using a high-pass hook, a broad-band aid can be adapted to produce an extreme high frequency emphasis. If a reverse 'ski-slope' loss is present, where residual hearing is markedly better in the high frequencies, a low-pass tone hook may be suitable. Very occasionally, hearing is normal around the 2 kHz region, but hearing at other frequencies is poor. If a conventional aid fitting is used it may lead to rejection, since the 2 kHz region is over-amplified. A notch-filter tone hook may provide a solution to the fitting problem. See Figure 4.12 for fitting ranges and Buerkli-Halevy (1987) for a more detailed review.

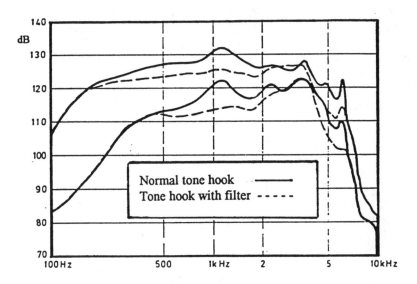

Figure 4.11 The effect of peak damping using a filtered tone hook

Hearing aid nomenclature

It is useful for the professional support team managing a child's hearing aids to remember that we can often establish an idea of the aid's performance simply by looking at the model name. A rough guide to the abbreviations commonly used is listed in Table 4.1. Therefore we might guess that a hypothetical aid known as a Phonovox PPCHD is a reasonably high powered aid with compression, high frequency emphasis and a directional microphone. Whilst this can be a useful guide, one should obviously check the manufacturer's data and specifications.

Table 4.1 Hearing aid nomenclature

If the aid has	it may refer to . . . .
PP	Push-pull amplification
L	Low frequency emphasis
H	High frequency emphasis
A	The option of direct audio input
C	Compression limiting
D	Directional microphone

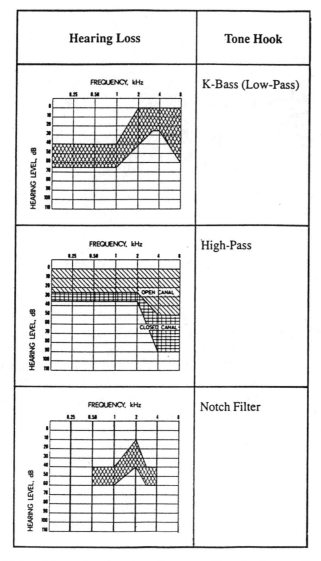

Figure 4.12 Special tone hook options for unusual hearing loss configurations

Types of hearing aid for children

Although all hearing aids perform a broadly similar function, they vary in format according to the needs of the user, and the range of aids now available for children is wide. Very few personal hearing aids have been designed specifically for children, since the paediatric market is relatively small. As a result, aids have historically been large and somewhat cumbersome in use, but with greater miniaturisation of components it is now possible to fit children with smaller instruments

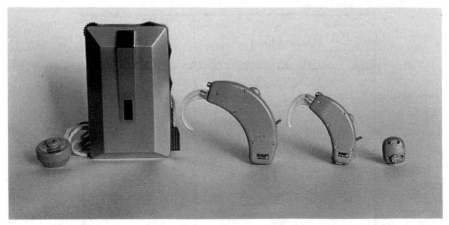

Figure 4.13 Types of air-conduction aid most commonly used by children

including in the ear aids. The types of air-conduction aid most commonly used by children are illustrated in Figure 4.13.

The conventional hearing aid consists of five discrete parts, and in the case of a BTE aid these could be illustrated in simple diagrammatic form as in Figure 4.14. It is vital that all of these component parts function properly for the sound signal to be delivered appropriately to the ear. The earmould should be considered as an integral part of the aid since it can radically affect the quality of the signal arriving in the auditory canal. Any supervision and routine testing of the hearing aid system should include a check of earmould function.

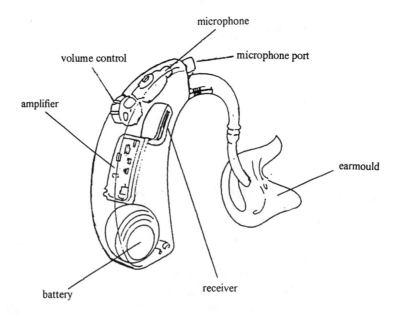

Figure 4.14 Components of a typical hearing aid

Behind the ear (BTE) aids

By far the majority of children are fitted with behind the ear aids. There is a wide range of BTE aids which are appropriate for children, and most have the facility to be compatible with systems for education. From an ergonomic point of view BTE aids are relatively small, light to wear and (in miniature format particularly) are easy to fit on young children. Some BTE aids are fitted with a tone hook allowing movement in three dimensions, providing a close fit for the aid against the child's head and reducing the risk of the aid slipping away from the back of the pinna.

In terms of performance many BTE aids are now able to deliver high levels of gain and output with the latest mini BTE aids providing over 80 dB gain and 140 dBSPL output. Low frequency emphasis has been available for some time on BTE aids in both standard and mini format, enabling children with only limited reserves of residual hearing to be fitted effectively when previously a body worn aid would have been required to meet their needs.

There are few external user-operated controls on most BTE aids, but frequently these would comprise a main power switch (often incorporating a telecoil switch), a volume control, occasionally an external tone control or noise reduction switch and possibly a directional microphone switch. For children in some situations it may be considered useful to be able to amplify sound from a frontal direction whilst suppressing noise from the background, and a directional microphone could be employed in such cases.

BTE aids are relatively robust and are less susceptible to damage than an aid worn on the chest by an energetic youngster. By placing the microphone of the aid close to the ear, a more natural sound field is created, and an improved ability to localise sound may be evident. The acoustic elbow or tone hook can be selected to influence the frequency response of the aid when worn, either by damping unwanted peaks in the output, or (with the introduction of sintered filters) by reducing the performance of the aid in specific areas of the frequency response.

In routine use, there are few problems with BTE aids; the battery drawers can be locked shut on most models and the volume controls can be covered with specially designed plastic fittings to make them tamperproof. Such features are useful in theory, but given that the aid is already very small, it becomes a challenging task for the parent or teacher to deal with minute control covers and screw-down battery drawers. However, with guidance, parents and teachers soon become expert manipulators of hearing aids and their controls, fitting and setting them quickly and efficiently.

The most common internal faults on high powered BTE aids include the failure of receivers after prolonged high-gain use, causing significant levels of low frequency distortion. Microphones are sometimes damaged if the aid is dropped, and moisture may migrate into the aid housing via the tone hook if the child tends to perspire. Moisture may also cause corrosion of the battery and rusting in the battery housing. Dogs seem to have a particular predilection for BTE aids, and many audiology departments have examples of dog-chewed aids. A sophisticated instrument can be reduced to a mangled twist of micro chips and wires in seconds by an exuberant pet. Parents should be encouraged to keep hearing aids beyond the reach of the family dog.

Hearing aid care kits have been produced for parents and teachers which contain all the essential items for routine management. These include 'dri-aid' crystals to reduce the build-up of moisture in the instrument, and a number of essential items including a stetoset for listening checks.

Body worn aids

The body worn (BW) aid remains a popular choice for some audiologists when fitting severely or profoundly hearing-impaired children. However, body worn aids are now less commonly used than previously, since in many cases the rapid development of high power BTE aids has largely closed the performance gap between the two types.

Body worn aids use penlite batteries, which account for most of the bulk of the system. The microphone is usually sited on top of the aid, where it is vulnerable to food and debris being dropped into it by the child. Plastic covers are often provided to protect the microphone without affecting the electro-acoustic performance of the aid; these covers also serve to prevent the child from adjusting the major controls on top of the aid. The aid itself is linked to the ear via a dedicated lead and button receiver feeding the acoustic signal through the earmould. The fact that the receiver is sited at some distance from the microphone of the aid may result in less acoustic feedback emanating from the earmould than might be the case with a BTE. It could be argued that the use of a BW aid provides a better ear–voice link for children who are in the early stages in the development of listening skills. However, there are a number of disadvantages to the use of BW aids by young children. In a survey of 1853 aids, Markides (1989) indicated that BW aids were less well used than BTE aids by the children under scrutiny. If protective covers are not used, the switches and controls can be easily knocked and changed by the child. They are susceptible to clothes rub where the frictional movement of clothes against the body and microphone of the aid is amplified and causes unwanted noise. The enhanced low frequency performance of a BW aid has been regarded as an advantage for some children, with body baffle effects playing a part (Erber, 1973). From a cosmetic point of view, a BW aid is bigger and less discreet than a BTE aid, and this may influence its acceptability by the parents and child.

Most BW aids would have the following external user-operated controls: main power switch, volume control (preferably separate), telecoil switch and occasionally an external tone control. In the case of young children, the fewer exposed controls on the aid the better, since an aid may be easily adjusted to an inappropriate setting or mode without the parent or teacher being aware of the change. Some BW aids can have blanking plates fitted by the supplier to prevent the child tampering with external controls.

Internally on conventional analogue aids there are often adjustable potentiometers for tone and output, with output control by peak clipping or compression. The tone control would be adjusted to accommodate the shape of the child's audiogram (within the limits of the aid's circuitry) matching frequency emphasis to hearing loss. Output limiting may be required to ensure that the output level does not exceed the child's loudness discomfort level whilst maintaining appropriate levels of amplification within the dynamic range of hearing.

Special BW/BTE systems

A few manufacturers have attempted to combine the advantages of a BW hearing aid with those of a BTE, developing a system which uses a chest-mounted microphone feeding the signal to a BTE aid by wire. The post-aural part of the instrument houses the receiver and uses conventional earmould tubing and coupling. An FM system can be coupled to the microphone if necessary. This approach was thought to combine the cosmetic advantages of a standard behind the ear aid with the increased gain available when the distance between microphone and receiver is increased. In practice however, such systems have not proved popular in the UK.

In the ear (ITE) aids

In the ear (ITE) aids and the smaller in the canal (ITC) aids have not been widely used for children in the past. These aids fit either entirely within the concha (ITE) or in the outer part of the auditory canal (ITC). This type of aid has only been appropriate for those with mild to moderate hearing losses since a high gain amplifier fitted in such close proximity to the microphone would lead to an increased risk of acoustic feedback. In the case of children, there has always been one particular drawback in the provision of ITE aids. Since a conventional ITE has the electronic circuitry bonded to the backplate/control panel of the aid and is housed in a custom-made shell, the aid would have to be remade each time the child grows. However, the recent and more widespread introduction of modular ITE aids (Figure 4.15) has resulted in effective fitting for children since the acrylic shell of the aid simply clips on to the aid housing and can be removed and exchanged just as a new mould is processed for a BTE aid. Figure 4.16 indicates the degree of loss for which ITE aids might be considered.

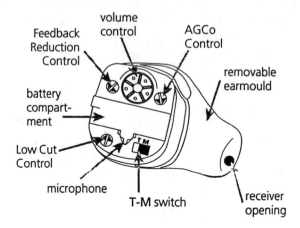

Figure 4.15 An example of a modular ITE aid with removable mould (Starkey, with permission)

The controls on an ITE aid are necessarily small and may be difficult for a parent or teacher to supervise, particularly if the child is very young. Since the microphone of an ITE is sited almost centrally within the concha, it provides perhaps the most natural sound field for the listener maintaining the frequency enhancement effects of the pinna.

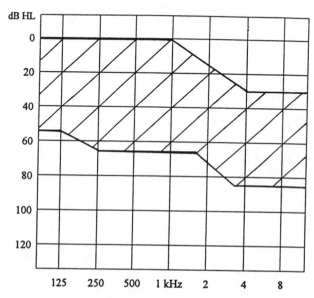

Figure 4.16 Typical fitting range of current modular ITE aids commonly used by children

ITE aids are now available with telecoil pick-up and some have the facility for direct audio input for personal FM systems. For youngsters with mild to moderate hearing losses the modular ITE aid may prove very suitable. It may provide a solution for hearing-impaired children who wear spectacles and find the combination of the arm of the spectacles and a conventional BTE too difficult to manage. Down's syndrome children who require an aid for a mild to moderate loss may find an ITE more acceptable since many find conventional aids difficult to site behind rather elastic pinnae. Youngsters with malformed outer ears but with near normal conchas may also benefit from the use of an ITE. Hearing-impaired children for whom the cosmetic appearance of the aid is a crucial factor in their willingness to use amplification may prefer an ITE (although in the author's experience many young people, when given the choice, have expressed a preference for a near transparent shell, or skeleton mould with a mini BTE which can be hidden under the hair).

Contralateral routing of signal (CROS/BICROS) aids

One option for children with a unilateral loss is the fitting of a CROS (contralateral routing of signal) hearing aid. Using this configuration a microphone is placed on the impaired side either in the temple of a spectacle frame or a conventional post-aural housing. The signal is amplified and converted into acoustic energy before being transmitted (via a flexible lead or electromagnetic radiation) to a receiver mounted in an equivalent housing on the opposite side. In this way, the wearer with a unilateral or significantly asymmetrical loss can use the good ear to hear sound from the impaired side. In general, if a severe unilateral loss is present, most children are thought to manage better without an aid, and the support of specialist teachers in advising mainstream professionals on classroom tactics is essential in such cases. The potential for confusion amongst young CROS hearing aid users is raised by Evans (1988), but he points out that despite this "the most appropriate candidate may be the very young infant who is assumed to be in the process of developing an auditory neural representation of the world". The CROS option remains popular for a few audiologists but it is not widely used with children.

For hearing-impaired listeners with a loss in both ears but with one unaidable ear, a BICROS system might be considered. This was first described by Fowler (1960) and developed by Harford (1966) as a system employing one complete hearing aid plus one additional microphone in an aid housing for the unaidable ear. Using this system, sound reaches the aidable ear by conventional amplification and the effect of head shadow is reduced with the use of the opposite microphone. As with CROS aids, these systems are not commonly used with children.

Bone conduction and bone anchored hearing aids

For some children a conventional air-conduction hearing aid may be unsuitable either because congenital abnormalities of the external ear preclude such a fitting or because the ear canal cannot be occluded. An absent or rudimentary pinna or meatal atresia will not allow the fitting of a conventional mould. Some children with recurrent middle ear effusions, which prove difficult to treat over time, experience more problems when the ear canal is occluded by a mould. The middle ear condition may be exacerbated by wearing a mould and further infection or discharge may result. Such a child with a significant conductive component in the hearing loss, and normal or near normal cochlear function, may benefit from a bone conduction hearing aid.

Originally bone conduction aids employed a standard vibrator unit and headband such as that used in bone conduction audiometry. The vibrator was attached to a BW aid via a lead, and the microphone of the aid was sited appropriately on the chest. This configuration is still used by some children, although it is becoming less common because of its bulk and inconvenience in everyday use. More recently, standard and mini BTE aids have been adapted to the same vibrator/headband arrangement and this has reduced some of the practical problems which accompanied the BW set-up (Figure 4.17).

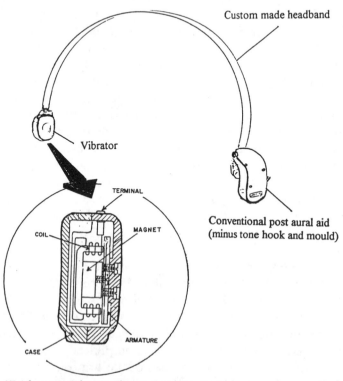

Custom made headband

Vibrator

TERMINAL

COIL

MAGNET

ARMATURE

CASE

Conventional post aural aid
(minus tone hook and mould)

Figure 4.17 A bone conduction hearing aid (post aural)

Despite the availability of BTE aids for bone conduction, there remain difficulties with siting the vibrator correctly on the mastoid and maintaining the headband position on the child. Whilst the transducer should be placed firmly against the skin of the mastoid process for the system to work effectively, this can cause skin irritation and headaches.

One solution to the drawbacks of headband bone conduction aids is the use of a bone anchored hearing aid involving the connection of the transducer to a titanium implant sited in the temporal bone. This direct anchoring of the transducer in the skull (established by Branemark et al., 1969 in dental surgery) permits excellent transmission of sound vibrations to the cochlea without the intervention of skin and soft tissue which would be present if conventional bone conduction aids were used. Implantation is not normally considered for children below the age of 6 or 7 years since the bone has to reach an appropriate thickness (Rothera, 1983). Bone anchored aids provide an alternative to extensive middle ear surgery, in which the operative risks may be higher and the success rate lower. Bone anchored hearing aids (BAHAs) may also provide a feasible alternative in a few cases of conductive or mixed loss when there is a skin reaction to any kind of earmould material (Snik, Mylanus and Cremers, 1995). There is a particular potential use for the BAHA with youngsters who have Treacher Collins syndrome.

Long term studies are now being reported outlining the effectiveness of bone anchored aids. Stevenson et al. (1993) outline the findings of a 4 year study of 12 children using BAHAs, and caution that only a small improvement in aided thresholds was noted, compared with their own previous bone conduction aids. However, subjective sound quality reportedly improved, and levels of satisfaction with the aid were high. Rothera emphasises that a percutaneous implant requires a strong commitment from the patient and his family. Careful monitoring of the implant site is essential, and an awareness of the delicate nature of the aid is important on the part of those involved in the management programme.

Analogue, hybrid and digital hearing aids

There have been rapid changes in hearing instrument technology in the recent past, and the development of fully digital hearing aids is one of the most significant. Analogue hearing aids are the most familiar type, still accounting for the majority of aids worn by children, and this is likely to remain the case for a few years. An analogue signal is the representation of a continuously changing variable such as sound by another physical variable such as electric current. The most common form of analogue signal is the sine wave. Analogue hearing aids process the sound signal via conventional input transducers (microphone, telecoil, etc.), filters, output limiters, amplifiers and output transducers. There are user controls and screwdriver operated potentiometers commonly for tone and output adjustment. It is suggested (Staab, 1990; Lyregaard, 1993) that analogue circuitry has almost reached maximum capacity in terms of hearing aid development and packaging.

Hybrid hearing aids use a combination of analogue and digital technology by processing the signal through analogue circuitry, with a digital system being used to extract key parameters. Noise reduction, digital feedback suppression and programmable memory modules are typical features of a hybrid aid.

Using digital technology, the signal is converted into a digital format, processed in a microprocessor and converted into an analogue signal. The operating characteristics of such hearing aids are determined by memory chips which hold data for a wide range of parameters, and can be programmed by computer. Digital hearing aid technology will soon be available to children on a wider scale, and the advantages of such digital aids could be summarised as follows:

- Programmable memory allows for almost infinite adjustments of the characteristics of the aid without having to compromise by using the pre-selected settings of a conventional instrument.
- Digital aids are likely to be more reliable in use since the circuitry is less likely to be affected by component variability and the electro-mechanical functions are automated.
- Such systems should improve the accuracy of the fit and consequently the likelihood of acceptance by the wearer.
- By including features within the system that can suppress feedback, reduce background noise and enhance desirable sound features in speech, there is greater potential for providing an extremely effective amplification system for everyday life.
- The advantage of being able to fine-tune the instrument whilst the hearing-impaired person is wearing it is a great boon for the audiologist, particularly since the earmould coupling will be integral to the listening experience. However, for those professionals involved in fitting young pre-lingual hearing-impaired children, the opportunity for meaningful feedback from the wearer remains elusive. Despite this we can be reassured that the aid remains flexible enough to be adjusted over time as the child's speech and language develop and his learning environment changes.

In future the time may come when a teacher in a unit or school for the deaf may teach a class of youngsters all wearing the same type of programmable aid but tailored to individual requirements. This should help particularly to alleviate the problems of keeping a wide range of spares if a hearing aid fails.

Several manufacturers are now producing hearing aids with some digital circuitry, allowing remote control of the aid from a hand-held unit (Figure 4.19). Some of these have been targeted at the paediatric market with the advantage for parents of very young children being able to adjust the aid by remote control without handling it. The potential exists therefore to adjust the memory of the aid to adapt to different environments, for example a quiet home setting, a long car journey or a noisy day nursery.

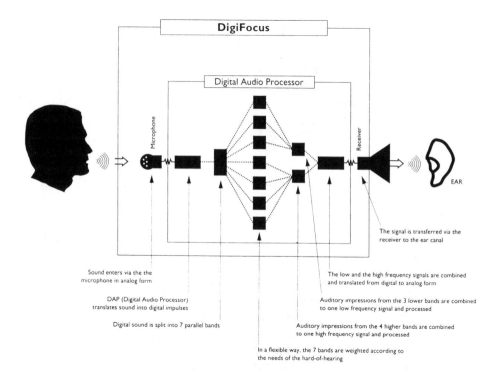

Figure 4.18 An example of digital processing courtesy of Otican A/S

Fully digital aids now form part of the range of aids available to the audiologist with digital BTEs and ITEs launched recently. Rapid progress has been made since the launch of the first wearable digital aid (Nunley et al., 1983) and the improvement in digital signal processing (DSP) chips has allowed the development of aids which are able to make decisions rather like a wearable computer.

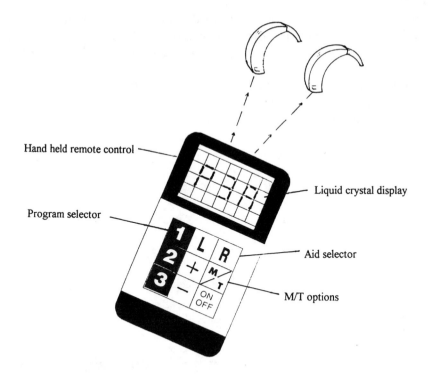

Figure 4.19 Schematic representation of programmable aids with a remote control system

Potential advantages of remote control programmable instruments for children

The advantages of digital technology in hearing aids have already been outlined but there are specific factors which may benefit children in the early years. The differences between ear canal volume and 2cc ear simulator couplers are well documented (see Stelmachowicz, 1991). The average real ear to coupler difference (RECD) changes significantly over the first five years as the child's ear canal develops to near adult size. The use of digital aids in conjunction with real ear measurement allows the audiologist to fine-tune the aid more precisely, taking into account the age-related RECD.

Optional programs for different listening situations may provide the child with an improved auditory experience according to the influence of noise and reverberation in the environment. Distance from the conversational partner will be a factor in determining the required level of gain for a young infant. An aid might be pre-programmed to accommodate the relatively high SPL of a parent's voice when holding a child close in the earliest stages of development. As the youngster moves to a more distant position in independent play, for example, a different aid program may be selected which automatically accounts for the slightly reduced voice level of the conversational partner. When remote control is linked to digital technology, there can be more precise control over the settings of the aids. Feedback can be a problem when a young infant rests his head against a parent's shoulder. Using remote control, an individual aid can be adjusted accordingly. Aids can be adjusted for gain either individually or in parallel. If an aid is set to receive remote control signals, an accidental movement of the volume wheel will have no effect. It is important, however, to know exactly how settings such as gain are being affected by simply pressing an increase/attenuation button, and this is where a display (e.g., liquid crystal) on the remote unit provides precise information on adjustments made.

Crucial to the success of implementing such technology is the appropriate training of the professional team, who can then advise parents and caregivers accordingly. The role of the informed teacher of the deaf at this stage is critical.

Potential problems with remote control programmable aids for children

With some early models of remote control hearing aid systems, there have been problems with efficient function when the aids were used in close proximity to the monitors of personal computers. Although the interference is not audible, remote systems use low power inductive transmission which can be adversely affected by radiation from monitors. Later versions of these systems will be higher powered and this should counteract the problem. If the remote control unit is required to switch on the aid and adjust the gain with no independent facility on the aid itself, a lost or malfunctioning remote control will render the aid useless. For adults, the auditory experience alone may be sufficient for hearing aid users to recognise which program is in use and whether the aid is appropriately and comfortably set. For children, however, some clear indication of the selected settings is required on the programmer to ensure effective use. It is important to remember that very few digital aids currently available have audio input facility, and this may be a critical factor in selection for children.

Frequency transposition aids for children

Frequency transposition is an attempt to render high frequency information audible to those with useful hearing only in the low frequency range. Transposition aids could be considered for those subjects with profound hearing impairment, who may be candidates for vibrotactile systems or cochlear implants. Those with left corner audiograms may also be potential candidates for aids which employ frequency transposition technology. Conventional high powered hearing aids, despite recent technical advances, typically have a narrower bandwidth than that of the acoustic speech signal. Boothroyd and Medwetsky (1992) highlight four main reasons for this:

1 It is difficult to produce output transducers which provide a combination of wide bandwidth, high output power and low distortion.
2 The coupling of the transducer to the ear canal introduces low-pass filtering.
3 The likelihood of increased acoustic feedback is greater when the upper frequency limit of the aid is extended.
4 A relatively low upper frequency limit has often been accepted in hearing aid technology as a result of early research that found such limits acceptable for normally hearing listeners when discriminating speech.

Extension of the high frequency response of conventional aids has been well documented (Harford and Fox, 1978) and attention to earmould acoustics (Killion, 1980, 1981) has contributed to shifting and preserving the upper limit of the available acoustic signal. However, for severely and profoundly hearing-impaired subjects where very high gain levels are required in the high frequency region, conventional techniques remain limited.

Early attempts to transpose high frequency information to the low frequency range were dependent on a transposition device developed by Johansson (1959). In the BW version, each signal in the 4–8 kHz region was fed into a distortion circuit, converting it into broad band noise and changing the spectral pattern. The band of noise below 1.5 kHz was then processed via a low-pass filter and added to conventionally amplified speech.

Some early attempts at frequency transposition simply shifted the high frequency components in the speech band by a fixed value equivalent to the modulating carrier's frequency. As a result, the product was non-proportionally transposed, so that not all the frequency components in the speech signal were shifted by the same ratio. This meant that the high frequency speech range was not genuinely compressed and led to an unnatural voice quality for the listener. By dividing the speech frequency band into several discrete bands using filters, the frequency of each band was shifted by a different amount. Thus the transposed frequencies were sometimes mixed with the original speech frequencies, leading to further unnatural qualities in the final speech signal.

Modern devices use real-time electronic processors to analyse the speech spectrum, cut the audio signal into discrete bands of information and divide the entire frequency spectrum by pre-selected factors. This audio signal is then reproduced within a narrower and lower frequency band which is determined by the audiologist to be within the listener's audible range (Figure 4.20). The transposition procedure occurs instantly and retains as much of the relative spectral information as possible. A further aim of the transposition process is that low frequency background noise may also be shifted low enough to be filtered out of the bandwidth of the instrument, rendering it inaudible to the listener.

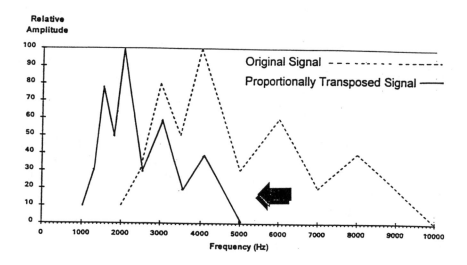

Figure 4.20 Proportional frequency transposition

Several studies have examined the effectiveness of frequency transposition with the hearing-impaired and the results have been variable (Foust and Gengel, 1973; Gustafsson, 1978; Velmans and Marcuson, 1983; Moore et al., 1992). Some researchers have focused in particular on the potential benefits of frequency transposition with congenitally deaf children (Velmans, 1975; Beasley, Mosher and Orchik, 1976; Rees and Velmans, 1993; Davis-Penn and Ross, 1993). The paediatric experience in frequency transposition is of most interest to those involved in the education of children with profound sensorineural losses. Beasley et al. (1976) examined the effect of proportionate frequency-shifting and time-compression, and compared this with speech intelligibility scores in an unmodified condition. Half of a group of 18 profoundly deaf children were presented with a transposed speech signal, whilst the other half were presented with an unmodified signal. By proportionately shifting frequency and using simultaneous temporal alteration, the aim was to preserve intelligibility and prosodic cues intact. After several auditory training sessions the subjects receiving the transposed signal showed improvements in speech intelligibility, and the implication is that a 'carry over' effect to normal speech may have occurred.

Rees and Velmans (1993) using a frequency recoding device (FRED) recently reported that a small group of hearing-impaired children demonstrated a significant enhancement in discriminating consonants in the high speech frequencies, without formal training. Davis-Penn and Ross (1993) report on clinical experience with a different frequency transposition device (Transonic FT40) and describe four successful fittings on children. Most authors agree that not all children within the potential fitting range will benefit from or accept frequency transposition instruments. By definition, those who might be considered as possible candidates for such devices are those who will be difficult to fit, deriving little or no benefit from conventional aids. However, it is also agreed that recent research into frequency transposition for children is providing more information as to the type of case where such devices will be useful.

New developments in BTE versions of frequency transposition aids will be watched with interest, since this is likely to make the systems more cosmetically acceptable to the young hearing-impaired child and his family. Frequency transposition may well play a significant part in future in the habilitative process for profoundly deaf children who fall within the narrow margins of benefiting from conventional amplification and cochlear implants.

Control of acoustic feedback

One major problem for hearing aid wearers when high levels of gain are required is the likely generation of acoustic feedback, the high pitched whistle present when the incoming signal is fed back through the amplifier and re-amplified. The suppression of acoustic feedback has preoccupied professionals since high gain aids were first introduced, and it is important for teachers and parents to recognise the commonest causes and potential cures. Acoustic feedback can often be overcome using relatively simple solutions. In many cases the child's ear may have grown, causing the mould to leak and allowing a feedback loop to be generated. In this situation a new mould should be processed without delay, and if the problem is very serious (resulting in the aid being turned down below the child's auditory threshold) then an instant temporary mould should be made.

Occasionally, feedback occurs when the mould tubing is either too thin-walled (Flack et al., 1995) or has cracked near the tone hook entrance or more commonly on the bend as it enters the mould. In such situations, the tubing should be replaced and regular tube replacement should be an integral part of the aid management programme. The state of the middle ear may be a factor in determining the cause of acoustic feedback. Where middle ear dysfunction has resulted in the tympanic membrane becoming highly reflective, then high levels of amplified sound may cause sound leakage from the acoustic coupling system, and feedback then occurs. For a fuller explanation of potential causes and cures see Nolan (1983).

A further potential cure for acoustic feedback is the development of digital circuitry which automatically suppresses the incoming feedback signal (Dyrlund et al., 1994). The digital suppression of feedback is likely to become a prominent feature in hearing aid design in future. Figure 4.21 highlights the possible causes of acoustic feedback and potential cures.

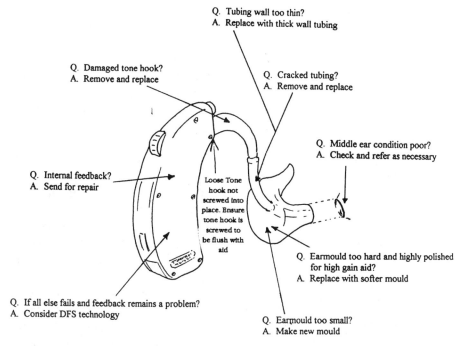

Figure 4.21 Possible questions and answers in the quest to rectify acoustic feedback problems

Hearing aid interference from mobile phones

The majority of hearing aids currently available are subject to interference when used in close proximity to digital mobile phones. The hearing aid industry representatives have voiced their concerns regarding this problem and a limited number of aids are currently available that are not susceptible to interference. The level of potential interference can be affected by the distance of the phone from the cellular transmitter; where the phone is close to the transmitter, the likelihood of interference is reduced, but as distance increases so too does the potential for difficulties for the hearing aid wearer situated close to the phone. This is not a major problem for hearing-impaired children, but as the use of mobile phones becomes more widespread the potential risks also increase.

Batteries

Most personal hearing aids for children are powered by disposable batteries, whilst FM systems are usually powered by rechargeable cells. Body worn aids normally use 'penlite' (IEC type LR6, DHS type CP6) batteries, which are manganese-alkali type with a nominal voltage of 1.5v. These are preferable to the carbon-zinc (IEC type R6) batteries, which have an inferior performance over time. Battery life will depend on the power demand of the aid (when a push-pull amplifier is used) and the amount of use made of the aid by the wearer.

Standard size BTE aids use a 'button' type (IEC type PR44, DHS type CP44) zinc-air cell. These are now widely used across the power range for BTE aids since improvements have been made to the casing of the cells. The wider availability of zinc-air and the decline in use of zinc-mercury is particularly important in the paediatric sector as the associated dangers of mercury ingestion can be avoided (Nolan and Tucker, 1981). It is important to seek medical attention if a child swallows any of these cells, although the zinc-air type is less toxic.

Smaller BTE aids commonly worn by children use the miniature button type (IEC type PR48, DHS type CP48) zinc-air cell. The latest range of modular ITE aids and most standard ITEs use the smallest button type (IEC type PR41, DHS type CP41) zinc-air cell. A summary of the types of batteries used for the hearing aids commonly available for children is illustrated in Figure 4.22.

Tamperproof battery drawers may be required for some younger children, and these are available on most commercial aids. On occasion, however, it may be necessary to tape the drawer in its closed position to prevent the child swallowing or losing the battery. If this is necessary, then an aid with a combined battery drawer and on-off switch is not appropriate. Later versions of such aids now have a separate on-off switch.

Most FM radio systems use rechargeable nickel-cadmium 9v cells although dry cells can be used in an emergency. The rechargeable batteries may be in a sealed pack (particularly for Type 1 systems - see later in this chapter), but are more convenient when they are removable from the system housing. Latest versions of Type 2 systems (see later in this chapter) will typically run for one week of classroom use before recharging is necessary. Older systems had batteries which required charging every night. The development of long life lithium cells for FM systems is a particular boon for the classroom management team.

Systems for education

Hearing aids have their limitations and there are some situations in which they function less than optimally. There are several well known enemies of the hearing aid, including background noise, reverberation

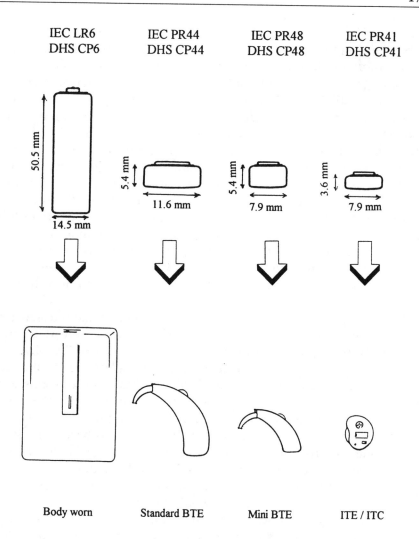

IEC LR6   IEC PR44   IEC PR48   IEC PR41
DHS CP6   DHS CP44   DHS CP48   DHS CP41

50.5 mm

5.4 mm   5.4 mm   3.6 mm

14.5 mm   11.6 mm   7.9 mm   7.9 mm

Body worn   Standard BTE   Mini BTE   ITE / ITC

Figure 4.22 Batteries commonly used for different types of aid

and distance from the sound source. It is the aim of all systems employed in the education of hearing-impaired children to reduce the effects of hostile listening conditions by providing an optimum signal regardless of the environment in which they are used. The options available as systems for education include: FM radio, loop, infrared and hardwire. These will be outlined with an analysis of their relative merits and disadvantages.

Infrared systems

Infrared light can be used in the transmission of acoustic signals and has some advantages over the more commonly used FM radio transmission.

Infrared light has a wavelength shorter than radio but longer than visible light. As the basis for a group hearing aid, infrared transmission found popularity in the late 1970s and 1980s in some special education settings, but is less commonly used now. Two basic types of system have been available for classroom use – one using a teacher-worn infrared transmitter providing a 'mono' signal, the other using hardwired free-standing microphones, angled to provide some localisation cues and a 'stereo' effect, and connected to a fixed infrared transmitter. Additional infrared transmitters can be fitted within the room to ensure an even coverage of optical signal. The signal is received by means of a photoelectric cell on the child's BW receiver. Early studies (Borrild, 1978) reported on the excellent fidelity of the signal, and this was certainly possible when broad frequency response headphones were used. It is possible, however, to use a variety of coupling systems including conventional button receivers and 'solid' style moulds; this configuration provided higher power but restricted the frequency response.

One principal advantage of infrared transmission is that the signal is restricted within the physical boundaries of the classroom, without the problems of over-spill which loop/FM systems introduce. This obviates the difficulties in allocating frequency channels in a large establishment for hearing-impaired children. There will be little or no transmission interference using infrared, but direct sunlight can adversely affect the signal (sunlight includes infrared frequencies which can overwhelm the transmitted infrared signal). Some schools for the deaf have attempted to overcome this problem by using reflective film on large window areas. A major disadvantage of such systems is the fact that infrared cannot be used outdoors. Youngsters who benefit from FM radio transmission on school field trips or similar outings would be unable to use infrared in the same way. Infrared systems available so far for classroom use have remained rather bulky and cumbersome for children to use, whilst the popularity of FM radio has resulted in greater efforts to make systems small, lightweight and cosmetically attractive.

In future this problem will be addressed. Berg (1993) reports that lightweight ear-to-mouth infrared transmitters are being developed with microphone and emitter attached to allow the teacher to transmit the signal to a base station. This in turn is re-transmitted to the class in which the children wear infrared receivers. The receivers pick up the signal, demodulate it and amplify it with final delivery via receivers or hearing aids to the ear.

Comparative studies have examined the relative merits of infrared compared with other systems for education, and the findings indicate that the high fidelity signal provided by infrared transmission is a very positive feature (Markides, Huntington and Kettlety, 1980; Beck and Nance, 1989; Beaulac, Pehringer and Shough, 1989). It is interesting to note in the Markides et al. study how auditory training units still provided the best acoustic signal in terms of the subject's speech discrimination ability under the conditions of different signal to noise ratios. The subject of auditory training units (ATUs) will be covered in more detail later.

FM radio systems

Anyone who has worked in a busy mainstream classroom will be aware of the high levels of background noise generated by routine activity. In general, the younger the class, the higher the noise levels are likely to be. Those working with hearing-impaired children in an outdoor setting will appreciate the ineffectiveness of conventional aids when the parent or teacher is at a distance from the child. Those involved in imparting information to hearing-impaired children in environments where the rooms are large and reverberant will appreciate the difficulties encountered by youngsters in attempting to discriminate speech. There is clear evidence that hearing-impaired listeners have disproportionately greater difficulty discriminating speech in poor listening conditions compared with their hearing peers (Finitzo-Hieber and Tillman, 1978). In summary, the combined effects of hearing loss itself, noise, distance and reverberation can have a devastating effect on the signal reaching the child's personal aids (Boothroyd, 1992). Efforts to combat these problems have resulted in the development of personal FM systems which have probably provided the most effective technological support in the integration of hearing-impaired children into mainstream schools.

The FM system provides a remote microphone worn by the signal deliverer (parent, teacher, friend, etc.) which transmits the required signal by radio waves to a receiver worn by the hearing-impaired child and linked to his personal hearing aids. In this way, the effects of background noise are reduced by the close voice-microphone link at the point of delivery, and the problems of distance up to 50–100 metres are counteracted.

Frequency modulation (FM) transmission involves the conversion of speech or other sound signal into an electrical signal superimposed on an FM radio signal by a microphone in a portable transmitter. Both transmitter and receiver have antennae. The radio signal is picked up by the portable FM receiver worn by the hearing-impaired user. The superimposed transmission is known as the modulated radio signal. A filter is used to select the transmitter frequency from the many other radio signals surrounding the wearer. On reception of the signal there is a corresponding separation of audio signal from radio signal known as demodulation. Finally amplification and connection to a hearing aid/earphone coupling restores the original sound signal and delivers it to the listener.

Principal types of FM system for education

FM systems used in homes and educational settings with hearing-impaired children in the UK fall into two main categories, commonly referred to by teachers and audiologists as Type 1 or Type 2.

Using a Type 1 system, the child's hearing aids and FM system are integrated into one BW unit. The hearing aid part of the system is set by the audiologist to accommodate the configuration and degree of hearing loss with the FM facility switched on or off according to need. Such systems usually have two independent inputs (environmental microphones) and two adjustable outputs with leads to button receivers. The potential market for Type 1 systems is smaller than that for Type 2 systems and this is reflected in the relatively limited choice of systems available.

Type 2 systems are often referred to as personal FM systems and are in much more widespread use. The hearing-impaired listener uses his own personal hearing aids, set and adjusted to suit his hearing loss according to audiologically determined criteria. The FM receiver is linked to the child's own aids either by direct input (a direct lead with audio input shoes connected to the aid) or by neck loop (with a mini loop worn around the neck and the personal aid set to pick up the signal on the telecoil setting). Other options in signal delivery are available, but are less commonly used than those outlined above (for a full description of these options see Thibodeau, 1992 and Berg, 1993). Direct audio input via dedicated leads or shoes provides a high quality replication of the desired signal. The use of a neck loop, however, has certain electro-acoustic disadvantages even though it may be more acceptable to the wearer from a cosmetic point of view. The orientation of the telecoil within the magnetic field of the loop can alter the strength of the signal. Therefore, if the child tilts his head to one side or at an angle to the loop field, there may be weak or dead spots in the signal. This can lead to an intermittent signal being delivered. The low frequency performance of the telecoil signal is generally poorer, and the levels of distortion when measured electro-acoustically are often higher. The new low frequency inductive coupling system described later may provide the answer to these problems.

There has been a significant move away from Type 1 systems over time with many more children now using Type 2 systems (Maxon, Brackett and van den Berg, 1991). The increasing number of hearing-impaired children integrated into mainstream settings has led to the development of less cumbersome and more cosmetically acceptable systems being developed, which can be removed when FM is not required. In addition, technology has been made available which allows more effective direct coupling between personal aids and FM systems. In the UK, the long awaited production of high quality NHS hearing aids with a direct input facility has finally come about, although the range remains limited at present. A summary of the commonly found features available in transmission and reception of the desired signal is outlined below in Figure 4.23.

FM Transmitter, common features and options

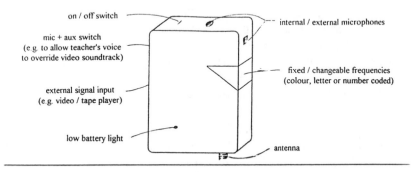

Type 1. FM Receiver, common features and options

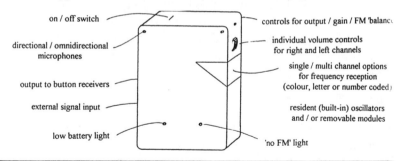

Type 2. FM Receiver, common features and options

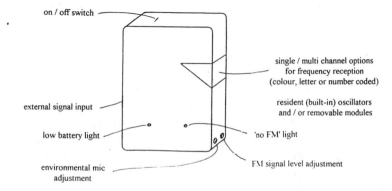

Figure 4.23 FM transmitter and receiver features and options

Radio frequencies

In the UK five primary frequencies are currently allocated for the sole use of FM hearing aid systems, with a further 15 available. Using these secondary frequencies, there is a possibility of some interference from other types of radio transmission system. In the US, most FM transmitters operate on one of 32 available discrete frequency bands between 72 and 76 MHz. An almost universal practice is to code the frequency being used by a colour, a letter or a number. Some manufacturers include both colour and letter coding to allow easy recognition of the carrier frequency. Most systems use either a built-in or a removable oscillator module for the carrier frequency, and in some cases both are used to allow dual frequency operation. There may be occasions when a group of hearing-impaired children within a mainstream setting are together for a joint activity and a common resident frequency is employed. As they return to their individual classes they can switch to the module frequency used by their individual class teacher. Recently, systems have been developed with three switchable frequencies to allow even greater flexibility. These operate on a user-programmable basis so that the teacher or audiologist can pre-select the desired frequencies using a set of binary coded sliding controls. By using frequency synthesis in such systems the need for removable oscillator modules is obviated. Other recent systems have introduced the feature of modules for the transmitter, allowing these to be easily changed and providing more flexibility in educational use.

Transmitter features and options

Type 1 and Type 2 transmitters operate similarly and in most situations (provided the frequency is matched) both will operate with either type of receiver. The transmitter generally has fewer controls than the receiver, and is designed to be simple to operate. There is a main power switch and often a low battery warning light. Some units incorporate the light into the power switch circuit to give the user an idea of the battery condition immediately the transmitter is switched on. Batteries used for FM systems are most commonly the RX22 9V cell, but some are housed in sealed packs that slide on and off the transmitter (or receiver) and require dedicated charging units. A few systems now operate on the smaller 'penlite' battery, allowing the system housing to be slightly more compact. Originally, batteries had to be charged every night after a day's use, but more recently circuitry has been developed which allows rechargeable cells to run for much longer. Many modern FM systems in regular use in schools in the UK only require a single weekly charge. The development of lithium batteries has also led to a much longer use before a battery change is necessary, although lithium cells remain relatively expensive.

Microphones in FM transmitters may be built into the transmitter housing, or in satellite format used high on the chest with the main instrument worn at waist level. The microphone may be directional (enhancing the sound source from the direction in which the microphone is pointing) or it may be omnidirectional (with no specific enhancement of sound from one direction). In some transmitters the antenna is built into the satellite microphone lead. Obviously where a built-in microphone is used, a separate antenna is required. It is extremely useful for the antenna to be of the plug-in type – teachers or parents often trap and damage the hanging aerial in desk drawers, etc., and easy replacement is essential. The transmitter usually has an input socket to allow external sound sources such as a television, radio or cassette player to be adapted. It should be remembered that the impedance of the input has to be matched to the transmitter to prevent overload or distortion; most manufacturers will provide dedicated leads and advice on input matching. In some situations it is desirable to have the teacher's microphone 'live' whilst a separate soundtrack is also being transmitted via the auxiliary input. A few systems operate this way, allowing the teacher's voice automatically to override the auxiliary input signal when he/she talks. This may be a useful feature when teachers wish to comment or expand upon a relevant point in a video or tape recording, for example.

Conference microphones (Figure 4.24) may also be used in conjunction with the FM transmitter via the auxiliary input socket. Using this facility, a hearing-impaired child may take part more easily in small group activity with his hearing peers. Provided the conference microphone is placed on a reflective surface centrally within the group, the wearer of the FM receiver will receive a satisfactory signal. The participants in the group discussion should remain within 3 to 6 feet of the microphone (see Figure 4.25).

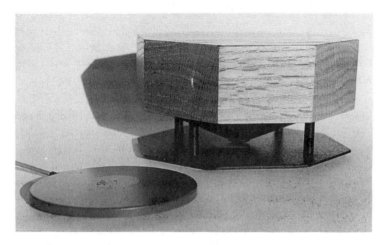

Figure 4.24 Examples of conference microphones

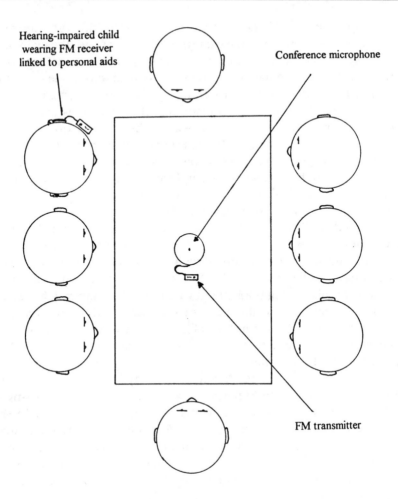

Hearing-impaired child
wearing FM receiver
linked to personal aids

Conference microphone

FM transmitter

Figure 4.25 A conference microphone in classroom use

Receiver features and options

Type 1 receivers commonly house dual frequencies with one on a removable oscillator module. There are individual volume controls for the two channels, and leads with button receivers to be coupled to the child's individual earmoulds. The receivers are available in different specifications to provide a range of frequency responses to suit the hearing loss, and selected in conjunction with the adjustable potentiometers on the aid for tone and output. The FM signal adjustment control is set by the audiologist to provide the optimum signal from the FM transmitter relative to the environmental microphones (procedures for setting this are outlined in Chapter 8). In some situations it may be preferable to mute the environmental microphones and allow the child to focus on the FM signal only. Most Type 1 receivers have the facility to do this. It is also possible to use the receiver simply as a powerful hearing aid by switching off the FM reception. An indicator light (no FM) is often incorporated to give a clear indication to the parent or teacher that the FM signal is not being received. A low battery warning light is a common and useful feature.

Type 2 receivers have fewer controls, since they are FM receivers only and not hearing aids. It is possible to use an external microphone as an input into the receiver, but this is not frequently employed since the child's own hearing aid microphone will usually be 'live' and would pick up environmental sound. However, any child using a neck loop with a personal aid that has no MT setting, will need an external microphone to monitor his own voice (this applies to some of the older model UK NHS aids). Potentiometers for adjustment of the transmitted FM signal and the external input signal are either manually or screwdriver adjusted. Some systems feature an environmental microphone muting/attenuation switch to allow the FM signal to take priority over the child's personal hearing aid microphones. The same specifications for batteries outlined above apply to Type 2 FM receivers. A summary of the different modes of FM reception is outlined in Figure 4.26.

Low battery lights

Although the presence of a low battery warning light on an FM system is desirable, experience has shown that they are not always reliable. The lights have to be visible to the teacher or parent, and the siting of the indicator on the system housing is important. If care is taken to keep the unit hidden beneath clothing or in a purpose designed bag or pouch to meet the parent's or child's wishes for discretion, then equal care should be taken to monitor the system's function. Worn externally on a belt or harness, the battery lights will be clearly visible. Manufacturers usually indicate in their specifications the level at which the low battery light is activated and in some early FM systems this was found to be beyond the point where the system functioned optimally. Recent systems are more reliable in this respect. Parents and teachers should always remember that the low battery light will not function if the cell is completely exhausted, nor will it work if the battery is incorrectly inserted in the housing. Again, some manufacturers have attempted to reduce the margins for error by designing systems that allow correct function regardless of the polarity position of the battery terminal.

New developments in FM systems

A recent addition to the range of FM systems available for the hearing-impaired listener is a new type of receiver which uses digital low frequency inductive coupling. The wearer uses a conventional aid with an audio input shoe to which a small inductive coupler is connected

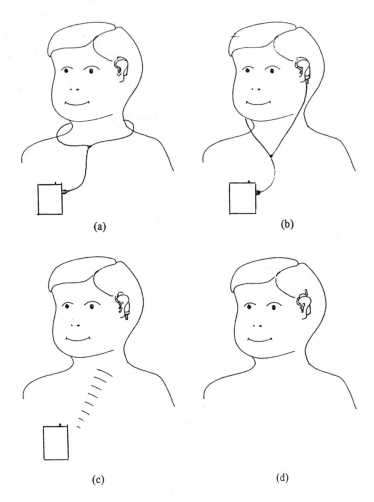

Figure 4.26 Different modes of FM reception; (a) neckloop with personal aids set to T or MT (b) direct audio input (c) digital low frequency inductive coupling (d) BTE FM receiver

(see (c) in Figure 4.26). The single receiver and transmitter unit worn by the child uses a digital processing system to receive the signal from the teacher/parent worn transmitter, then transmit the signal across the short distance from the receiver to the aid. The system is reported to manifest none of the potential disadvantages of the established neckloop systems, giving a received signal equal in quality to direct input.

Recently available in the US, and a possible development in the UK, is a BTE FM system in which the radio receiver is housed within the BTE aid casing. The reception range of the system is approximately 30 metres, and the receiver can be used with any compatible conventional transmitter. It can also function as a stand-alone hearing aid. At the moment, the differences in legislation for authorised FM transmission preclude its use in the UK but development for the US market is well established. A further configuration has been developed and will be available for the UK market, which has the FM receiver housed entirely in the direct input shoe.

Hardwire systems

The rapid increase in the use of personal FM as the primary system for education has been matched by a concomitant decline in the use of hardwire headphone-based auditory training units (Figure 4.27). With more hearing-impaired children integrated into mainstream, the need for discreet and aesthetic systems has grown, although we should be careful not to disregard the considerable merits of the traditional auditory training unit (ATU). The market for hardwire systems remains small and the level of current research and development in the field is limited. However, in some situations the ATU is an ideal hearing aid, providing a high fidelity signal across a wide frequency range whilst maintaining a consistent speaker to microphone distance.

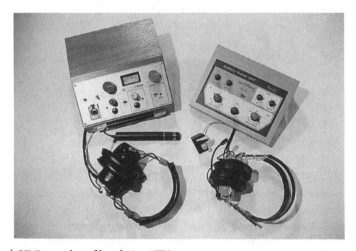

Figure 4.27 Examples of hardwire ATUs

Few studies have examined the relative advantages and disadvantages of systems for education, but Markides, Huntington and Kettlety (1980) highlighted the clear superiority of the ATU compared with FM, infrared and personal hearing aids using various signal to noise ratios. A later study by Flexer et al., (1987) attempted to compare classroom effectiveness of hardwire, FM and personal hearing aids for college students with moderate losses. In this report, the FM unit gave the best overall performance, although the hardwire system used was technically very inferior to the ones available specifically for auditory training use with hearing-impaired children. It has long been recognised that hardwire systems are particularly useful for younger children (Ross, 1981; Hawkins, 1984), but they should not be confined in their use to those in the early stages of language development. The continued use of hardwire systems in many special schools with a reputation for developing intelligible speech in profoundly deaf pupils is testimony to this (Clark, 1989; Shaw, 1995). Modern ATUs have changed little in their outward appearance over the years, but internally make use of the latest silicon chip technology. Teachers who are in a position to influence the purchase of equipment for education should continue to bear in mind the following advantages of a hardwire unit:

* Large circum-aural headphones with wide range speakers provide an excellent quality signal.
* The broad frequency response of the system is superior to that available through earmoulds.
* A boom microphone allows the child consistent monitoring of his own voice while the teacher uses a hand-held or remote microphone.
* Background noise is effectively reduced.
* High levels of gain/output are available.
* The option of FM transmission for the teacher is available to provide mobility.
* When linked together to form a group hearing aid system, the ATU provides excellent child-to-child communication, which is unaffected by the distance between the listener and his peers in the group.

The obvious primary disadvantage is that such units are large and rather inconvenient to use compared with FM systems. With careful classroom management, particularly in unit or special school settings, the hardwire system still has a valuable place. For teachers withdrawing children for one-to-one work from a mainstream class, there may be opportunities to use the ATU. It does seem regrettable, however, that in this, the generation of the Walkman, we still do not have a system which is powerful, high fidelity and yet compact, lightweight and attractive to the young hearing-impaired listener.

Conclusion

Experienced teachers working with severely and profoundly hearing-impaired children will have already witnessed many advances in technology that have benefited the youngsters in their care. The development in hearing aid design and the spin-off in the paediatric market continue apace. In 1993, Lyregaard predicted some trends in technological development that were likely to be available by the end of the decade (Table 4.2).

Table 4.2 Trends in hearing aid technology - Lyregaard, 1993

System	Improvements	New technology
Microphones	75% smaller	Silicon-based
Receivers	25% smaller	
Electronics	500% increase in density	Digital
Batteries	100% increase in capacity	Lithium-based
User controls	200% increase in reliability	Electronic
Adjustment control	50–100 controls	Digital
Earmoulds	5 minutes to make	In situ production

There are clearly uncertainties as to the rate of development of component improvements, but the overall trend indicates a move towards greater miniaturisation and markedly improved reliability. The arrival of smaller digital hearing aids allows greater accuracy in fitting, provided of course that the training of professionals responsible for fitting and management is accordingly updated and effective.

In classroom-based systems, developments may not be so rapid, since the market is so small. However, with personal aids, the potential for amplifying even minimal cues to a young hearing-impaired listener has improved enormously over recent years. If such progress continues alongside the development in implantable devices and with high quality training in aural habilitation techniques, the prospects of children born with a significant hearing loss acquiring intelligible spoken language are brighter than ever.

References

Beasley DS, Mosher NL, Orchik DJ (1976) Use of frequency-shifted/time compressed speech with hearing-impaired children. Audiology 15: 395-406.

Beaulac DA, Pehringer JL, Shough LF (1989) Assistive listening devices: available options. Seminars in Hearing 10(1): 11-30.

Beck LB, Nance GC (1989) Hearing aids, assistive listening devices and telephones; issues to consider. Seminars in Hearing 10(1): 78-89.

Berg FS (1993) Acoustics and Sound Systems in Schools. San Diego, California: Singular Publishing Group. p 132.

Boothroyd A (1992) The FM wireless link: an invisible microphone cable. In Ross M (Ed) FM Auditory Training Systems, Characteristics, Selection and Use. Maryland: York Press.

Boothroyd A, Medwetsky L (1992) Spectral distribution of /s/ and the frequency response of hearing aids. Ear and Hearing 13(3): 150-157.

Borrild K (1978) Classroom acoustics. In Ross M, Giolas T (Eds) Auditory Management of Hearing-Impaired Children. Baltimore: University Park Press.

Branemark PI, Adell R, Breine V (1969) Intraosseous anchorage of dental prostheses; 1. Experimental Studies. Scandinavian Journal of Plastic and Reconstructive Surgery 3: 81-100.

Buerkli-Halevy O (1987) Hard to Fit Clients - Special Fitting Solutions via the use of Response Modifying Tone Hooks (and 1989 revision). Phonak Focus 4. Stafa: Phonak AG.

Carlson EV (1988) An output amplifier whose time has come. Hearing Instruments 39: 10.

Clark MH (1989) Language Through Living for Hearing-Impaired Children. London: Hodder and Stoughton.

Davis-Penn W, Ross M (1993) Paediatric experiences with frequency transposing. Hearing Instruments 44: 26-32.

Dreschler WA (1992) Fitting multichannel compression hearing aids. Audiology 31: 121-131.

Dyrlund O (1988) Some relationships between hearing aid frequency response and speech discrimination of profoundly deaf children. Scandinavian Audiology 17: 201-205.

Dyrlund O, Heningsen LB, Bisgaard N, Jensen JH (1994) Digital feedback suppression (DFS): Characterisation of feedback margin improvements in a DFS instrument. Scandinavian Audiology 23: 135-138.

Erber NP (1973) Body baffle and real ear effects in the selection of hearing aids for children. Journal of Speech and Hearing Disorders 38: 224-231.

Erber NP (1982) Auditory Training. Washington DC: Alexander Graham Bell Association.

Evans PIP (1988) Hearing aid systems in paediatric audiology 0-5 years. In McCormick B (Ed). Paediatric Audiology, 0–5 years. London: Taylor and Francis. p 276.

Finitzo-Hieber T, Tillman T (1978) Room acoustic effects on monosyllabic word discrimination ability for normal and hearing-impaired children. Journal of Speech and Hearing Research 21: 440-458.

Flack L, White R, Tweed J, Gregory DW, Qureshi MY (1995) An investigation into sound attenuation by earmould tubing. British Journal of Audiology 29: 237-245.

Flexer C, Wray D, Black T, Millin J (1987). Amplification devices - evaluating classroom effectiveness for moderately hearing-impaired college students. Volta Review, December: 347-357.

Fortune TW, Preves DA, Woodruff BD (1991) Saturation-induced distortion and its effects on aided LDL. Hearing Instruments 42(37): 40-41.

Foust KO, Gengel RW (1973) Speech Discrimination by sensori-neural hearing-impaired persons using a transposer hearing aid. Scandinavian Audiology 23: 161-170.

Fowler E (1960) Bilateral hearing aids for monaural total deafness; A suggestion for better hearing. Archiver of Otolaryngology 72: 57-58.

Franck B (1991) Low Frequency Emphasis Hearing Aids for Profoundly Deaf Children. Phonak Focus 13. Stafa: Phonak AG.

Geers A, Moog J (1989) Factors predictive of the development of literacy in profoundly hearing-impaired adolescents. Volta Review 91(2): 69-86.

Gustafsson A (1978) Experience with transposer hearing aids. Scandinavian Audiology 8: 48S-53S.

Harford E (1966) Bilateral CROS. Archives of Otolaryngology 84: 426-432.

Harford ER, Fox J (1978) The use of high pass amplification for broad-frequency sensori-neural hearing loss. Audiology 17: 10-26.

Harrison D, Simpson P, Stuart A (1991) The development of written language in a population of hearing-impaired children. Journal of the British Association of Teachers of the Deaf 15(3): 76-85.

Hawkins DB (1984) Comparisons of speech recognition in noise by mildly to moderately hearing-impaired children using hearing aids and FM systems. Journal of Speech and Hearing Disorders 49: 409-418.

Johansson B (1959) A new coding amplifier system for the severely hard of hearing. In Proceedings of the Third International Congress on Acoustics, Stuttgart. pp 655-7.

Killion MC (1980) Problems in the application of broad band hearing aid microphones. In Studebaker, Hochberg GA, Acoustical Factors affecting Hearing Aid Performance. Baltimore MD: University Park Press. pp 149–168.

Killion MC (1981) Earmould options for wide band hearing aids. Journal of Speech and Hearing Disorders 46: 10-20.

Knowles Technical Bulletin TB 21 (1989) EB Directional Hearing Aid Microphone Application Notes. Knowles.

Lewis S (1994) The reading achievements of a group of hearing-impaired school leavers educated within a Natural Aural Approach. Journal of the British Association of Teachers of the Deaf. 20(1): 1-7.

Lyregaard P (1993) Hearing instruments from present to future. Proceedings of the 15th Danavox Symposium, Scanticon, Kolding, Denmark. pp 39-54.

Markides A (1989) The use of individual hearing aids by hearing-impaired children; a long term survey 1977-1987. British Journal of Audiology 23: 123-132.

Markides A, Huntington A, Kettlety A (1980) Comparative speech discrimination abilities of hearing-impaired children achieved through infrared, radio and conventional hearing aids. Journal of the British Association of Teachers of the Deaf 4: 5-14.

Maxon AB, Brackett D, van den Berg SA (1991) Classroom amplification use; a national long term study. Cited in Ross M. FM (1992) Auditory Training Systems, Characteristics, Selection and Use. Timonium, Maryland: York Press.

Moore BCG, Johnson JS, Clark TM, Pluvinage V (1992) Evaluation of a dual-channel full dynamic range compression system for people with sensori-neural hearing loss. Ear and Hearing 13: 349-70.

Nolan M (1983) Acoustic feedback – causes and cures. Journal of the British Association of Teachers of the Deaf 7: 13-17.

Nolan M, Tucker I (1981) Health risks following ingestion of mercury and zinc-air batteries. Scandinavian Audiology 10: 189-191.

Nunley J, Staab W, Steadman J, Wechsler P, Spencer B (1983) A wearable digital hearing aid. The Hearing Journal 36: 29-31.

Punch JL, Beck LB (1986) Relative effects of low frequency amplification on syllable recognition and speech quality. Ear and Hearing 7: 57-62.

Rees R, Velmans M (1993) The effect of frequency transposition on the untrained auditory discrimination of congenitally deaf children. British Journal of Audiology 27: 53-60.

Ross M (1981) Classroom amplification. In Hodgson WR, Skinner RH (Eds) Hearing Aid Assessment and Use in Audiologic Habilitation (2nd Edition). Baltimore, MD: Williams and Wilkins. pp 234-257.

Rothera M (1983) Implants and artificial ears. Talk 131: 20-21.

Shaw A (1995) A new digitally controlled group hearing aid system. Paper presented at the 1995 International Congress on the Education of the Deaf, Tel Aviv, Israel.

Snik AFM, Mylanus EAM, Cremers CWRJ (1995) Bone-anchored hearing aids in patients with sensori-neural hearing loss and persistent otitis externa. Clinical Otolaryngology 20: 31-35.

Staab WJ (1990) Digital/programmable hearing aids: An eye towards the future.

British Journal of Audiology 24: 243-256.

Staab WJ, Lybarger SF (1994) Characteristics and use of hearing aids. In Katz J (Ed) Handbook of Clinical Audiology. Baltimore: Williams and Wilkins.

Stelmachowicz P (1991) Current issues in paediatric amplification. In Stelmachowicz P, Feigin (Eds) Proceedings of the 1991 National Conference. Boys Town: Boys Town National Research Hospital.

Stevenson DS, Proops DW, Wake MJC, Deadman MJ, Worrollo SJ, Hobson JA (1993) Osseointegrated implants in the management of childhood ear abnormalities: The initial Birmingham experience. The Journal of Laryngology and Otology 107: 502-509.

Studebaker GA, Cox RM, Formby C (1980) The effect of environment on the directional performance of headworn hearing aids. In Studebaker GA, Hochberg I (Eds) Acoustical Factors Affecting Hearing Aid Performance. Baltimore: University Park Press.

Sung RJ, Sung GS (1982) Low frequency amplification and speech intelligibility in noise. Hearing Instruments 33: 20-47.

Thibodeau LM (1992) Physical Components and features of FM transmission systems. In Ross M (Ed) FM Auditory Training Systems, Characteristics, Selection and Use. Maryland: York Press.

Valente M, Fabry D, Potts LG (1995) Recognition of Speech in Noise with hearing aids using dual microphones. Phonak Focus 19. Stafa: Phonak AG.

Velmans M (1975) Effects of frequency 'recoding' on the articulation learning of perceptively deaf children. Language and Speech 18: 180-194.

Velmans M, Marcuson M (1983) The acceptability of spectrum-preserving and spectrum-destroying transposition to severely hearing-impaired listeners. British Journal of Audiology 17: 17-26.

Walker G, Dillon H (1982) Compression in hearing aids: an analysis, a review and some recommendations; NAL report No 90. Canberra: Australian Government Publishing Service.

Chapter 5
Earmoulds

R BRETT and A JOSHUA

Photography by R. Brett

Introduction

The earmould, though not the most glamorous part of the hearing aid chain, is of the utmost importance in the system. Despite this importance it remains the bane of teachers' and parents' lives. It is often difficult to fit, and initially it may be the cause of frequent visits to the audiology clinic for re-makes. It can make the ear itch, become sore and may even cause ear infections. Nevertheless it remains the conduit through which the child is able to gain access to a world of speech and language. The hearing aid's strengths and weaknesses rest with the quality of the earmould produced.

The earmould may make the difference between the child's acceptance or rejection of the hearing aid provided. It can alter the child's perception of his own voice in a way that may cause him to discard or accept the hearing aid, and it is likely to be the restraining influence upon the amount of gain that the hearing aid is able to provide for the child. The earmould is responsible, in part, for the frequency characteristics of the hearing aid. It has a profound influence on the overall performance of the hearing aid system at every level and it is, therefore, vital that the best possible earmoulds are always provided for the child and that professionals involved do not accept poor quality of product or service.

This chapter aims to provide the reader with the fundamentals of earmould technology, to review past and present developments, and to outline the impression-making procedure and the manufacturing process. It also aims to consider the types of earmoulds available and their effect on the hearing aid system in terms of frequency response and comfort and quality of sound received from the hearing aid fitted.

History of earmoulds

The history of the earmould is a comparatively short one. It was not until the 1920s that the earmould, as we know it today, came into use. It is a spin-off from the world of dentistry, the aim of both practitioners being to obtain an accurate cast of a part of the human anatomy. Initially this meant using plaster of Paris to take an impression of the mouth or ear. A couple of decades later, as technology advanced, more manageable materials were utilised for this process, notably polyethylmethacrylate.

It should be remembered than in the early days of audiology, only body worn (BW) hearing aids (Figure 5.1) were available. It was the advent of the transistor and much later silicon chip technology, which changed the shape and the size of the hearing aid instrument and led to the possibilities we have today, such as behind the ear (BTE) (Figure 5.2), in the ear (ITE), and completely in the canal (CIC) systems. The potential for the earmould, at this time, was limited because amplifier design was primitive. An earmould was manufactured in order that a receiver, from the BW hearing aid, could be attached to it. This imposed restraints upon the type of material which could be utilised in the earmould manufacture – retainer rings, to hold the receiver, could not be attached to soft materials and there was no expertise available to conjugate hard and soft materials.

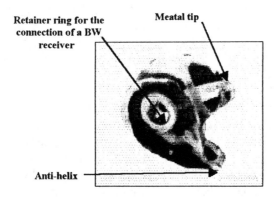

Figure 5.1 Body worn earmould

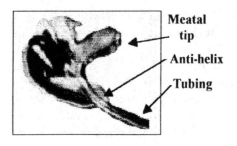

Figure 5.2 BTE earmould

Inevitably the earmould evolved, not initially for cosmetic reasons, but because of its acoustic properties. It was discovered that certain modifications made to the earmould were able to provide the listener with a different experience of sound. When the BTE hearing aid became available, the physical link required between the earmould and the hearing aid brought with it new possibilities for earmould development. This link, between ear and receiver, was no longer an electrical one, i.e., a wire, but a tube. The fact that the length and diameter of a tube alters frequency characteristics was very quickly applied to earmould technology as a means of making further adjustments to the response available from the hearing aid system as a whole. Notable in this history of earmoulds, for these modifications and developments, are Lybarger, Killion and Macrae. Their names remain associated with earmoulds to this day.

A nomenclature for classifying moulds and tubing soon evolved and in 1962 the National Association of Earmould Laboratories (NAEL) laid down a specification for earmould type, tubing size and earmould materials. Table 5.1 shows earmould sizes recommended by NAEL (1979).

Table 5.1 NAEL guide to earmould tubing

NAEL size	Type	Inside diam. (mm)	Outside diam. (mm)
9		3	4.01
12	Standard	2.16	3.18
13	Standard	1.93	2.95
13	Medium	1.93	3.1
13	Thick	1.93	3.3
14	Standard	1.68	2.95
15	Standard	1.5	2.95
16	Standard	1.35	2.95
16	Thin	1.35	2.16
13	Double wall	1.93	3.61
15	Thick wall	1.5	3.56
1/32 in.		0.75	2.39

Earmoulds are available now in a bewildering array of shapes and sizes, but essentially they can be divided into four main categories: solid earmoulds (rarely used today for BW hearing aids – see Figure 5.3), the shell earmould, the skeleton/frame earmoulds, and the open/non-occluding earmoulds. For a typical range of moulds see Figure 5.4.

The solid earmould (Figure 5.4a) is used with BW hearing aids. The earmould fills the concha bowl entirely. The meatal tip extends into the ear canal. A retainer ring is fitted to the body of the earmould in order

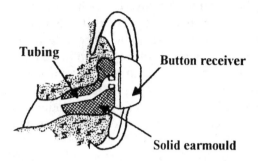

Figure 5.3 Solid earmould with receiver attached

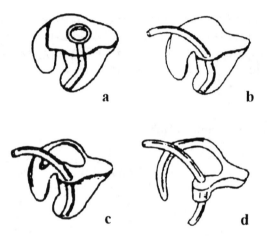

Figure 5.4 Four main types of earmould: (a) the solid earmould, (b) the shell earmould, (c) the skeleton earmould, (d) the open/non-occluding earmould

that a receiver can be clipped on to it to make the link between the hearing aid and the earmould. Like the majority of earmoulds, it locks into the ear with a hook which fits under the anti-helix of the ear. The shell earmould (Figure 5.4b), unlike the previous earmould type, is used with tubing attached to it. This earmould fills the concha bowl and ear canal, forming an hermetic seal. Unlike the shell earmould the skeleton earmould (Figure 5.4c) is essentially a minimum frame which will effectively hold the meatal tip and the tubing in the ear. It is designed primarily with comfort in mind. This type of earmould can prevent the ear from sweating and rubbing. The earmould is limited in its application as, although the meatal tip seals tightly to the wall of the ear canal, the hearing aid is generally less able to make use of high gain output before acoustic feedback occurs. The open/non-occluding earmould

(Figure 5.4d) does not, by design, form an hermetic seal. It is similar in design to the skeleton earmould in that it is a minimum frame. This frame, however, is only required to hold in place a tube which projects into the ear canal. Gain output and frequency range are severely restricted by this type of earmould. It has a specific application; it was originally designed for use with patients having a unilateral hearing loss. Sounds are routed transcranially from the bad to the good ear, via a CROS (contralateral routing of signal) hearing aid, to eliminate a head-shadow effect. The normal or near-normal ear is fitted with an open earmould in order that sounds can continue to enter this ear unimpeded without passing through an amplifier stage. The open earmould is now often used with mild high frequency hearing losses.

In the 1960s a one-stage earmould was developed – i.e., an earmould which is actually the impression. The one-stage process does have the obvious inherent advantage that no further processing is required once the impression is taken. A number of resins were tested. The first was an auto-polymerising acrylic (ADI Plastics, 1967). This material proved to have a number of deficiencies that are well documented in the literature (Bulmer, 1973). The next development was based on a room temperature vulcanised silicone (Tucker et al., 1978). Both these materials had the advantage of maintaining their shape over time whilst being acceptable to hearing aid wearers. In practice, however, it was not possible for the material to support a conventional retainer ring for a body worn hearing aid. The earmoulds also tore easily.

Further attempts were made at developing an 'ideal earmould material'. Tucker et al (1978) developed a composite earmould, consisting of a silicone rubber interior (Silisoft) with an acrylic backplate. A clinical trial was carried out and it was possible to conclude that the composite earmould performed better than all earmould materials hitherto used. Why do we not see this product used today? Unfortunately the effective bonding of silicone to acrylic has not been fully achieved, and the tear resistance of this type of earmould remains unsatisfactory.

Other products have been developed in a number of countries, but unfortunately similar failings to the above apply to these also. These include Insta-Mold (USA) and, more recently, Otozen (Denmark). A soft one-stage material called Otana (Okpojo, 1990) which seeks to overcome these limitations has now been developed and patented.

Impression-taking considerations

All earmoulds, regardless of their type, must take into account the individual shape and size of the child's ear canal and external auditory meatus (EAM) and ear flap (pinna). In order to obtain an earmould which is a comfortable fit and an accurate representation of the dimensions of the child's ear, it is first necessary to take an accurate impression or cast of the ear. This is achieved by investing a material that will set or cure, with the aid of a syringe, into the child's ear canal and concha bowl (Figure 5.5). Before this is done, however, it is important that the EAM is sealed off to ensure that any impression material does not find its way to the eardrum or to the middle ear if there is a perforation. It is possible to seal the EAM off with the aid of a cotton or foam tamp (Figure 5.6). This is positioned in the canal beyond the cartilage/bone junction with the aid of a light-pen. It is important that the resultant earmould, when it returns after manufacture, does not have a tip that goes beyond this junction, or the child will almost certainly experience discomfort, particularly when moving his jaw to talk or eat, unless the tip is tapered. The tamp does have an additional function and that is to ensure that the impression material fills the canal completely and affords an accurate impression.

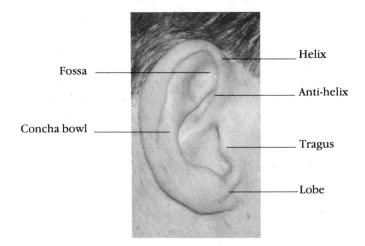

Figure 5.5 The pinna and its landmarks

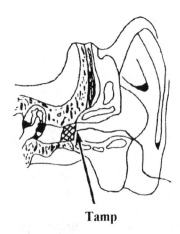

Tamp

Figure 5.6 Location of tamp within EAM

There are certain landmarks that are of importance when an impression is taken, and when an earmould is worn. These are identified in Figure 5.5. It is crucial that the earmould fits snugly into the ear, but without discomfort. A poor seal may result in acoustic feedback – that is, a high-pitched whistling from the hearing aid, due to the output being picked up at the input stage and amplified repeatedly. Feedback will result from the smallest of gaps or irregularities around the periphery of the earmould.

In order to ensure a good fit it is necessary to insert the earmould correctly into the ear. The helix/anti-helix is worthy of a special mention here as this is the part of the ear which locks the earmould in place. It is also the part that the child and parent will find the most difficult to insert correctly into the ear. A good fitting method is to insert the meatal tip of the earmould into the canal first, then to rotate the earmould to place the anti-helix hook under the flap on the pinna. This procedure is difficult, but most parents very quickly get the hang of it. Let us consider the impression-taking process in more detail.

There is some current debate as to which professionals should take ear impressions (Annear, 1995). Although, in an ideal world, this procedure should perhaps only be carried out within the structure of an efficient audiology department, there are many teachers of the deaf (TOD) who find themselves to be the only professionals in a position to provide this service. Many TODs visit children who reside in remote, rural areas, where the parents find it difficult or impossible to meet appointments. The children may have additional needs which make provision within a hospital department woefully inadequate. The TOD will make visits to the home on a regular basis and will know that the well-being of the hearing-impaired child rests with his having good quality earmoulds on a regular basis. This is a professional dilemma.

An impression is needed not only for an earmould, but also for building ear canal hearing instruments, swim plugs, and noise-protection moulds. It is the quality of the impression that determines, to a great extent, the accuracy of the finished product. Besides the choice of suitable impression-taking material and suitable impression-taking tools, the person taking the impression will need to be familiar with the relevant parts of the ear that are involved in impression-taking, and with the actual techniques employed in the process.

Equipment

The following equipment is required (Figure 5.7a):

- box for impression,
- otoscope,
- light-pen,

- tamps/otostops,
- impression material,
- spatula/measuring spoon/mixing slab,
- syringe,
- forceps/tweezers,
- blunt-ended scissors,
- assorted toys!!

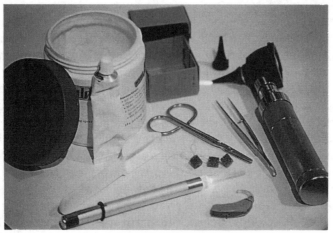

Figure 5.7 a

Impression materials

The range of materials used for impression-taking varies considerably from one country to another and from service to service within countries. For example, in the USA, pre-measured powder-liquid acrylic is widely used, whereas in the UK, bulk silicone-based putty impression material finds widespread application. Each of these materials has limitations, as both have the potential to affect adversely the final product if not used carefully.

Unfortunately, many clinicians are not aware of the limitations of impression-taking materials. However, the results of recent studies (for example, McHugh and Purnish, 1984; Nolan and Combe, 1985) provide basic information on the properties of various impression-taking materials. McHugh and Purnish (1984) investigated the degree to which impression materials retained their shape and size (dimensional stability). They looked at two impression materials: the acrylic powder-liquid (polyethylmethacrylate) and a silicone-based material (polydimethylsiloxane), over time and using three experimental temperatures (optimum – 22 C, cold – 18 C and hot – 38 C). They found that under cold temperature conditions both polyethylmethacrylate and polydimethylsiloxane impressions showed negligible changes in size over a period of one month. However, under optimum temperature conditions, shrinkage occurred in all samples over the experimental period. The acrylic material exhibited a linear shrinkage of 1.86%, whilst the silicone material also shrank, with a slightly lower mean shrinkage of 1.7%. In the hot temperature, McHugh and Purnish found that the silicone material did not show any gross changes, but rather followed the shrinkage pattern exhibited under optimum conditions. On the other hand, the acrylic material underwent gross dimensional change. These findings concur with the contention from some laboratories in the USA that more earmould and ITE hearing aid remakes are required during the summer months, due to the effects of the summer heat (Curren, 1989).

Interestingly, the work of McHugh and Purnish has offered some practical clinical suggestions for the handling and shipping of earmould impressions. These include:

• Never expose a polyethylmethacrylate earmould impression to high heat, such as leaving the impression in the sun, next to a heater in the office or in the car on a hot day (especially on the dashboard).
• If a plus-24-hour time delay is anticipated before mailing the earmould impression, consider storing the impression in the refrigerator.
• A silicone-based impression material is advisable during the summer months to limit possible distortion from heat exposure during shipping.
• A silicone-based material is advisable if dispensing in the 'Sun Belt' states or if mailing impressions to a laboratory located in those states (McHugh and Purnish, 1984; p 15).

Addition and condensation silicones

There are two distinct types of silicone – condensation silicone and addition silicone. It is important that these materials should not be allowed to interact. The platinum catalyst present in the addition silicone will be corrupted in the presence of the condensation silicone hardener. This will result in the addition material not curing properly. Contamination can result through shared syringes or other equipment; therefore two completely separate sets of equipment should be utilised. Condensation silicones are not mixed in a 1:1 ratio. They are generally purchased in the form of a tub of paste and a tube of hardener. Addition silicones are mixed in equal quantities.

A similar study to that of McHugh and Purnish was carried out in the UK. Nolan and Combe (1985) compared selected properties of the two different types of silicone impression-taking materials, condensation (Amsil) and addition-cured (Otoform A/K).

The condensation silicone widely used in the UK for ear impression-taking was criticised on the following grounds:

1 The lack of batch numbers makes it difficult to determine the shelf
   life of the material.
2 Inadequate mixing instructions often lead to poor determination of the
   base:hardener ratio in practice, resulting in poor dimensional stability.

Nolan and Combe, therefore, recommended the use of the addition-
cured (Otoform A/K) impression-taking material as an alternative
because of its minimal shrinkage and perhaps also because of its specified mixing base:hardener ratio, which reduces mixing errors considerably. This choice is further supported by recent clinical data provided by
Parker et al. (1992).

An alternative

In some countries, dental-based impression-taking materials are being
used for audiological application – with little or no empirical data on
their suitability. The choice of impression-taking materials, therefore,
should be given further consideration.

Impression-taking procedure

The procedure below should be followed:

Step 1

Make sure that all the equipment is set out and ready to use. The impression material can be measured out (but obviously should not be mixed
at this stage).

Step 2

The ear should be examined carefully before any impression is
attempted. An impression should not be attempted if :

i)   there is any sign of infection - i.e., the ear canal is wet or fetid,
ii) the eardrum is hyperaemic (red and sore looking),
iii) there is an otitis externa (outer ear infection),
iv) the canal is inflamed or sore,
v)   there are any foreign bodies in the ear,
vi) there is impacted wax, or wax occluding the canal to the position
     where the tamp will be inserted.

In the event of any of the first four situations arising, a referral should
be made to the child's general practitioner and in the event of the last
two, to an ENT department. The ear should not be syringed to remove
wax by a practice nurse or GP, if the eardrum is perforated or a grommet
is in situ.

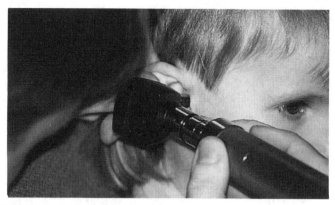

Figure 5.7 b

Step 3

A tamp of an appropriate size should be chosen for the child. It may be necessary, when dealing with a small baby, to trim even the smallest tamps. Care should be taken, if this is done, to ensure that the string remains firmly attached to the tamp so that it is not lost in the ear canal. A tamp may be lost in this way for reasons beyond control, for example, if the child pulls the string when the tamp is in situ. Foam tamps can usually be removed from the ear canal quite easily with a pair of angled forceps, as the surface of the tamp is rough. If this is not possible a referral should be made to an ENT specialist.

With the aid of a light-pen, the tamp should be advanced beyond the second bend, i.e. to the position indicated in Figure 5.6, whilst keeping hold of the string on the tamp to ensure that it sits squarely in the canal. It may be necessary to be quick when doing this as many children and babies object! Often the child will cough with this procedure. The reaction may be more pronounced; he may sneeze, his eyes may run, he may gag or even vomit. This is because Arnold's branch of the vagal

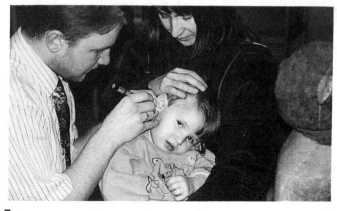

Figure 5.7 c

nerve (Xth cranial) runs close to the surface of the canal and can be very sensitive to tactile stimulation.

If a baby is having the impression taken, he should be sitting on the parent's lap, side-on with head leaning against the parent's chest. One arm should cuddle the infant whilst gently holding down its hand. The other hand should be lightly placed on top of the baby's head in order to prevent a sudden movement. A parent or assistant should try to attract the baby's attention and entertain him whilst the impression is being taken. This is more likely to succeed if it is the parent/partner affording the distraction. At a later age a puppet or other bright toy may be utilised.

If an infant, or a developmentally delayed child of similar developmental age, is having an impression taken, it is advisable to have a large and friendly teddy bear sitting close at hand, together with a spare syringe and tamp. One will find that the infant will often comply after the procedure has been carried out on the bear. To restrain a child physically is a mistake. It will not work! The child will be coming back again, sooner rather than later, and the next time he will be more unhappy, frightened and bigger!

In some instances, if the child is physically handicapped and has no control over head movement, it may be necessary to lay him down with his head on a pillow, whilst the impression is being made. Considerable reassurance and patience may be necessary.

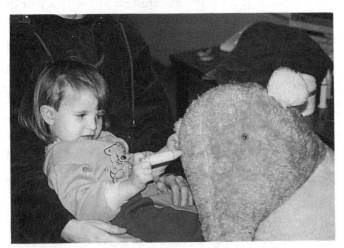

Figure 5.7 d

Step 4

Repeat for the other ear.

Step 5

Mix the impression material, following the manufacturer's instructions. Quantities and materials vary considerably.

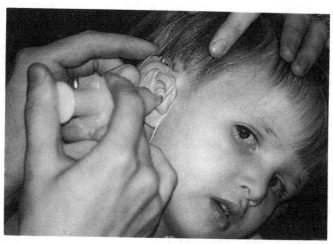

Figure 5.7 e

Step 6

Place the child's hearing aid behind the child's ear (and one behind Teddy's). This is to ensure the correct positioning of the pinna. Very often a BTE hearing aid will move the pinna out slightly. If a hearing aid is not positioned behind the child's ear, a poorly fitting earmould may result.

Step 7

Ensure that the syringe used has a suitably sized tip. These are not easy to acquire. The syringes that are retailed for impression-making generally have tips which are far too broad for babies' ears. A dental syringe can often be better – the tips interchange rather like the nozzles on an icing bag.

Step 8

If the child is aware of the syringe, make sure that he knows that it has no needle before proceeding any further. Fill a syringe for the child, if appropriate, and let him syringe Teddy's ear with your help.

In order to ensure that the impression does not have any holes in it due to trapped air, carefully advance the tip of the nozzle up the ear canal towards the tamp, squeeze the barrel and wait for the impression material to come back over the tip of the syringe. Continue to fill the concha bowl ensuring that the tip of the syringe is at no time allowed to come out of the impression material.

Step 9

Repeat for the other ear.

Step 10

Entertain the child while the impression material cures. Allow the child to check Teddy's ears.

Step 11

The impression can be removed from the ear when a fingernail pressed into the material does not leave a mark. If the impression is being taken from a young baby or a Down's syndrome child, it should be remembered that they have narrow ear canals. It is better to allow the impression material to cure for a longer period since the narrowness of the canal impression can easily be distorted if the material is a little too soft.

Step 12

To remove the impression, peel the top of the pinna back with one hand, and holding the impression between finger and thumb of the other hand, carefully ease it out of the ear. In this way, a partial vacuum will not be created in the ear canal and cause discomfort or damage to the child. Do not be tempted to remove the impression by pulling on the string attached to the tamp!

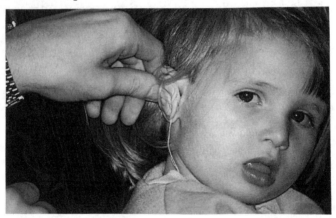

Figure 5.7 f

Step 13

Remember that the tamp cannot be included in the earmould as part of the impression, so if the impression is too short it will be necessary to repeat the whole procedure. If the tip is too long, either cut the impression to the required length, or mark the impression with an indelible marker pen.

Step 14

Remove any wax on the mould.

Step 15

The impression should be placed in a rigid box with a separate box for each ear. The impression must be glued to the base so that the meatal tip does not make contact with any of the surfaces of the box. No other material should be placed around the impression.

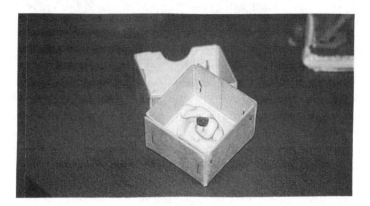

Figure 5.7 g

Step 16

The box should be clearly labelled with the name of the centre, the child's name, the date, 'left' or 'right', the type of mould (number), indication of any special finishes or tubings required on the earmould and the clinician's initials.

Manufacturing process

There are two main approaches to earmould manufacture, the 'one-stage' approach and the 'two-stage' approach.

The one-stage approach

The one-stage or direct approach is rarely used in developed countries. In the direct approach, an impression of the ear is taken in the clinic. The impression is then used as the final earmould. The process is quicker and cheaper, in terms of materials and time, than the two-stage approach. However, in the UK, for example, it has been reported (Evans et al., 1989) that 'instant' earmoulds are used only in situations where the patient is seriously ill, when an earmould is required only for short term use, and in an emergency when an earmould has been lost or damaged.

The direct approach does not require specialised equipment, a laboratory infrastructure, or the expertise needed in the two-stage approach. Indeed, one-stage earmoulds could even be made on school or clinic premises – providing a 'quick remake' service that could be vital for child users of hearing aids. There would, of course, be considerable financial implications for earmould manufacturers if the one-stage process were to be developed and utilised to any significant degree.

A further reason for the demise of the direct approach earmould material is the availability of pre-formed earmoulds, for example, Doc's Promolds and Comply Tips. These are discussed later.

The two-stage approach

In the two-stage approach, an impression of the ear is taken in a clinic as detailed above. The impression is then sent to a specialised laboratory where it is processed. The finished earmould is then returned to the clinic for fitting. This indirect approach requires dedicated, specialised laboratory equipment and technical skills akin to those needed for the fabrication of dentures. In addition, good communication and efficient transportation between the clinic and the laboratory are essential for the success of this approach. At present, the two-stage approach is the most widely used (and most easily abused) method of earmould manufacture.

At the factory

Due to wide variation of techniques used in the making of an earmould by the two-stage approach, it is not feasible to provide step-by-step details here. Instead, a list of the stages in the process is provided, with brief comments on steps that may be considered as potential sources of problems in the fabrication process.

The stages in constructing an earmould are:

1 The impression is numbered and trimmed (if necessary).
2 The impression is then wax-dipped to smooth out irregularities.
3 The impression is invested in a matrix medium to form an inverse mould.
4 The original impression is removed.
5 The cast created in the matrix medium is then used for the manufacture of the final earmould.
6 The earmould material is poured into the cast and processed to the cured state.
7 The earmould is then removed from the matrix medium, drilled, bevelled and polished.

Trimming

It is recommended that the impression is marked with an indelible marker pen or actually trimmed before it is despatched to the laboratory for processing. For a reason known only to the audiologist, the meatal tip may need to be a specific length. The tip length does affect the frequency response of the hearing aid. It may also be useful to mark where the emerging tube is required in the meatal tip.

Wax-dipping

This is a technique whereby the impression is coated with heated wax before the fabrication process begins. The main objective of this technique is to correct flaws in the impression – from either poor impression-taking technique, poor handling of the impression, inherent properties of the impression material (for example, shrinkage), and/or to compensate for dimensional change introduced during drilling, bevelling, and polishing of the finished earmould.

Boothroyd (1965) reported that the thickness of wax layer on an impression is a variable, depending on the temperature of the molten wax, the thermal capacity of the impression, and the length of time for which the impression is left in the wax. These findings therefore indicate the need for the use of a consistent wax-dipping technique, and the importance of accurate temperature control in order to obtain an even coating of wax of the required consistency.

Unfortunately, many manufacturers have no established procedure for wax-dipping, with the result that variability in the uniformity and thickness of wax coating may occur, causing an oversized earmould. Another current challenge to earmould manufacturers is the lack of wax types that are compatible with silicone impression-taking materials (Nolan and Combe, 1985).

Processing

Processing can also have a significant influence on the quality of the finished earmould. For example, poor drilling would affect the acoustic characteristic of the sound passing through the earmould, whilst poor bevelling and polishing could cause the earmould to be undersized or could leave a rough surface, leading to possible problems with feedback, retention of the earmould in the ear, and discomfort for the wearer.

Materials used in earmould manufacture

At present, a wide range of products is used to manufacture earmoulds. These include hard acrylic, soft materials (flexible acrylic, polyvinyl chloride (PVC), silicone), and polyethylene. It has been reported that the choice of earmould material is one of the major factors contributing to inaccuracy in the two-stage approach to earmould manufacture (Nolan and Combe, 1989). It may be that the visible-light curing resins, which have recently become available for audiological application, will prove to be better suited to earmould technology than existing materials.

In order to aid appreciation of the considerations needed in the selection of earmould materials some of the more common materials and reasons for their selection are detailed below.

Hard acrylic

Polyethylmethacrylate ('Lucite') is the most widely used earmould material. It is non-porous and can be buffed to form a very smooth surface. It has been found to be more comfortable to wear in hot weather (Skinner, 1988), is more durable, generally non-allergenic, and can be modified more easily than soft materials. For children with severe or profound hearing losses it may however be inappropriate, since it does have limited gain handling capacity before acoustic feedback occurs.

Soft materials

These materials (for example, flexible acrylic, PVC, silicone) are often used for earmoulds for young children. These materials do have significant advantage over hard acrylic in that their use prevents injury if the ear is banged during play. A further major advantage is that generally a tighter acoustic seal is obtainable. It is therefore possible to achieve high levels of gain in the ear for those children with severe to profound hearing losses. Skinner (1988) believes that this seal is possible because the wearer's body heat causes the material to expand slightly.

There are disadvantages too, however, and most soft earmould materials, as mentioned previously, will not effectively support a lock-spring for body worn hearing aids. Furthermore, PVC tubing discolours and hardens when used with soft materials, and the tubing is then prone to sliding out of the earmould. It has, additionally, been noted that the earmould tubing shrinks and collapses, particularly when used in silicone materials (Evans et al., 1989). Flexible acrylic does shrink sufficiently to cause problems with acoustic feedback, and it becomes sufficiently brittle with time for parts to crack and break off.

If soft materials are used it is therefore important that impressions for new earmoulds are taken on a regular basis.

Polyvinyl chloride (PVC)

Polyvinyl chloride (PVC) is pliable and relatively durable, but limited in that it hardens with age. It is, therefore, necessary to repeat the impression-taking procedure on a more regular basis if this material is used rather than hard acrylic (McHugh and Morgan, 1988).

Polyethylene

Polyethylene ('Polythene') is a semi-hard material and is often used for patients with severe allergy to hard or soft acrylic materials. Polyethylene is considered to be the least durable of all earmould materials (Skinner, 1988). Polyethylene moulds can appear quite obtrusive and are often brightly coloured. It has also been noted that both polyethylene and silicone have less cosmetic appeal than acrylic earmoulds and that they have been shown to be very difficult to modify and re-tube (McHugh and Morgan, 1988).

The development of the one-stage material

There is no doubt that the driving force behind efforts to develop materials for the one-stage approach in earmould manufacture has been the problems of technique and materials inherent in the two-stage approach.

A one-stage material needs to combine some of the qualities of existing impression materials with those of the earmould materials. If we look at some of our requirements, we can see the problems which exist in finding a suitable one-stage earmould material.

It must i) be non-toxic to the ear, ii) have similar handling characteristics to conventional impression materials, iii) be capable of retaining the shape and size of the ear once cured, iv) be durable and resilient in differing environmental conditions, v) be cosmetically acceptable, vi) be comfortable to wear and easy to fit, vii) be capable of handling high acoustic output, viii) be compatible with commercial hearing aids and ix) be readily available.

Dimensional accuracy

It has been demonstrated under laboratory conditions (Nolan and Combe, 1989) that the dimensional accuracy of a range of hard and soft polymeric earmould materials is a function of the choice of material, the processing equipment, the curing cycle, the time elapsing after processing and the choice and storage time of the impression material. These workers also noted that the overall shrinkage of an earmould produced by the two-stage method is approximately equal to the sum of the impression shrinkage plus processing shrinkage. Recent clinical data on the assessment of real ear performance of earmoulds, as a function of material accuracy and flexibility (Parker et al., 1992), have shown that the choice of impression material made a significant difference to earmould performance.

Parker et al. (1992) recommended that where very high gain is required without acoustic feedback, as would be the case for children with a severe to profound hearing impairment, the best strategy to adopt, when using existing, commercially available materials in the two-stage approach, is to use an addition-cured silicone impression-taking material and to prepare the earmould from a flexible, soft, rubber-like material, such as Molloplast B, a modified silicone.

Factors in earmould design

Effects of earmoulds on frequency characteristics of hearing aids

There are several ways in which the response of a hearing aid can be affected by its transmission route – the transmission route of concern here being the earmould and its plumbing. The fidelity of the sound produced in the child's ear should be of a high order – there should be as little as possible added or taken away from the original signal. Why worry about the slight fluctuation in the frequency response caused by the earmould and its plumbing? Bücklein (1962) demonstrated, using normally hearing listeners, that peaks of 10 dB could be identified by all listeners in the 3 kHz range. Interestingly, a 10 dB dip in the response could only by recognised by 10% of the group studied. It is assumed, therefore, that hearing aid users will also be affected by fluctuations in response and perhaps to a keener degree if they are recruiting.

The BTE hearing aid has a very complex transmission route, and this route will introduce distortion to the system at a number of levels. The reverse side of this coin is that, with a BTE hearing aid, there are more possibilities for making adjustments to the frequency response of the system available to the audiologist. A BW hearing aid does not have any plumbing to introduce distortion, but neither does it have the possibility of making adjustments to the frequency response of the hearing aid system at this level. This is the case with CIC hearing aids. With respect to the earmould and tubing alone, the frequency response may be altered at five distinct levels – by venting, damping, horning, adjusting tip length and by the provision of 'special' earmoulds.

Venting

The earmould is available in three distinct types – solid, skeleton and open. Essentially an open earmould is a form of venting. Venting is the action of making or leaving a hole in the earmould so that air can pass to the EAM. The solid and skeleton earmoulds, though not naturally vented, can be modified to take advantage of a vent.

Vents are provided for three main purposes: 1) to ventilate an ear – a child may have repeated infections caused or exacerbated by the sealing off of his outer ear, 2) to reduce low frequency (LF) amplification – to allow LF sound to pass to the ear through the vent and to amplify high frequency (HF) sound (this will also require a suitably set hearing aid) and 3) to improve the quality of sound perceived.

In the first case, ventilating the ear, a hole of 0.5mm may be drilled in the earmould without any significant effect upon the frequency characteristics of the hearing aid within the speech spectrum. This will allow air to pass into the EAM and may prevent problems occurring. A vent of 1mm would be too large and would begin to have an effect upon the frequency response of the hearing aid within the speech range.

In the second case, to reduce LF amplification, a sufficiently large hole will effectively allow LF sounds into the meatus 'normally', i.e., provided that a suitable hearing aid is selected and set, the LF sounds will not be amplified by the hearing aid. A vent can be made in a non-occluding earmould in three ways – parallel, 'Y' or diagonal, or external (Figures 5.8, 5.9 amd 5.10). It is generally considered that the parallel

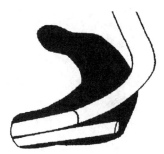

Figure 5.8 Parallel vent

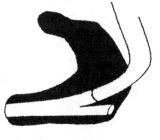

Figure 5.9 'Y' vent

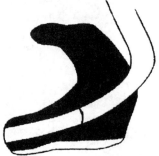

Figure 5.10 External vent

vent provides the most satisfactory solution to allowing LF sound into the EAM naturally. A 'Y' vent is used only when size is a constraining issue within the earmould and it is not possible to provide a parallel vent. It very often poses problems with acoustic feedback, and it does reduce HF sound. The parallel vent does not reduce HF sound but does effectively succeed in reducing LF energy. The third option, the external vent, is a 'V' shape cut into the outside of the earmould. This is a further compromise on the parallel vent and is intended to reduce possible feedback problems that may occur with the parallel vent.

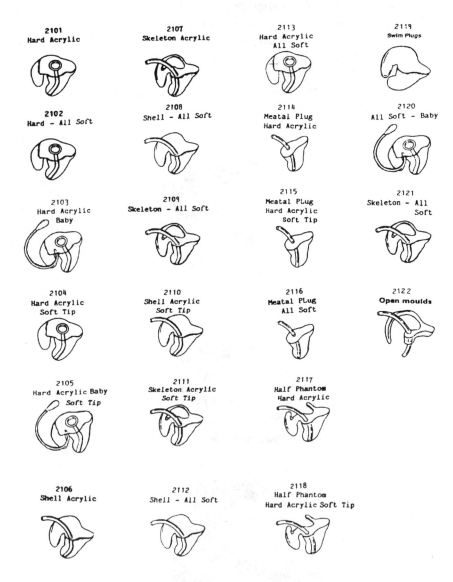

Figure 5.11 Examples of earmoulds – by DHSS code number

If the child has a HF hearing loss and normal hearing in the LF range, a wide vent or non-occluding earmould may be useful. The HF sounds can be amplified by the hearing aid and directed into the meatus in the normal way. Referring to Figure 5.11, note that a 2122 gap earmould consists simply of a frame which holds the tube only in the ear canal. An open earmould will make little difference to the frequency response developed in the EAM above 2 kHz. There may be a small resonant peak around the 3 kHz range. See Figure 5.12 (Lybarger, 1980).

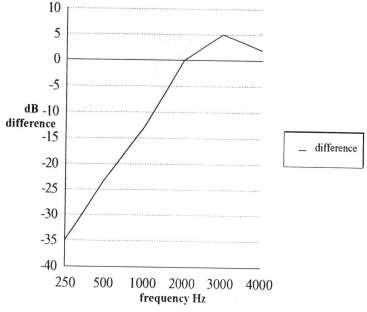

Figure 5.12 Closed vs. open earmould – differences in response with a wide-band receiver

Allowing the low frequencies into the EAM through a vent is not always a solution. There is a limitation on the degree of gain that it is possible to provide with an open mould, since acoustic feedback results beyond a certain point. As a general guide, the author uses the rule that if the hearing loss at 4 kHz is less than 50 dBHL, then it may not be possible to provide sufficient gain without the hearing aid feeding back.

In the third case, namely that of improving the quality of the sound for the user, improvements can sometimes be made to the quality of sound perceived by the user through the introduction of a vent. Users often complain that they are unhappy with the sound of their own voices when they are wearing a hearing aid. This may be caused by LF sounds being made more intense and slightly delayed. Furthermore, the occlusion effect, which causes an apparent increase in loudness for bone conducted sound, results in the user's voice sounding out of balance with other sounds, which are air-conducted. A vent may improve the situation significantly if this is the case.

It is often difficult to establish the exact size of vent required for a child before fitting. With this in mind, earmoulds are available which have adjustable vent sizes. A channel in this earmould allows the fitting of a range of inserts with vents of varying sizes (Figure 5.13). This facility allows the audiologist to choose an appropriate vent for the level of LF attenuation required by the child.

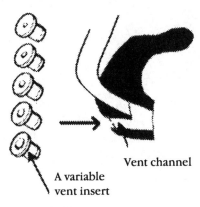

Figure 5.13 Variable vent earmould

The length of the tubing and its diameter both make a considerable difference to the characteristics of the sound received from the hearing aid. The general rules are:

- The longer the tubing, the greater the increase in low frequency sounds (under 750 Hz).
- The shorter the tubing, the greater the increase in HF sounds (above 3 kHz).
- The greater the internal bore of the tubing, the greater the increase in HF sound.
- The narrower the internal bore of the tubing, the greater the decrease in HF sound

Tubing size is specified by number according to the dimensions laid down by the National Association of Earmould Laboratories (NAEL) (see Table 5.1 p. 191). The earmould tubings alone make a clear difference to the overall frequency response.

These different tubings can also be connected together in series to produce special acoustic effects. Perhaps the most notable of the special tubing designs is the Libby horn – named after its developer. The term horn is used in a descriptive capacity, as the tubing is made to increase in diameter along its length. This increase in size is carefully and specifically controlled. The specifications for a 4mm Libby horn are to increase the earmould tubing from 1.93mm internal bore, a standard No.13, to 4.3mm in a 43mm length (Figure 5.14).

The resultant effect of this tubing change is to enhance HF sounds. This is achieved by moving the resonant peak towards the upper end of the frequency response. The Libby horn is able to do this quite successfully. The effective gain can be calculated by the increase in diameters of the tubing. There are disadvantages with these horns, as far as children are concerned; they can be too large and bulky for their ears and they attract moisture.

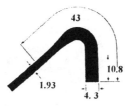

Figure 5.14 The Libby horn

Insertion depth

It is important to obtain the correct insertion depth of the tubing into the ear canal when fitting an earmould. This is particularly important when fitting a vented earmould. When an open earmould is utilised, the degree of gain available in the HF range is governed to a significant degree by the insertion depth of the tubing. The difference between a tube inserted to a

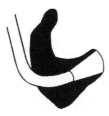

Figure 5.15 Bell canal on earmould

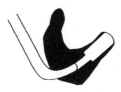

Figure 5.16 Stepped canal on earmould

depth of about 15mm and one barely inserted is some 7 dB at 2 kHz (Lybarger, 1980). Applying a half gain rule, this is equivalent to another 14 dB of hearing loss. In Figure 5.18, the differences between the two depths of insertion are clear. There is an increase from 3 kHz downwards.

Damping

Hearing aid systems do not produce 'smooth' frequency responses. Undesirably peaky signals occur at various points along the frequency

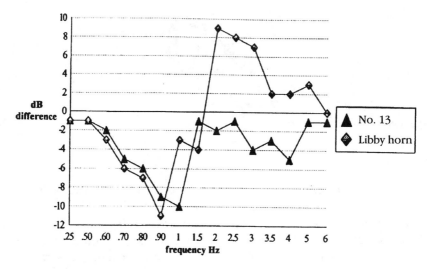

Figure 5.17 Libby horn effect compared to No.13 tubing – both 43mm. Lybarger (1980)

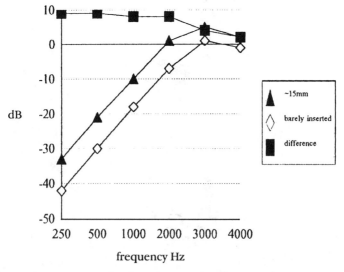

Figure 5.18 Insertion depth – 15mm vs. barely inserted

response (see Figure 5.19). These peaks can be related to receiver-earmould effects. Two main peaks can easily be identified in a response; one corresponds to the receiver diaphragm/reed, and the other to the length and diameter of the earmould tubing. A hearing aid is often purchased with a damper already positioned in the acoustic elbow to damp the known receiver resonance. A damper works by providing a resistive path to sound. If a tube is closed at one end, its fundamental resonant frequency is 1/4 wavelength. If it is closed at both ends then the fundamental frequency is 1/2 wavelength. Smaller resonances will occur at odd and even harmonics of that fundamental frequency. However when a tube terminates in a cavity, such as the ear canal, a further 'reactance resonance' occurs. These resonances are dependent upon the size and shape of the cavity. Energy, which builds up in the tubing, can be dissipated by making the air move backwards and forwards within a damper. Dampers generally take the form of a sintered metal plug or a fine fused plastic mesh, and can easily be seen within the earmould or acoustic elbow. They may sometimes contain an organic material such as cotton, but the disadvantage of this material is that it traps moisture, which can significantly affect its efficiency within the system.

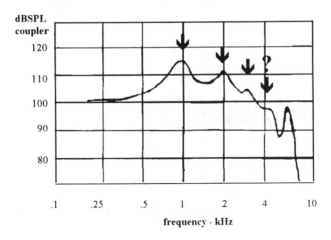

Figure 5.19 An undamped response using a 43mm length of tubing

The mechanical problems caused by the receiver diaphragm are generally dealt with, but the length of the tubing presents problems because there are individual differences in requirement. The earmould tubing creates a peak in the response as it resonates at a frequency that is dependent upon its length and diameter, i.e., a standing wave will be created within the tubing. Whilst making adjustments to the length and the diameter of the tubing has an effect upon the frequency response, it is, in practice, only feasible to make adjustments to the diameter of the tubing, since the tubing length is governed by the size of the child.

Figure 5.19 illustrates the resonant peaks in a 43mm length of No.13 tubing. If the energy creating these peaks is to be dissipated, it is necessary to place a damper at a point along the tubing that corresponds to that of maximum air movement.

This point of maximum air movement occurs at the tip of the earmould. Placing a damper at this position, however, presents problems to the user as it may become blocked with wax or debris. It may also accidentally be removed when the earmould is cleaned, or become so loose as to fall out into the ear canal. In practice, a damper is usually placed 20mm back from the tip. Note the effect in Figure 5.20 of placing a 680 Ohm damper and a 2 kOhm damper at the beginning of the tubing furthest from the meatal tip. The dampers have both succeeded in smoothing out the resonance around 1 kHz, but neither has reduced the 2 kHz peak. The damping effect would have been more pronounced had the filter been placed at the meatal tip end of the tubing. Observe the difference in damping obtained with 680 and 2000 ohm filters. A filter in the range 680 to 1500 ohms is generally sufficient for smoothing the mid frequency range response. Beyond this resistance the overall mid frequency response tends to be reduced too dramatically thereby reducing speech intelligibility.

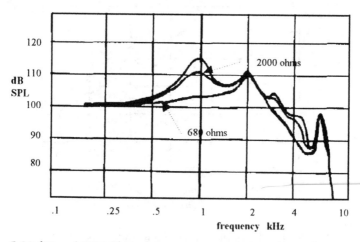

Figure 5.20 680 and 2000 Ohms dampers – top curve is undamped response

The diagram, Figure 5.21, summarises how venting, damping and horning can be used across the speech frequency range. In addition to the above combinations, there is a range of earmoulds worthy of mention, developed by Mead Killion. Killion, through his work in 1970s, brought about a new understanding of earmould design, particularly with reference to insertion gain measurements. He continues to lead the field today with fresh ideas on amplification. His range of earmoulds are referred to by numbers which logically indicate the function of the earmould. Table 5.2 summarises some of the Killion range of earmoulds and their function.

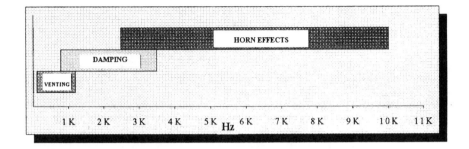

Figure 5.21 Summary of venting, damping and horning

Table 5.2 Some of the Killion range of earmoulds

Earmould number	Function	Response
6R10	Rising HF	Rising HF response 10 dB above 1 kHz to 6 kHz
6R12	Rising HF	Rising HF response 12 dB above 1 kHz to 6 kHz
8CR	Canal resonance compensation	Rising HF response to 8 kHz
6AM	Acoustic modifier	No LF amplification Peak to 6 kHz
6B	Boost	Increases the HF response above 2 kHz
6C	Cut	Decreases the HF response above 2 kHz
6EF	Originally designed to be used with the Knowles EF receiver	The meatal tip end of the mould can be fitted with a range of different sized tubings to size No. 19 (1mm) – these successively cut the HF response when used. Significantly, a 20 dB drop at 5 kHz is obtained between the unmodified No. 9 tubing (3mm) and the No. 19.

Earmould maintenance

A child's earmould should be checked on a daily basis to ensure that it is not split, sharp, cracked, dirty or blocked. The child should be made to be responsible for his own earmould maintenance and hygiene from an early age. When a hearing aid is prescribed, a 'kit' should be given to the child/parent in order that they can maintain the hearing aid system effectively. The kit might include the following:

- information sheet *re* hearing loss
- contact numbers and addreses — local and national
- pack of batteries
- battery book (for obtaining future supplies)
- instructions on how to use hearing aid including battery locks if used
- screwdriver for battery locks — if required
- stetoclip
- puffer
- spare tubing
- threader
- pipe cleaners
- small brush/tooth brush

The last six items are of importance for the maintenance of the earmould. It should now be clear how important the earmould is in the hearing aid chain. It is therefore paramount that the earmould is kept in good working order. The child should be shown how to use the puffer and how to clean his earmoulds, as well as how to put them in and take them out independently. It should become part of the morning and bedtime routine. The earmould is best washed at night times as it then has time to dry thoroughly before being used again in the morning. When the child cleans his teeth at night he should, by habit, clean his earmoulds.

A brush is very useful for cleaning earmoulds, particularly hard earmoulds, otherwise plain soapy water and a wipe will suffice. Children who are prone to ear infections can leave their earmoulds in a sterilising solution — the type used for sterilising babies' bottles and teats. These children should have hard earmoulds. If this procedure is followed it should be noted that the earmoulds may not last as long as they would otherwise, and they will need to be re-tubed on a more regular basis.

Water and debris can be removed from the earmould tubing with a pipe cleaner provided there are no dampers in-line. Alternatively a puffer/air-blower can be attached to the tubing and air blown through. The puffer is also a good way of checking that the tubing is not blocked or split at any point. One of the most common reasons for the hearing aid system not functioning properly is that the earmould and/or its plumbing are damaged or worn. There may be a build-up of wax in the tubing which has occluded the tube, or the tubing may be twisted or collapsed. There might be condensation in the tubing blocking the sound intermittently. Alternatively, the tubing may be split and the sound escaping, giving rise to acoustic feedback. These problems can be identified simply with the aid of a puffer.

Below is a check-list to help identify any problems with the earmould and what to do if any are found.

Earmould maintenance flowchart

1. REMOVE THE HEARING AID FROM THE CHILD'S EAR
2. DETACH THE EARMOULD FROM THE HEARING AID
3. IS THE CHILD COMPLAINING ABOUT THE EARMOULD?
   N ↓ Y → 15
4. LOOK CAREFULLY AT THE EARMOULD
5. IS THE EARMOULD SHARP, SPLIT OR DAMAGED?
   N ↓ Y → 22
6. SWITCH THE HEARING AID ON & TURN THE VOLUME FULL UP UNTIL THE HEARING AID WHISTLES
7. ATTACH THE EARMOULD TO THE HEARING AID
8. DOES THE HEARING AID STOP WHISTLING?
   N ↓ Y → 26
9. DOES THE HEARING AID STOP WHISTLING WHEN THE EARMOULD TIP IS COVERED WITH A FINGER?
   Y ↓ N → 38
10. LISTEN TO THE HEARING AID AT A COMFORTABLE LEVEL, WITH THE AID OF A STETOCLIP, THROUGH THE EARMOULD (STETOCLIPS CAN BE PURCHASED WITH ATTENUATORS FOR LISTENING TO THE CHILD'S HEARING AID AT USER SETTING)
11. IS THE SOUND QUALITY GOOD?
    Y ↓ N → 24
12. IS THE EARMOULD CLEAN & DRY?
    Y ↓ N → 34
13. IS THE EARMOULD WHISTLING WHEN WORN AT THE APPROPRIATE USER SETTINGS FITTED TO THE CHILD?
    N ↓ Y → 32
14. END
15. IS THE EARMOULD INSERTED PROPERLY?
    N ↓ Y → 17
16. INSERT PROPERLY
    → 3
17. IS THE TIP TOO LONG? (DOES IT EXTEND BEYOND THE SECOND BEND OR IS THE CHILD SAYING IT HURTS DOWN HIS EAR CANAL?)
    N ↓ Y → 21
18. IS THE EAR VISIBLY SORE?
    Y → 36 N → 22
19. ADVISE THE CHILD/TEACHER/PARENT TO LEAVE THE EARMOULD OUT & TO REFER TO GP VIA PARENT
20. END
21. IS IT A SOFT EARMOULD?
    N ↓ Y → 41
22. ARRANGE FOR NEW IMPRESSIONS TO BE MADE
23. END

24. IS ANY SOUND PRESENT?
    N ↓ Y → 42
25. CHECK THE HEARING AID
26. REMOVE THE EARMOULD FROM THE HEARING AID
27. CAN YOU BLOW AIR THROUGH THE TUBING WITH THE PUFFER?
    N ↓ Y → 42
28. TRY TO CLEAR ANY BLOCKAGE WITH THE PUFFER OR A PIPE
    CLEANER—BEWARE OF ANY FILTERS/DAMPERS WHICH MAY BE
    DELIBERATELY IN THE PLUMBING
29. CAN YOU BLOW AIR THROUGH THE TUBING WITH THE PUFFER?
    N ↓ Y → 6
30. IS THE EARMOULD TUBING TWISTED?
    Y ↓ N ↓
31. RE-TUBE THE EARMOULD USING THE SAME TYPE AND SIZE OF
    TUBING
    → 6
32. IS THE EARMOULD FITTED PROPERLY?
    N ↓ Y → 22
33. FIT THE EARMOULD PROPERLY
    → 32
34. CLEAN THE EARMOULD WITH AN ULTRA–SONIC
    CLEANER/BRUSH/ALCOHOLIC WIPE/PIPE CLEANER
35. DRY EARMOULD THOROUGHLY
    → 13
36. ADVISE THE CHILD/TEACHER/PARENT TO LEAVE THE HEARING
    AID OUT
37. END
38. RE-TUBE THE EARMOULD
39. DOES THE HEARING AID STOP WHISTLING NOW WHEN THE
    EARMOULD TIP IS COVERED WITH A FINGER?
    Y → 10 N → 49
40. END
41. TRIM THE TIP OF THE EARMOULD—A LITTLE—VERY CAREFULLY
    → 3
42. IS THERE ANY CONDENSATION IN THE EARMOULD TUBING?
    Y ↓ N → 44
43. USE THE PUFFER TO CLEAR THE TUBING
    → 11
44. IS THE TUBING TWISTED?
    N ↓ Y → 47
45. IS THE TUBING BLOCKED?
    N ↓ Y → 48
46. THERE IS MOST PROBABLY A HEARING AID FAULT
    → 6
47. RE–TUBE THE EARMOULD
    → 10

48. TRY TO UNBLOCK THE EARMOULD TUBING— BEWARE OF ANY
    FILTERS/DAMPERS WHICH MAY BE DELIBERATELY IN–LINE
49. IS THE TUBING CLEAR?
    Y → 10 N → 47
50. THERE MAY BE A FAULT WITH THE HEARING AID—PROBABLY
    THE ACOUSTIC ELBOW/RECEIVER
51. END

It is suggested, at certain points in the flowchart, that the earmoulds
should be re-tubed. This is an easy process which can be learned by
anyone. A number of items from the 'kit' are required. In order to re-
tube an earmould one will require

- earmould tubing — of the same size as that already in the earmould.
  The child should have been provided with this. Look carefully as the
  tubing may be different for each ear.
- a tubing threader
- a scalpel/hobby knife
- possibly a reamer
- possibly earmould glue.

Re-tubing an earmould

1. Remove the old tubing from the earmould. If the old tubing has
   been glued in place it may be necessary to pull this out with pliers or
   forceps and then to use a reamer to clean out the channel. The use
   of a reamer is not usually necessary for soft earmoulds. If a reamer is
   used care should be taken not to alter the diameter of the channel
   through the earmould.
2. Clean the earmould. This can be done with soap and water, with an
   alcoholic wipe or with a proprietary spray or wipe. The latter are
   advertised as being unscented, disinfecting and quick drying. They
   are useful, not essential and quite expensive for a Service to
   purchase. If the earmould is wet inside the channelling, it is possible
   to dry it out by carefully pulling through a dry pipe cleaner.
3. Insert the nylon hoop of the tubing threader through the earmould,
   starting at the meatal tip.
4. Ensure that the new tubing is of the correct size and type. It should
   be provided specifically for the child by the audiologist. It should
   preferably be pre-bent tubing.
5. Place the end of the earmould tubing under the loop of the
   threader. It is best if the tubing has been cut at an angle. If it has not,
   cut it at an angle with a scalpel or hobby knife.
6. Determine the angle required for the tubing and position it under
   the threader loop in this position. It will not be possible to twist the
   tube once it is inserted through the earmould.

7. Carefully pull the tubing through the earmould holding the meatal tip stationary, with respect to the body of the earmould, as the meatal tips on soft earmoulds easily split and tear away.

8. Stop when the tubing is at the correct position. If the tubing is pre-bent this is easy to determine as the tubing will stand up at > 90° with respect to the back of the earmould.

9. Place the excess tubing at the meatal end of the earmould on a table top, place thumb on top and stretch the tubing. With a scalpel or sharp blade cut the tubing close to the meatal tip of the earmould. Once the tubing is cut, the end of the tubing should spring back into the earmould. Tubing should never be allowed to protrude beyond the end of the earmould tip.

10. Check that the air-way through the earmould is unobstructed by blowing air through with a puffer.

11. Position the hearing aid, minus the earmould, behind the ear. Insert the earmould. Cut the tubing to the desired length. If the tubing is left too long it may twist or collapse and thus prevent sound from reaching the ear. If the tubing is cut too short then the hearing aid will not sit comfortably behind the ear. If you are not sure cut a little off first and then try again!

Problems with earmoulds

Earmould does not fit

- problem at manufacturing stage
- problems due to no tamp/syringe used
- tamp is positioned incorrectly
- problems with transportation and communication
- hearing aid not positioned post aurally during impression taking
- impression material not hardened before removal
- other reasons for poor impression
- earmould inserted incorrectly

Problems with feedback

- earmould is a poor fit due to one of the problems above
- meatal tip is too short
- earmould inserted incorrectly
- venting is inappropriate
- wrong type of earmould
- impacted wax
- a convoluted ear canal/sound outlet positioned incorrectly
- tubing split or wall too thin

Problem with comfort

- earmould is a poor fit, as previously listed
- earmould is not in the ear properly
- meatal tip is too long
- grommet/grommet wire is in the canal
- requires a comfort vent
- earmould dirty
- wrong type of earmould

Earmould does not fit

Problem at the manufacturing stage

A non–fitting earmould can be the result of the manufacturing process. A good quality impression may have been provided and received by the laboratory but a poor quality earmould produced. Generally this is a result of the wax dipping and finishing stages, where the earmould may become over or under sized. Most earmould laboratories return the ear impression together with the earmould. Compare the two for obvious differences and obtain a complimentary re–make if they differ significantly.

Problems due to no tamp/syringe used

Usually the poorly fitting earmould is a result of a poor impression. A survey of earmould provision in the UK (Evans et al., 1989) took the form of a questionnaire, directed to earmould manufacturers, hospital services, educational services, and hearing aid users. The survey provided information on various procedures for ear impression–taking, for example, for hospital services. Only 73% of the centres included in the survey always tamped the ear before investing material and an additional 21% sometimes did. In 6% of cases no tamp was employed.

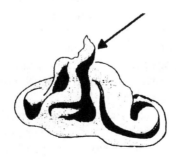

Figure 5.22 Poorly formed meatal tip — no syringe used

Additionally, 81% of the centres included in the survey reported that a syringe was always used to invest material into the ear, a further 13% used a syringe sometimes and 6% of centres did not use a syringe at all, stating the material was invested manually.

Tamp positioned incorrectly

Even when impression-taking procedures are well defined, other sources of error in the process may be traced to poor skills on the part of the impression-taker. For example, the recommended position for the tamp is just beyond the boundary of the cartilaginous and bony sections of the meatus (Brooks and Nolan, 1984), two-thirds of the way down the meatus or beyond the 'second bend'. However, in practice this position seems difficult to locate, especially if one is not very familiar with the anatomy of the relevant part of the ear. As a result, ear impressions with either too short or too long tips are produced. A long tip is not a problem for the earmould manufacturer as it can be trimmed back but a tip which is too short cannot be built up.

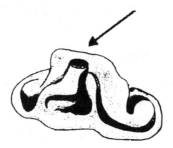

Figure 5.23 Meatal tip too short

Problems with transportation and communication

If the two-stage approach is used, the impression needs to be transported safely to a specialised earmould laboratory. Often these laboratories are only to be found in large, city areas and the transportation of the ear impression from the clinic to the laboratory constitutes a very weak link in the two-stage approach to earmould manufacture. Recent investigations into earmould provision in the UK (for example, NDCS, 1985; Evans et al., 1989) have reported dissatisfaction with the arrangements and have highlighted some consequences of sending impressions away for earmould manufacture. These include: i) poor packaging of impression, causing damage to it; ii) loss of the impression in transit, leading to unforeseen delay in the entire manufacturing process; iii) extended delays for the earmould wearer.

Other problems include: impressions being sent away with inadequate paperwork (e.g., omitting details of style of the earmould and the materials to be used). In addition, whilst some clinics specify the type of earmould required, others do not; some trim or mark impressions before despatch, others do not. In general, therefore, the clinic–manufacturer communications are far from satisfactory at present and this does not facilitate the effective provision of earmoulds for hearing aid users.

Hearing aid not positioned post-aurally during impression taking

An easily resolvable source of error in the impression-taking procedure is that of not positioning the post-aural hearing aid behind the ear before taking the impression. This may result in a poorly fitting earmould since a post-aural hearing aid can significantly alter the whole positioning of the pinna and its associated anatomy. The pinna may undergo a significant lateral displacement when a post-aural hearing aid is in position. The result will be that the impression, although an accurate representation of the un-aided ear, will be the wrong shape when the hearing aid is fitted.

Impression material not hardened before removal

If the impression material is not allowed to harden sufficiently before it is removed from the meatus then it is very unlikely that a well-fitting earmould will result. The impression must be allowed to cure completely before removal. This may prove to be a very trying time during the impression-making procedure, as a child will probably need considerable distraction in order to persuade him to keep his hands away from the impression. It is vital that the impression material sets totally.

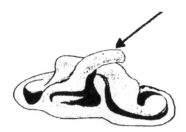

Figure 5.24 Earmould with deformed meatal tip

Other reasons for poor impressions

Earmould laboratories criticise impressions forwarded to their laboratories on the following additional grounds (Sneyd 1985):

i) pieces of impression material are often added onto an impression once the syringe has been emptied into the ear canal. These pieces later break off in the processing;

ii) the concha bowl is often not filled entirely, giving the laboratory no idea of the depth of the earmould required;

iii) 'walnut whip' earmoulds are often received.
These are impressions which result from allowing the syringe to drift randomly in the ear. The resulting impression contains gaps and inadequately represents the shape of the ear;

iv) often impressions are trimmed back too far along the meatal tip.

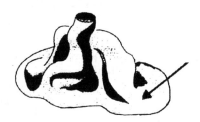

Figure 5.25 Earmould with no anti–helix

Earmould not inserted correctly

A hearing aid will whistle if the earmould is not inserted correctly in the ear. It is important that the anti-helix/helix portion of the earmould is 'locked' into place and that the earmould is flush in the concha bowl. Children, when they are first learning to insert their earmould, often do not manage to lock the earmould in place under the anti-helix. This not only gives rise to acoustic feedback and sore ears but may tempt a teacher to turn down the volume of the hearing aid.

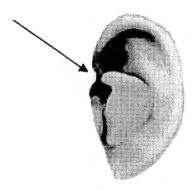

Figure 5.26 Earmould not fitted properly

Earmould inserted incorrectly

See section **Earmould does not fit**

Problems with feedback

Earmould is a poor fit due to one of the problems above

Acoustic feedback can, of course, result from a poorly fitting earmould due to any of the above factors since feedback occurs when there is an air-gap at some point around the earmould. The usual causes for feedback are as follows.

Meatal tip is too short

If the meatal tip is too short it is almost invariably a direct result of poor impression. Either the tamp has not been positioned correctly, no tamp has been used or the meatal tip has been trimmed too short before dispatching to the laboratory.

If a soft earmould is required for the child it is invariably best to err on the side of caution when taking the impression, that is, take an over-long impression rather than one too short. A soft earmould tip can easily be trimmed back, without giving rise to any discomfort problems, when it arrives back from the earmould laboratory. To shorten a tip on a hard earmould requires specialist grinding and buffing wheels and is not recommended without appropriate machinery.

Venting is inappropriate

Feedback will occur if the earmould has a vent and the child is using the hearing aid at a volume in excess of that prescribed. A correct volume for the child should be established. If the child's hearing loss as indicated on a pure-tone audiogram is ~50dBHL or greater at 4KHz then venting may not be appropriate. If a child consistently turns the volume up on his hearing aid then a further hearing test should be arranged.

Wrong type of earmould

If the child has an open earmould/non-occluding earmould and the loss at 4kHz, as indicated on a pure-tone audiogram is ~50dBHL or greater, then this type of earmould may not be appropriate. The open earmould may cause the hearing aid to whistle. Similarly if the child turns the volume control beyond the position required then feedback may also result. If a child consistently turns up the volume on his hearing aid then a further hearing test should be arranged.

Impacted wax

Impacted wax can cause acoustic feedback. Normally, sound is directed towards the eardrum which, if compliant, absorbs the sound. If the sound is made to strike the hard wax within the EAM, it may rebound back and cause feedback. The solution to the problem is to have an ENT consultant remove the wax. This may need to be done on a fairly regular basis for some children and it is therefore important that a good working relationship is established with the local ENT department. The removal of ear wax should not be performed via syringing. A consultant will hook out the wax.

A convoluted ear canal/sound outlet positioned incorrectly

If the sound outlet at the tip of the earmould is made to point other than towards the eardrum a similar situation to one of impacted wax can result. Sound is made to hit the ear canal wall, to rebound off it and give rise to acoustic feedback. Where there is an unusually convoluted EAM the position of the tubing on the tip of the earmound impression should be clearly marked before dispatching to the earmould laboratory. A solution to the problem may be to flare the meatal tip of the earmould so that the sound is not directed at an adjacent wall.

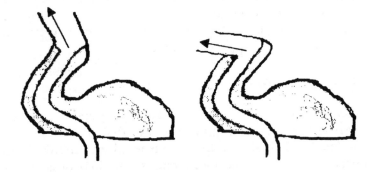

Figure 5.27 Flaring of meatal tip to alter direction of the sound pressure

Tubing split or wall too thin

Acoustic feedback will occur if the tubing is split as sound will leak out through the hole. Less obvious is that if the wall of the earmould tubing is too thin sound may also leak out and result in acoustic feedback. This will be a potential problem where high output is required from a hearing aid.

Problem with Comfort

Earmould is a poor fit as previously listed

Discomfort can arise because the earmould is simply a poor fit due to reasons aforementioned. This may cause rubbing in the canal or concha bowl or under the anti-helix. It is possible to mark the area giving rise to discomfort with an indelible marker and arrange for it and the impression to be returned to the manufacturer for a re-make. If it is a soft earmould a re-make will be necessary. If it is a hard earmould it will be ground down. The manufacturers will ensure that if an earmould is ground down it is buffed up again until completely smooth. These modifications should not be made 'in-house' unless the appropriate equipment and expertise are available. This equipment includes diamond cutters, polishing stones and mops, polishing powders and assorted drills and burrs.

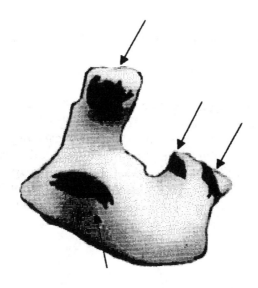

Figure 5.28 Problem with earmould comfort

Earmould not inserted correctly see p. 226.

Meatal tip is too long

If the meatal tip is too long on an earmould, it can cause considerable discomfort to the child, caused by the tip length extending beyond the cartilaginous region of the EAM. When jaw movement takes place, the EAM changes in shape and volume causing the earmould to move and rub. This is because the condyle of the temporal mandibular (the end of the jaw bone) joint lies inferior to this region. It has been reported that the anterior movement of the condyloid process of the mandible during speech can be as much as 14.4mm with vertical movement of up to 4.2mm. This movement is greater during mastication (Edwards and Harris, 1990).

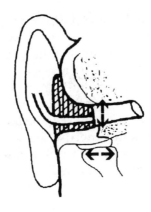

Figure 5.29 Jaw movement and earmould fit

Grommet/grommet wire in canal

If a child has undergone middle ear surgery and had grommets inserted there can be problems with the wearing of an earmould. Some grommets have wires attached to them, for ease of removal. These lie along the EAM. The wire, as the grommet extrudes, can make contact with the earmould and in turn push the grommet against the eardrum, thus causing considerable discomfort. Here, too, it is useful to have good relations with the local ENT consultants as it is possible for them to insert grommets without wires attached, if asked.

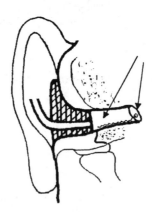

Figure 5.30 Problems with grommets

Comfort vents

An older child, who has had some auditory experience pre-hearing aid, may reject the aid on the basis that it makes his own voice sound strange. Usually the voice is made to sound louder and slightly delayed. This can be a result of occluding the ear canal. A simple remedy is to vent the earmould. A comfort vent of 0.5mm should be used. This will not affect the frequency response of the hearing aid within the speech frequency range.

Earmould dirty

A build-up of wax and grease on the earmould can result in an uncomfortable fit. It may also result in acoustic feedback. Earmoulds should be cleaned on a daily basis.

Wrong type of mould

Children can develop or have allergies to foreign materials which come into contact with their body. This includes earmould material and the hearing aid plastics and plasticisers. If allergy is suspected, a referral should be made, via the GP, for testing. Testing can be done through the application of scrapings, under a patch, of the suspected material to a sensitive part of the body—usually the inside surface of the arm, or a shoulder. The area under the patch will become swollen or red by the next day if there is a problem.

There is a range of non-allergenic earmould materials available which are relatively inert. The most popular of these is Molloplast. In extreme cases, where the wearing of a hearing aid is impossible on a long term basis due to allergy, a gold coated earmould may solve the problem.

In addition to allergies to earmould material, children can develop an otitis externa, an infection in the ear canal, due to the permanence of an earmould. The earmould precipitates the infection by causing the ear canal to get hot and moist. It may have a rough surface. These factors can give rise to infection. In these cases, acoustics permitting, it is sensible to try a smaller earmould or venting. A canal earmould or skeleton earmould will reduce the surface area covered by the earmould and allow air to pass freely over more of the canal and concha bowl. Venting the earmould will allow air into the canal and promote a more healthy environment. In chronic cases, after unsuccessful medical intervention, the gold coated earmould can be a solution to this problem since it has an extremely smooth surface, is inert and is cooling to the ear. Additionally it is advisable, where children are prone to this type of problem, that they wear ear plugs when swimming.

Other useful developments in earmould technology

There have been some new developments in recent years in terms of hardware available for the impression–taking procedure, short term earmould solutions, recommendations for combinations of materials to be used for special earmould fittings, and the development of a new one-stage impression material.

Pro-molds

Pro-molds are temporary earmoulds made from soft, clear hypoallergenic Kraton. They are available in six sizes from tiny to extra large (Figure 5.31). They are useful in the clinical setting for hearing aid trial or as a temporary measure when a child loses or damages his earmould. They are not designed to be used long term with a child. Pro-molds can be used with BE hearing aids, with conventional tubing, or BW hearing aids with a receiver adapter unit which attaches to the earmould tubing and fits behind the ear. They have limitations. Some regular hearing aid users comment that they do not like the feel of these earmoulds. They can be customised to a limited extent. Venting can be achieved through inserting No.13 tubing a short distance (1–2mm) into the channelling on the Pro–molds thereby providing a stepped horn. The earmould material, Kraton, has a good 'memory' for shape and contour of the individual concha bowl and it is possible to obtain a seal suitable for use with a severe to profound hearing loss. The manufacturers state that these earmoulds will fit 95% of ears.

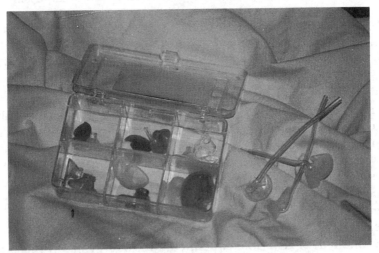

Figure 5.31 Pro-molds

Foam inserts

Foam inserts consists of earmould tubing, pre–bent or with a right–angled elbow, attached to an expanding foam insert. They are similar to foam inserts used on the probe tips of otoacoustic emission machines or, as noise attenuators. Whilst the foam inserts do not provide an alternative for an earmould, they may be useful in cases where no earmould is available for a child and where he would otherwise be without amplification. They have obvious limitations as they become dirty very quickly and cannot be cleaned successfully. They may not provide a sufficient acoustic seal for a high gain hearing aid and they do provide a 'horn' effect which may be either advantageous or disadvantageous.

Two-cartridge injection gun

Two-cartridge injection guns are now available for impression-taking purposes (Figure 5.32). The impression gun loads with a dual cartridge, filled with impression base, polyvinyl siloxane and a platinum hardener. When a trigger is squeezed the two materials from the cartridges 'spiral' together and mix prior to being ejected through a disposable canula.

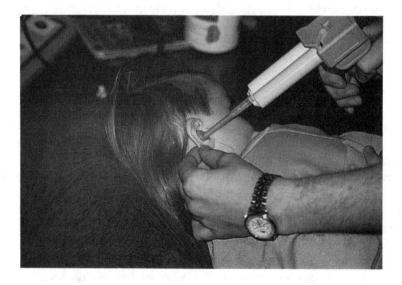

Figure 5.32 Two-cartridge injection gun

Some advantages to this system are clear: there is no messy mixing, the materials are measured in the correct quantities and standards of hygiene are high since a new canula is used for each child. The material has good dimensional stability. Furthermore, the impression material used, prior to set-up, has a low viscosity. This means that it is capable of forming an accurate impression of the ear without causing displacement. With some high viscosity materials 100% displacement can occur of the ear canal. The contra-point to this advantage is that, because the material is a low viscosity silicone, it does make handling of the impression difficult during set-up. It is necessary for the child to position his head on its side on a pillow or the side of the table, otherwise the material runs out of the ear. This may be very difficult to achieve with some children. Additionally there is a distance of some 20cm between trigger and canula. This makes control of the tip difficult since any small movement of the handle and trigger is magnified at the tip end. A further problem is that the hardware is large, 37cm when extended, gun-shaped and frightens some children. It is also very cumbersome to use with tiny babies.

Aerating tamps

Aerating tamps have been designed to release the air in the EAM thus preventing a partial vacuum from occurring. It is particularly important to bear this in mind when a deep impression is required. The aerating tamp consists of a flexible aerating tube with a flanged end, fabricated from silicone, which is attached to a foam tamp. This aerating tube, apart from releasing air pressure, makes it possible to position the tamp more easily in the canal square. The tamp has a plug at the far end which is cut off before removal of the impression to release the pressure.

Two -layer impression technique

A technique has been developed for taking aural impressions using two different silicone rubbers with different properties. The technique is of primary benefit for those wearers of deep-fitting canal instruments — peritympanic or CIC — but it is also advocated for those patients who require high gain hearing aid fittings, or for those whose outer ears are hard, crooked or inflexible. This procedure prevents the ear from being stretched and/or distorted and results in the final earmould being more comfortable and a better fit (Martin, 1995). Staab and Martin (1995), who developed the technique, suggest that the use of today's materials for impression-taking may be the reason for many poorly fitting earmoulds. They advocate a two-layer impression technique.

The rationale behind this technique is based on the premise that the ear canal consists of two distinctly different regions — the cartilaginous, flexible outer region and the bony, inflexible inner region. They suggest that this merits the use of impression materials with differing viscosity. The cartilaginous region requires a material which is flexible since the EAM can be quite flaccid. It is reported by Termeer (1994) (in Staab and Martin, 1995), that impression material can cause this region to expand 100%. Staab and Martin (1995) state that a low viscosity silicone should be used in the bony region as it is quite rigid and requires an impression material which does not cause additional pressure in the canal during setting or removal. The material is additionally required to have good elongation properties i.e. properties which allow it to compress to a degree, without final deformation, when pulled through a narrow ear canal.

Staab and Martin use Philips XP-Ear Impression Material 9022 909 48049 AD948/04 for the canal and Silhouette from Siemens which has an end Shore hardness between 30 and 40 Shore. These silicones bond well together.

One–stage impression material—Otana

One-stage impression materials, or earmoulds made by the direct method, have been available for some time. They have the obvious advantages of minimising waiting time for the child and reducing the risk of a poor fitting earmould through processing error. Very stringent demands are required of a material which will take both a successful impression and produce a quality durable earmould. Silicones have been used in one-stage materials since the late 1970s. They have many advantages over previous acrylic cold–curing methods but they have exhibited low shear strength properties — i.e. the earmoulds have torn easily and hence they have not proved to be durable enough for the paediatric population. This problem was overcome, to some extent, by the composite one-stage earmould which had an acrylic backplate and a silicone interior.

Okpojo (1990), concerned with meeting the amplification needs of hearing-impaired children in developing countries, considered criteria that would guide the development of a one-stage (instant) earmould material which would, additionally, be suitable for use as an impression for the two-stage process. In 1992 a successful product was produced and patented (Okpojo and Braden, 1993).

Conclusions

This chapter has sought to provide professionals, who work with deaf children, with an overview of the essentials of earmould technology by considering the current modus operandi together with the relevant past and present developments within the field. The chapter has considered the salient features of impression-taking and earmould manufacture, the role of the earmould in controlling frequency characteristics of a hearing aid system, earmould maintenance and problems encountered when working with children who use earmoulds. The reader interested in the 'classical' earmould articles and more detailed background information is directed to Recommended reading (p. 237).

References

ADI Plastics Limited (1967) Cold Cure Ear Inserts, Guidance Note, Blackpool, England.

Annear P (1995) Ear Moulds. Audiology and Education Technology Committee, British Association of Teachers of the Deaf Magazine, May 4.

Boothroyd A (1965) The provision of better earmoulds for deaf children. Journal of Laryngology and Otology 79: 320–335.

Bücklein R (1962) Hörbarkait von Unregelmässigkeiten. Frequenzgangen bei akustischer Übertagung Frequenze, 16: 3, p103.

Bulmer D (1973) Cold cure acrylic moulds. British Journal of Audiology 7: 5–8.

Brooks DN, Nolan M (1984) Good Fitting Earmoulds. In The Earmould, Current Practice and Technology. Hearing Aid Audiology Goup, British Society of Audiology, Reading.

Curren J (1989) Personal communication. Cited in Okpojo A (1990) Investigations into relevant earmould technology for developing countries. PhD Thesis, University Manchester, Manchester, UK.

Edwards J, Harris K S (1990) Rotation and translation of the jaw during speech. Journal of Speech and Hearing Res 33: 550–562.

Evans V M, Nolan M, Combe EC (1989) The Provision of Earmoulds in the United Kingdom: Results of a Survey. Department of Audiology, Education of the Deaf and Speech Pathology and the Biomeaterials Science Unit of the Department of Restorative Dentistry, University of Manchester.

Lybarger SF (1980) Earmoulds venting as an acoustic control factor. In: Studebaker GA and Hochberg I (eds) Acoustical Factors Affecting Hearing Aid Performance. Baltimore: University Park Press.

Martin RL (1995) A new technique for taking better ear impressions. The Hearing Journal 48(5).

McHugh ER, Morgan R (1988) Earmould/ITE Shell Technology and Acoustics. In Pollack MC (Ed) Amplification for the Hearing-Impaired (3rd Edition). Hemel Hempstead: Grune & Stratton.

McHugh ER, Purnish MA (1984) Evaluating the accuracy of earmould impression materials. Hearing Instruments 35, (12), 14, 15, and 60

Morgan R (1987) The foundation of a good impression. Hearing Institute 38(4): 20–24, 57.

National Deaf Childrens Society (NDCS), (1985) Earmoulds: fitting problems undermine the work of the hearing aid. Talk 117: 14–17.

Nolan M, Combe EC (1985) Silicone materials for ear impressions. Scandinavian Audiology 18: 35–39.

Nolan M, Combe EC (1989) In vitro considerations in the production of dimensionally acurate earmoulds – 1. The ear impression. Scandinavian Audiology 18: 35–41.

Okpojo AO (1990) Ph.D Thesis, Faculty of Medicine, University of Manchester.

Okpojo AO (1990a) Meeting the Amplification Needs of Hearing-Impaired Children in Developing Countries: The Earmould Factor. A paper presented at the 17th International Congress on Education of the Deaf, Rochester, New York. The Congress Proceedings, p 121.

Okpojo AO (1990b) Provision of Effective Services for Hearing-Impaired Population in Developing Countries. A paper presented at the Meeting of WHO working group re: Consultation on Evaluation of Low Cost Hearing Aids – EURO, WHO Regional Office, Copenhagen, Denmark.

Okpojo AO, Braden M (1993) Development of a novel audiological clinical material.

Biomaterials 14(1).

Parker D J, Okpajo AO, Nolan M, Combe EC, Bamford JM (1992) Acoustic evaluation of earmoulds in situ: comparisons of impressions and earmould materials. British Journal of Audiology 26: 159–166.

Skinner MW (1988) Hearing Aid Evaluation. Englewood Cliffs: Prentice Hall.

Staab WJ, Martin RL (1995) Mixed-media impressions: A two-layer approach to taking ear impressions The Hearing Journal MA 48(5).

Tucker IG, Nolan M, Colclough RO (1978) A new high-efficiency earmould. Scandinavian Audiology 7, 225.

Recommended reading.

Berger KW (1976) The earliest known custom earmoulds. Hearing Aid Journal 29, 5, 10, and 35.

British Society of Audiology (1994) Current Practice and Technology 1994 Hearing Aid Audiology Group British Society of Audiology.

British Society of Audiology (1986) Recommended procedure for taking an aural impression. British Journal of Audiology 20: 315–316.

Combe EC, Nolan, M (1989) In vitro consideration in the production of dimensionally accurate earmoulds - II. The earmould material. Scandinavian Audiology 18: 67–73.

Correl IC (1983) Notes from Oticon. Information Department, Oticon International, Copenhagen.

Fidield DB, Earnshaw R, Smither MF (1980) A new impression technique to prevent acoustic feedback with high powered hearing aids. Volta Review 82: 33–39.

Krough HJ (1975) Placing the receiver in the earmould. Scandinavian Audiology Supplement 5, 113–122.

Libby ER (1985) Earmould modification by special bores and dampers, particularly in relation to the need and high frequency range. Audiology in Practice II, 5–7.

McVey E, Grier AM (1983) A survey of 3,392 earmoulds in Scottish schools by the Scottish Association for the Deaf. Health Bulletin 41(6): 305–309.

Macrae J (1984) Earmould venting. Audiology in Practice 1: 7–8.

Macrae J (1989) The Acoustic Seal of Earmould. Unpublished Ph.D Thesis, NAL, Australia.

Mahon W J (1984) Earmould remakes: The bottom-line causes. The Hearing Journal 37: 7–10.

Morgan R (1987) The foundation - A good impression. Hearing Instruments 38(4): 20–24, 57.

Muriithi CG (1989) The Factors Influencing Dimensional Changes of Ear Impression Materials. Unpublished M. Ed Dissertation, University of Manchester.

Mynders JM (1985) Human acoustic couplers. In Sandlin R (Ed) Hearing Instrument Sciences and Fitting Practices. NIFHIS.

Nolan M (1985) The earmould: variations in the transmission curve of a hearing aid as a Result of changes in the sound bore diameter and length and venting. Audiology in Practice II 1–4.

Nolan M (1988) Earmoulds. In McCormick B (Ed) Paediatric Audiology. London: Taylor and Francis.

Nolan M, Combe EC (1987) Dimensional Accuracy and Stability of Materials and Techniques Associated with Audiology. Report of Research Conducted for the Department of Health and Social Security (1986–1987). Biomaterials Science Unit and Department of Audiology, Education of the Deaf and Speech Pathology,

University of Manchester.

Nolan M, Elizemethy S, Tucker IG, McDonough DF (1978) An investigation into the problems involved in producing efficient earmoulds for children. Scandinavian Audiology 7: 231–237.

Nolan M, Hostler M, Taylor IG, Cash A (1986) Practical consideration in the fabrication of earmoulds for young babies. Scandinavian Audiology 15: 21–27.

Nolan M, Tucker IG, Colclough RO (1979) Instruction Manual on the Production of the Composite Earmould. Department of Audiology, Manchester: University of Manchester.

Rice SL (1984) NAEL fitting facts, Part V: Remakes and how to prevent them. Hearing Instruments 35(2): 6–7, 51.

Schier BA (1933) Retentive auditory prosthesis. Dental Items of Interest 55: 783–796.

Schier BA (1941) The earpiece - in testing for and fitting hearing aids. Laryngoscope 51: 52–60.

Schier BA (1945) Clinical phenomena in conductive media: the individual earpiece. The Journal of the Acoustical Society of America 17(1): 77–82.

Shah V (1980) Hearing Aid Dispensing in India. International Hearing Aid Seminar, San Diego, California.

Sneyd A (1985) EMTEC Earmould Handbook. Letchworth: EMTEC.

Takinishi K, Itedan I (1984) A new earmould tubing to reduce moisture problems. Hearing Instruments 35: 32, 60.

Chapter 6
Cochlear Implants

S ARCHBOLD

Introduction

Paediatric implantation has been the subject of great controversy, but has also been described as the single most important development in the audiological management of deaf children in recent years. In a comparatively short time, paediatric implantation has become a widespread procedure for profoundly deaf children, both those born deaf and those with acquired hearing losses. Most teachers of the deaf, whether in the UK or elsewhere, can now expect to work with children using cochlear implant systems during their careers. It is therefore imperative that teachers in training and those seeking to update their professional expertise, should ensure that they are aware of the issues concerning cochlear implantation.

This chapter begins by describing the development of cochlear implant systems, the essential components of a cochlear implant, and the current systems in use. It goes on to describe currently accepted criteria and assessment procedures, specialist paediatric practice, rehabilitation and outcome measures. The educational implications are discussed, with particular reference to the role of the child's teacher of the deaf, and the responsibilities of the implant centre teacher of the deaf. Some ethical questions raised by the deaf community are considered, and the parental responsibilities in the decision making process and long term care are described. Finally, some of the questions which remain are raised, and long term responsibilities of teachers of the deaf with regard to the day-to-day management of implanted children are outlined.

Development of cochlear implant systems

Cochlear implantation aims to stimulate the auditory nerve directly, to give a sensation of hearing in those unable to benefit from conventional hearing aids. Several histories of cochlear implantation have been written (House and Berliner, 1991; Mecklenburg and Lehnhardt, 1991; Clark, 1997) for those interested in reading further. Following encouraging results in adults, the first child was implanted with a single-channel cochlear implant by William House in 1980, and in 1985 the first child was implanted with the Nucleus 22 channel device. Paediatric implantation began with very conservative criteria, with those children with acquired losses, most commonly from meningitis. It remains a controversial subject, but encouraging outcomes are now well documented (Osberger et al., 1991a; Osberger et al., 1991b; Osberger et al., 1993; Waltzman et al., 1994; Miyamoto et al., 1995; Waltzman et al. 1995: Dettman et al., 1995). It is now considered that children born deaf may do as well over time as those deafened below the age of three (Waltzman et al., 1994; Dettman et al., 1995) and may do better (Summerfield and Marshall, 1995). 2500 children under the age of 10 have been implanted to date world-wide, and are likely to be the major source of demand for cochlear implants in future (Summerfield and Marshall, 1995).

Cochlear implant systems

A cochlear implant is an electronic device, providing direct electrical stimulation to the cochlea via surgically implanted electrodes. Although there are several implant systems in use, varying in the number and position of the electrodes, and in the strategy used to process the incoming signal, there are several common features. All implant systems consist of internal and external parts, as illustrated in Figure 6.1:

- The internal parts: receiver and electrodes, surgically implanted.
- The external parts: microphone, speech processor and transmitter.

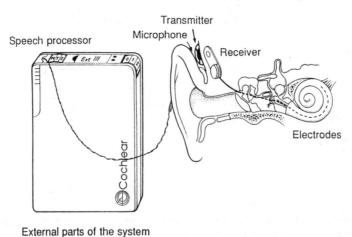

Figure 6.1 A typical implant system, showing internal and external parts

The microphone collects the acoustic signal at ear level, and the signal is then converted within the speech processor into electrical signals that are conveyed via the transmitter through the skin to the implanted receiver and then to the electrodes. The transmitter and the receiver are most commonly held in opposition to each other by magnets placed in each of them (transcutaneous transmission). The electrical signal is relayed by radio-frequency transmission through the intact skin, without the need for internal power supply. Signal transmission may also take place by means of a percutaneous plug through the skin (percutaneous transmission), but this is not usually considered appropriate for children. Implant systems may vary as to whether they use:

- single- or multi-channel electrodes,
- intra- or extra-cochlear electrodes, or
- an analogue or feature extraction speech processing strategy.

Single-channel systems deliver the signal to one electrode inside or outside the cochlea, while multi-channel systems deliver the signal to a number of electrodes, with the aim of imitating the tonotopic organisation of the cochlea. Currently, most implant centres use an intra-cochlear, multi-channel device as the system of choice, with the evidence being that better results are achieved (Tyler, Moore and Kuk, 1989; Cohen, Waltzman and Fisher, 1991, 1993; Waltzman et al., 1992). However, there is still debate about which processing strategy is most effective. Analogue systems provide the entire acoustic signal, while feature extraction strategies process the signal and deliver those features of the signal considered the most important for the recognition of speech to the electrode array within the cochlea. The interested reader is referred to Wilson (1993).

Research continues in cochlear implant technology; reviews of developments are given by Tyler and Tye-Murray (1991), Mecklenburg and Lehnhardt (1991), Summerfield and Marshall (1995) and Patrick, Seligman and Clark (1997) amongst others. A new processing strategy was introduced for the Nucleus device called S-PEAK (McKay et al., 1991) conveying spectral peaks in the signal, rather than the feature extraction strategy of the previous processor, the mini speech processor (MSP), and the Nucleus C1-24 M system has recently been developed, offering further options. Devices such as the Clarion and Medel Combi-40 utilise the continuous interleaved sampling (CIS) strategy, which presents the compressed analogue signal at a very fast pulse rate to the electrodes in order to avoid interactions between electrodes. These three devices plan to introduce an ear level processor for suitable users. The newer generation of implant, offers more flexibility and choice in tuning the system; however, in considering the choice of device with children, it is important to look at reliability, which is lower for children than adults (Parisier et al., 1995; Ajayi et al., in press) as well as potential benefit. In choosing a cochlear implant for children, the following issues need to be considered:

- The long term reliability of internal and external parts.
- The use of the latest, proven technology.
- The long term technical support from the manufacturer.
- An effective interface with FM systems.
- The possible use of future developments in technology.
- The limitation of use of magnetic resonance imaging (MRI) following implantation.
- Ease of identification of technical problems, for example with the use of telemetry in the newer devices.
- Practical features for use with very young children; for example, size and robustness.

Having described the essential components of an implant system, it is important, before discussing the process itself, to consider the ethical issues and concerns raised by the deaf communities around the world to the procedure.

Ethical issues

Much of the publicity about cochlear implantation has supported the myth of the 'bionic ear' as a cure for deafness (Power and Hyde, 1992; Laurenzi, 1993). This promotes the medical model of deafness; members of the deaf community, however, view themselves as those with a cultural and linguistic identity, rather than those with a medical condition to be 'treated'. Many advocates of implantation have shown little understanding of the views of the deaf community, and have excluded deaf people from discussion about the implications of cochlear implantation (Lane, 1994). Cochlear implantation has thus been seen as a threat to this cultural identity, and there have been many protests world-wide from deaf associations about what is seen as experimentation on children who are unable to decide about cochlear implantation for themselves. As increasing numbers of young children are being implanted, deaf communities question the right of hearing parents to make this decision, with its long term implications, on behalf of their deaf child. The statements of the deaf associations about cochlear implants reflect these concerns; for example, the consensus view of the British Deaf Association expressed in their policy on cochlear implants (BDA, 1995) is that they feel unable to support implants for deaf children. Similar statements have been published by other deaf associations around the world.

In addition to the social and ethical objections to implantation, concerns have been expressed about the scientific validity and objectivity of the results presented about cochlear implantation. To date, much of the published data come from the vested interests of implant programmes or manufacturers, and there have been criticisms that the published material is biased and has not been subject to rigorous scientific scrutiny (Lane, 1994). Additionally, much of the work has concentrated on measures of speech perception, largely ignoring the areas of social adjustment, quality of life, and language. An essential achievement of early childhood is the acquisition of language. In the case of profoundly deaf children this may be a visually based language, that is sign language, rather than an auditory based spoken language. The ongoing argument is that language development has, as yet, not been proven to be effective via audition through a cochlear implant system.

Another major concern about cochlear implantation is the time and money that has been spent on the implantation of comparatively few individuals, with concerns that implanted children receive more input from rehabilitation professionals than their hearing aided peers. These are very real concerns for which cochlear implant programmes bear the responsibility for providing some of the answers. Tyler (1993), in asking if resolution of the conflict is possible, suggests three ways forward: interaction between implant teams and the deaf community; fair and accurate counselling of parents, and acceptance of diversity in the deaf and hearing cultures. This requires that cochlear implant programmes work with the deaf communities, providing objective, accessible outcomes on all implanted children. Parents need to be fully counselled as to the implications of implantation for their child's future; it is not a single audiological or medical process, but one that has life-long implications for the child. A cochlear implant may extend educational and communication options for a profoundly deaf child, but as a technical device, the implant itself will need life-long monitoring and maintenance.

The responsibility for ensuring that these criticisms are addressed lies with paediatric implant teams, which must include personnel conversant with these issues.

The specialist paediatric cochlear implant team

Any paediatric cochlear implant team must be established with a range of professionals experienced with deaf children (Deguine et al., 1995). The team, in its planning, must consider:

- the complexity of paediatric implantation,
- the numbers of people involved in the process,
- the differing professional groups involved,
- the variability in outcomes, and influences on progress,
- the long term implications for staffing and funding,
- the long term implications for maintenance.

Descriptions of the staff required and their roles are given by Fraser (1991), Tye-Murray (1993) and Archbold (1994a); as illustrated in Table 6.1, the complete implant team must include those at the child's home and school, as well as those at the implant centre. Liaison between the implant centre and the family and local professionals is vital and must begin prior to the first appointment, with the co-ordinator ensuring that it continues during the assessment period and throughout the ongoing care of the child.

Table 6.1 The complete paediatric cochlear implant team

The local team at the child's home	The team at the implant centre
Parents	Co-ordinator/ administrator
Family	Surgeon
ENT consultant	Nursing staff
Audiological scientist	Paediatric audiological scientist
Teacher of the deaf	Medical physiscist
Other educators	Teacher of the deaf
Speech and language therapist	Speech and language therapist
Educational psychologist	Educational psychologist
Social worker for the deaf	Social worker for the deaf
Other carers	Technician

One way of illustrating this co-operation is shown in Figure 6.2; this triangle of support demonstrates the way in which family, local professionals and implant centre must work together on behalf of the child.

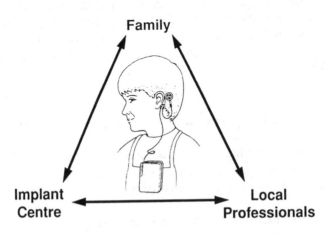

Figure 6.2 The triangle of support needed for an implanted child

Before the first appointment, the co-ordinator should send out information for the child, family and professionals (Archbold, 1992; Tye-Murray, 1993). This information may cover the implant systems, the process of implantation, and the implications and commitment required, and should be accessible to all groups and cultures. In addition, information should be obtained from the local team to begin to obtain a picture of the child's functioning, so that children are not subject to unnecessary assessment procedures.

The process of implantation

The process of implantation is usually divided into four areas: assessment, surgery and initial tuning, rehabilitation and finally the maintenance phase, which lasts for the entire period of implant use. The following are the guidelines for suitability for implantation given by Staller et al., (1991a):

* Bilateral profound deafness.
* Age 2-17 years.
* No radiological contraindications.
* No medical contraindications.

    In addition, children should:

* demonstrate little or no benefit from conventional amplification,
* receive educational support which includes a strong auditory/oral component,
* be psychologically and developmentally suitable,
* have appropriate family and educational expectations and support.

Although still generally accepted, these guidelines are being challenged in several ways as experience grows with implantation; the audiological guidelines are relaxing, as discussed later, children younger than two are now increasingly being implanted, and children with other handicaps may be considered appropriate in some instances.

Assessment

It is important that, although much information may be passed to the implant centre by the child's referrer, the professionals at the implant centre carry out their own assessments with their knowledge of cochlear implantation. The implanting surgeon carries legal responsibility for the care of the child, and needs to be involved in the full process of assessment, so that the decision to implant is an informed one by all concerned. At each stage of assessment, full discussion must take place with the parents, and child if appropriate, about the implications of implantation, including the possibility of device failure. There should be opportunities to discuss alternative ways of management for the child, and to meet parents of both implanted and non-implanted children, deaf adults, and adult deaf implant users. At all times of the assessment phase both parents and implant team must feel able to decide against implantation for the child.

The assessment protocol used by the author's team is given in Figure 6.3. The process of assessment includes audiological, medical, speech and language, and educational evaluations in addition to assessments of family expectations and commitment. The initial visit is for the audiological evaluation, unless the child has been deafened by meningitis. In this case, a radiological evaluation will be carried out first to ascertain whether there is ossification (the growth of bone) taking place in the cochlea.

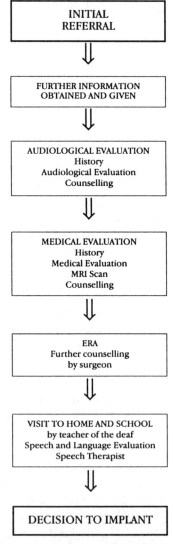

Figure 6.3 The assessment protocol of the Nottingham programme (Reproduced with permission from Archbold, 1994a)

The first audiological criteria were stringent, reflecting caution; accepted audiological guidelines are now average aided thresholds of greater than 60 dBA across the speech frequencies (McCormick, 1994). These may be interpreted flexibly, the essential criterion being that the child does not demonstrate a potential to understand spoken language via conventional hearing aids. Summerfield and Marshall (1995) consider that, with the latest technology, children with average hearing losses of 95 dBHL are likely to achieve better outcomes in terms of auditory reception with cochlear implants than with hearing aids. The audiological evaluation should be carried out by experienced paediatric audiological scientists, in the absence of a conductive element, with well fitting earmoulds, and after a reasonable trial with appropriate hearing aids. The recording of otoacoustic emissions (OAEs) and brainstem evoked responses should be included as part of the audiological assessment (McCormick, 1994; Mason, 1994).

The medical assessment includes consideration of the following factors:

- The degree of deafness.
- The aetiology of the deafness.
- The otological assessment (including diagnosis and treatment of other factors contributing to the deafness), radiological assessment, and genetic family history.
- The general medical evaluation including an assessment of such factors as general developmental progress and general medical conditions which may affect outcome.
- The overall interpretation of the audiological and other data resulting from the assessment process.
(Gibbin and O'Donoghue, 1994)

The otological evaluation will particularly consider the presence of active middle ear disease which may need treating before a full audiological evaluation can take place, or before implantation is possible. Careful consideration of the history of the child is essential to attempt to rule out the possibility of implanting a child with no potential to benefit from implantation – for example, a child with an absent auditory nerve. The general medical assessment should ensure that the child is fit to undergo anaesthesia, and for children with other medical problems which may complicate surgery, or those with developmental delay, it will be necessary to liaise with other specialists (Gibbin and O'Donoghue, 1994). Experienced implant centres are now implanting those children with other disabilities (Lesinski et al., 1995); Usher's syndrome children in particular may be considered to be priority cases (Young et al., 1995).

Computed tomography (CT) is used to image the inner ears and brain, although magnetic resonance imaging (MRI) is increasingly useful to provide more detailed imaging of the neural anatomy and cochlear fluids. Approximately one third of children deafened by meningitis will have new bone growth in the cochlea, and radiology may provide evidence for one ear being more favourable for the insertion of an implant than the other. In congenitally deaf children, radiology may reveal congenital abnormalities which may be contraindications to cochlear implantation.

Assessments of speech and language are carried out by implant centre speech and language therapists and teachers of the deaf both at the implant centre, and at home and school. Speech and language therapists look at the child's linguistic functioning at the levels of communication, receptive and expressive language, and voice and speech (Dyar, 1995). Teachers of the deaf working on the implant team visit the school and the home in order to provide information on cochlear implants and describe potential benefits or problems, assess the child's functioning compared with his peers, and assess the level of appropriate support should implantation proceed (Nevins and Chute, 1994; Nevins and Chute, 1996; Archbold, 1994a). A psychological report may be helpful to assess whether there are any other learning difficulties present which may hinder the development of spoken language following implantation. This stage of assessment may be stressful for the family, and the child, and it is essential that the local professionals, on whom a great deal of responsibility will fall should implantation proceed, are involved as fully as possible.

When all the assessments have been completed, a useful means of considering the issues covered was developed at the Children's Institute, Manhattan Eye, Ear and Throat Hospital in the form of the children's implant profile (ChIP) (Hellman et al., 1991). The ChIP is used to guide the decision making process, to ensure that all these areas have been covered, and that potential areas of difficulty have been anticipated, and where possible addressed.

Surgery and initial tuning

Once the decision to implant has been made, the child, parents and local professionals should be prepared as fully as possible for the operation, with written materials where appropriate. The operation itself takes about three hours, including the measurement of stapedius reflex thresholds, recording electrically evoked brainstem responses (EABR) and integrity testing of the device. Prior to the operation, the EABR can be evoked by promontory stimulation as a means of attempting to assess the number of surviving neurones in the cochlea. This may help to decide which ear to implant if there are no other audiological, medical or radiological indications as to choice of ear (Mason et al., 1995). The shape of the incision may vary according to the choice of the surgeon; a typical incision is shown in Figure 6.4. Following the operation, the child will wear a large pressure bandage for 24 hours, and receive antibiotics for several days. Parents find it helpful to have the reassurance which can be given following the intra-operative electrical testing, that the device itself is indeed functioning. Children are usually active the following day and home within 2–3 days. Cochlear implantation has been found to be a safe procedure (Clark, Cohen and Sheppard, 1991; Staller et al., 1991a; Summerfield and Marshall, 1995) when carried out by experienced surgeons, and complications are rare.

Once the wound has healed, usually some four weeks after surgery, the child returns to the implant centre to receive the external parts – microphone, transmitter and processor – and for the initial stimulation of the system. Compared with the huge dynamic range of the auditory system, the dynamic range between threshold of sensation and discomfort for electrical stimulation is narrow; it is equivalent to less than 15–20 dB (Patrick and Clark, 1991). The electrical dynamic range for each individual, and for different positions in the cochlea, differs. Setting the implant system to maximise the use of the dynamic range for each electrode is called 'programming', or 'tuning', or 'mapping'. Particularly with young children, unable to comment on the sensations they receive, the electro-physiological measurements taken during the operation are useful to set initial levels with the least risk of presenting unpleasant sensations (Mason et al., 1995). It will be some time before the child is able to receive optimum settings; the scientist is faced with choices of strategies to use, and a young child may be unable to give responses which enable the scientist to tune the device optimally. Tuning the implant system usually necessitates return visits to the implant centre over a period of time, although some centres offer the possibility of tuning in the device within the child's school. Fuller discussions of tuning procedures are available elsewhere for the interested reader (Roberts, 1991; Tye-Murray, 1993; Sheppard, 1994; Rance and Dowell, 1997); Figure 6.5 shows a child with his mother during a tuning session.

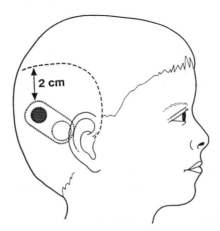

Figure 6.4 A typical incision for a cochlear implant

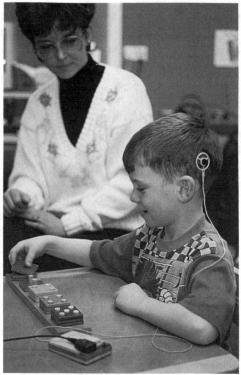

Figure 6.5 A child with his mother during a cochlear implant tuning session

Rehabilitation and evaluation

The rehabilitation period necessarily includes the regular reprogramming of the implant system as the child's ability to listen to sound develops, and involves considerable teamwork. Unless the device is appropriately tuned for the child, then rehabilitation activities designed to help the child attach meaning to sound will be ineffective. Similarly, reports from rehabilitation staff may influence the tuning of the device and the programming decisions of the scientists. Children should be wearing the implant system all their waking hours, in good working order and at appropriate settings. They also need to experience good listening conditions, and opportunities conducive to the development of communication skills and spoken language.

These needs are very similar to those of conventionally hearing aided children, but there are some differences. The complexity of tuning the device, and of monitoring its functioning, necessitates close assessment of the child's developing listening skills, particularly in the early stages. A child receiving a cochlear implant may well be listening for the first time after a period of some years with little or no useful hearing; the style of management which may have been appropriate prior to implantation may not be appropriate after implantation with the new emphasis on the use of audition, and it is important that the child experiences activities which will enable it to make sense of the new signals as quickly as possible. Additionally, there will be access to mid and high frequency information, which is not usually achievable in the profoundly deaf using conventional hearing aids. There must be expectation of the use of this information in the development of listening and spoken language skills.

Although there is a continued debate as to whether specific rehabilitation activities are needed for implanted children, the theoretical frameworks for rehabilitation with children with cochlear implants are described elsewhere (Eisenburg, 1985; Cooper, 1991; Somers, 1991: Tye-Murray, 1993; Archbold and Tait, 1994). As the age at implantation is lowered, the emphasis on rehabilitation taking place at the implant centre is being replaced by an emphasis on giving the skills in managing an implant system to the parents and local professionals, and influencing the everyday activities of the child so that they are productive in encouraging spoken language.

However, before we can begin any activities, the child must be wearing the processor happily; children may not enjoy the first sensations of sound, and need some time using the device at conservative settings to adjust to the new sensations. Fryauf-Bertschy (1992) gives some practical ideas for encouraging the wearing of the processor; Figure 6.6 illustrates a child wearing an implant system. With the child wearing the system comfortably, we can begin by aiming to encourage early responses to sounds, both environmental and speech, in order to develop the discrimination necessary to identify sounds.

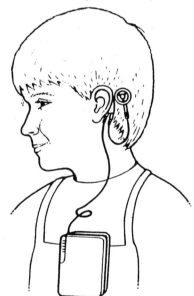

Figure 6.6 Wearing a cochlear implant system

For some, environmental sound discrimination may not be an important aim for cochlear implantation, but many parents mention this for safety reasons (Eisenburg, 1985), and some of the first reactions may be to environmental sounds. Gradually, early responses will develop so that the child is able to identify many of the sounds in the environment, and to ignore those which are not relevant. At a time when evidence of progress may be slight, questionnaires showing progress in listening to environmental sounds may be helpful to parents. Following the initial responses to environmental sounds, musical instruments, sound makers, and speech sounds, the children learn to attach meaning to these sounds through play at home and at school.

However, in children, the major aim of cochlear implantation is to provide audition by which a child can acquire speech and language. Initially there were more cautious aims, but the outcomes currently documented and described later indicate that it is possible for young children to acquire intelligible spoken language via audition following implantation. For the child with no spoken language skills prior to implantation, we are aiming to develop the early communication skills of turn-taking, autonomy, eye-contact and auditory awareness (Archbold and Tait, 1994). Eye-contact and turn-taking may be developed through the use of partner and parallel play, familiar formats and shared activities. The development of auditory awareness of spoken language can be encouraged through games with animal sounds, the use of appropriate books, singing and games which involve the child's response to speech. Response to, and discrimination of sounds will be followed by identification and comprehension, following Erber's categories (1982), including single words, phrases, sentences and connected speech. With older children, activities may be more structured, involving the use of stories and poems, written language and taped materials. At all times, the aim is not to 'train' the child in specific skills, but to ensure that the adult structures the learning experiences for the child, bearing in mind the likely sequence of development of auditory skills and leading the child on to the next stage of development (Webster, 1992). The ultimate aim is the integration of the hearing provided by the implant into the development of communication and spoken language skills; those activities found to promote the development of spoken language in both deaf and hearing children are equally important for an implanted child.

Educational implications

A study of European and UK implant centres revealed that appropriate educational support was viewed as a major problem, following funding (Archbold and Robinson, 1997; Archbold and Robinson, in press).

However, Geers and Moog (1995) comment that the educational implications of cochlear implantation should be negligible since teachers of the deaf have long been responsible for the education of children with access to sound from conventional hearing aids. Cochlear implantation has added a new dimension to these responsibilities, but, as described above, many of the activities which are used with hearing aided children are suitable for those with cochlear implants. Implanted children do not present entirely new problems; they are children who have useful audition following implantation, as do many hearing aided children (Geers and Moog, 1995; Tyler, 1993). Are there any implications for teachers of the deaf in practice?

Geers and Moog (1995) suggest that there are three implications: expectations, teaching and costs. There should be changed expectations of the use of audition, and this may influence teaching. Teachers should be able to interpret tuning reports from the audiological scientists at the implant centre and understand some of the implications for the child's listening abilities in the educational setting. There are training and cost implications for teachers to acquire an understanding of the implant system, to become familiar with its daily management and for the supply of spares. Much of the long term responsibility for managing the implant system falls on the child's own teacher of the deaf (Geers and Moog, 1991; Somers, 1991; Nevins and Chute, 1996); teachers must be able to monitor its functioning, so that any faults in the functioning of the internal or external parts are identified as soon as possible. It is vital that teachers are fully supported in their role by the implanting centre. The House Ear Institute initiated the School Contact Program in 1982 (Selmi, 1985) and the Cochlear Implant Center at the Manhattan Eye, Ear and Throat Hospital appointed the Educational Consultant Model to facilitate communication between the centre and school (Nevins and Chute, 1994; Nevins and Chute, 1996). Other implant teams in Australia, the USA, the UK and the Netherlands have developed close links with teachers in their classrooms. The Network of Educators of Children with Cochlear Implants gives a forum for the dissemination of practical information in the USA, and in the UK the British Association of Teachers of the Deaf has encouraged teachers to access useful information. There is still a need, however, for direct contact between implant centre, and home and school; each child has different needs, and each educational setting and communication style varies (Archbold, 1994a).

In the UK, most implant centres have developed educational outreach programmes, with rehabilitation staff from the implant centre making regular visits to the child's home and school (or to the teacher of the deaf if the child is at the pre-school stage). It has been calculated that children spend 1% of their waking hours in the first year after implant in the implant centre; the other 99% are spent at home and at school (Archbold, 1994a). In order to influence the use of the implant system during these hours, and to use the existing skills of local professionals and adapt them to use implant technology, implant centre staff focus on working with educational staff, speech and language therapists, and families during outreach visits. In order that consistency of support provided by implant centres throughout the UK can be encouraged, guidelines have been developed for implant centre teachers of the deaf (BATOD, 1995) and are currently being drawn up for implant centre speech and language therapists. Guidelines for the corresponding responsibilities of local teachers of the deaf are also currently being discussed. In addition to written and telephone communication, the minimum levels of direct support are illustrated in Figure 6.7.

EDUCATIONAL OUTREACH PROGRAMME

Visits to home and school by rehabilitation staff

Year 1 : Monthly

Years 2 & 3 : Bi-monthly

Year 4 onwards : Annually

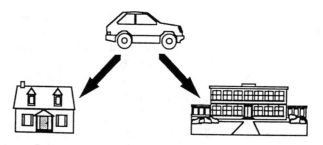

Figure 6.7 The suggested minimum educational outreach visits to home and school

At the author's centre, the aim of the visits is the support of the local team and parents, although some time may be spent with the child, monitoring progress, and demonstrating activities to families and professionals (Lutman et al., 1996). The responsibilities of the implant centre teacher of the deaf include:

- taking part in the assessment of candidates,
- liaising between implant centre and home and school,
- counselling and advising children, families and local professionals,
- supporting parents during assessments and hospital stay,
- providing feedback to team members involved in the tuning process,

- providing appropriate rehabilitation and advice on rehabilitation,
- assessing progress in the use of the system,
- providing advice on the use of the radio hearing aid system,
- establishing long term maintenance of the system,
- providing long term support to children's families and teachers.
  (BATOD, 1995)

The responsibilities of the local teacher of the deaf prior to implantation include participation in assessment, acquisition of knowledge of implantation and the preparation of the child, family and peer group. In order to be able to fulfil these responsibilities, the teacher needs to acquire knowledge about:

- the differences between hearing aids and cochlear implants,
- reasonable expectations from the device,
- the basics of the tuning process,
- using and monitoring the system,
- trouble-shooting the system,
- what to do, and who to contact, should a problem occur.

Following implantation the child's teacher should be able to:

- carry out a daily check on the system and monitor any changes in listening skills,
- trouble-shoot the device,
- provide good listening conditions; including other assistive devices, such as an FM system,
- provide appropriate rehabilitation activities,
- support the child and family, particularly if progress is slow, or there are any problems,
- liaise between home, school and implant centre,
- participate in obtaining outcome measures.

The provision of an FM system is worthy of further comment; in the UK particularly, there have been considerable problems with connecting the speech processor to an FM system. At the time of writing, effective connecting leads appear to have been produced, but caution is still expressed about the use of FM systems until the child has become a good listener with the implant system, and able to report any interference.

While the responsibilities outlined may appear considerable, all deaf children should be the subject of specialist educational provision, and it may well be that, following implantation, the child does not require more time from his educators, but the focus of the time may be different – that of developing good listening skills.

In the UK, and elsewhere, decisions about communication modalities to use with deaf children and about educational placement may not be based on the children's needs or parental wishes, but on local policy. It is considered that, if children with cochlear implants are to develop intelligible spoken language through the implant system, then a strong auditory/oral component is essential with the emphasis on learning to speak, whatever the educational setting (Cooper, 1991: Somers, 1991; Tye-Murray, 1993; Summerfield and Marshall, 1995). Dettman et al. (1995) found that an oral educational setting was favourable to the development of speech perception in children with cochlear implants. In addition to deciding what mode of communication to use with a deaf child, decisions need to be made as to what type of educational placement is appropriate. Throughout the world, the trend has been for children to be placed in mainstream settings, and in the UK most profoundly deaf children are educated in integrated settings. Children with cochlear implants, implanted early and with appropriate educational support, are likely to move towards less restrictive educational environments (Nevins and Chute, 1994), but will continue to need appropriate support from a teacher of the deaf and other professionals, particularly in the long term monitoring of the system.

Monitoring progress in young children

With increasing numbers of younger children being implanted, there are three particular challenges to be faced: accurate assessment of audiological status, tuning in the device optimally and monitoring progress.

Audiological assessment and tuning of the system should be carried out by experienced paediatric audiological scientists; objective measures being developed should assist in optimum setting of the device. It is essential that, however young the child, progress is assessed in order to monitor the functioning and tuning of the device, and the appropriateness of the management of the child. There have been few measures available to assess progress in the pre-verbal deaf child. Video analysis measures developed with young conventionally aided children (Tait, 1987) have proved useful with children with cochlear implants (Tait and Lutman, 1994; Lutman and Tait, 1995). Other measures include the McCormick toy test (McCormick, 1977); the low-verbal version of the Early Speech Perception test (Geers and Moog, 1989) and the Discrimination After Training (DAT) test (Thelemeir, 1984). These all involve some use of language; Listening Progress (LiP) was designed as a profile of early listening skills to obtain evidence of progress in pre-verbal children particularly in the first year after implantation (Archbold, 1994b). Other tools that may be used include the Meaningful Auditory Integration Scale (McConkey Robbins et al., 1991), the Nursery Behaviour Checklist (Dyar, 1995) and the Pragmatics Profile of Early

Communication skills (Dewart and Summers, 1988). An example of assessments developed with this young age group in mind is given in full in McCormick et al. (1994).

Outcome measures

In addition to monitoring progress as outlined above, outcome measures are important to enable us to compare the functioning of different devices, to answer the ethical questions being asked about implantation and its effectiveness, and to produce accessible outcomes for parents, professionals and purchasers.

One of the criticisms that has been made of paediatric implantation in particular is the lack of objective, independent measures of outcome (Lane, 1994; Vernon and Alles, 1994). The difficulties in controlling for the variables in measuring progress in young deaf children are well known (Boothroyd, 1991; Osberger et al., 1991a; Staller et al., 1991a), but this does not remove the responsibility for ensuring that the procedure of cochlear implantation is evaluated in all children as fully and objectively as possible.

Early studies (Staller et al., 1991a) concluded that the device was safe with children; this has since been confirmed by others (Clark, Cohen and Sheppard, 1991). Its effectiveness has been the subject of many studies (Staller et al., 1991a; Cohen, Waltzman and Fisher, 1991; Osberger et al., 1991b; Tobey et al., 1991; Miyamoto et al., 1995). Several studies that have been carried out to compare groups using hearing aids or tactile aids give favourable results for children using cochlear implants (Osberger et al., 1993; Tait and Lutman, 1994; Miyamoto et al., 1995).

In the UK, the Department of Health established a multi-centre objective study of cochlear implantation reported by Summerfield and Marshall (1995). This only looked at one paediatric centre but recommended that paediatric implantation should continue in the UK, considering it likely to become routine to implant children between the ages of two and three. Summerfield and Marshall recognised that children who were born deaf or who were deafened before the acquisition of spoken language have been able to perceive spoken language through audition after implantation; although older pre-lingually deaf children have received some benefit from implantation, they found that the development of auditory receptive abilities in children was particularly linked to length of use of the device.

Waltzman et al. (1994, 1995) and Dettman et al. (1995) found encouraging results for speech perception in young children. Waltzman found high levels of speech understanding without lip reading in congenitally deaf children implanted before the age of five, and all children were using oral language to communicate. Dettman et al. (1995) found that, with young children, the only factor affecting speech perception was experience; with older children, speech perception was influenced by duration of deafness, age at onset, and educational placement. Using a behavioural measure of benefit (Meaningful Auditory Integration Scale), Quittner et al. (1991) found that length of time using the device, and educational setting, were positively related to the meaningful use of sound.

An upper age limit for children has not been determined, although congenitally deaf teenagers may produce disappointing outcomes and need careful selection (Chute, 1993), and Osberger et al. (1993) found that children with early onset of deafness implanted after the age of 10 had less intelligible speech than those implanted younger. Beiter et al. (1991) reported that pre-lingually deafened children implanted before the age of seven were more likely to achieve open-set auditory recognition than those implanted later.

In summary, congenitally deaf children and those with early onset of hearing loss can acquire spoken language via audition and learn to use oral language as their means of communication. Although early implantation appears linked with the greatest progress in spoken language following implantation, older children have the potential to benefit, although the degree of benefit may be less. Particularly for older children, the number of years using the implant is significant in development of benefit, and children continue to progress for several years after implantation. Implanting children before the age at which decisions are made about school placement may be sensible so that these decisions can be made in the light of the functioning of the child.

These measures of benefit have concentrated on measures of speech production and perception; there is an increasing interest in looking at measures of language development, educational achievement, and at broader psycho-social issues (for example, Quittner et al., 1991). However in considering published outcomes from paediatric implantation, there is little that is accessible to parents, the non-specialist, or to purchasers. One measure which was designed with this purpose is Categories of Auditory Performance (CAP); this is an index of readily understood categories that can be used as a global measure of outcome whatever the child's level of functioning (Archbold, Lutman and Marshall, 1995). Table 6.2 shows the results in the author's programme from the first 89 children, born deaf or deafened before the age of three; it illustrates the time-scale over which benefit develops. The more demanding skills, which require linguistic competence, develop between one and two years after implantation; three years after implantation 92% of the children were able to understand conversation or common phrases without lip reading.

Table 6.2 Categories of auditory performance (CAP, Nottingham)

Category of performance	Number of children achieving each stage			
	Before implant	*12 months*	*36 months*	*60 months*
Use of telephone with known speaker	0	1	1	2
Understanding of conversation without lip reading	0	2	10	2
Understanding of common phrases without lip reading	0	7	12	0
Discrimination of some speech sounds without lip reading	0	50	2	1
Identification of environmental sounds	0	2	0	0
Response to speech sounds (e.g., "go")	4	0	0	0
Awareness of environmental sounds	8	0	0	0
No awareness of environmental sounds	77	0	0	0
Total number of children	89	62	25	5

Influences on progress

The question needs to be asked: why do some children not do so well as others? There is huge variation in outcomes amongst cochlear implant wearers and particularly amongst children; what has been found to influence progress? Some of the factors that may be significant have been mentioned in the previous section: age at onset, duration of deafness, length of use of the system, educational management. There are other factors which reside in the child, including medical factors, learning style, personality and the presence of other learning difficulties. There may, however, be other factors, related to the device itself: whether the device is worn, device functioning (internal and external hardware) and device programming. For benefit to be achieved the device must be worn consistently. Rose et al. (1996) report an incidence of 47% non-use in their study in the USA. In the author's study there are no cases of poor or non-use and it is important for teachers to encourage consistent use. These may, however, be device problems. In any sizeable paediatric programme there are likely to be some children underachieving because of problems with the internal or external devices. Processors must be monitored carefully, particularly before the child is able to listen and report any problems, and teachers and parents must be vigilant about daily checks of the system. There may be a problem with the internal device which may be more difficult to detect, especially if it is intermittent. The failure may be sudden, or there may be problems with electrodes happening over a period of years or months. It is vital that all teachers of the deaf are aware of this possibility and are able to monitor even subtle changes in listening skills which may reflect a potential problem with the device. It is equally vital that they, and parents, are in contact with an experienced centre which can identify and deal with the problem swiftly and sensitively. Experience indicates that re-implantation is likely to be possible and successful, and that the child should quickly achieve the levels of functioning previously attained.

The future

Although there is evidence of both the safety and efficacy of cochlear implantation, there remain questions and concerns to be answered. Amongst the questions are the ability to predict outcomes from implantation for children, to determine which tuning strategies and devices are the most effective, and the level and type of rehabilitative support which is appropriate. The concerns include:

- long term technical problems,
- long term funding arrangements,
- long term monitoring of device functioning,
- the availability of experienced staff and centres.

Cochlear implantation is an expensive procedure; Table 6.3 shows the prices of the Nottingham programme for the financial year 1997/98. It includes the costs of all spares and maintenance, and upgrading as necessary for external and internal parts. With growing demands on services, health-care purchasers are demanding information about the cost-effectiveness of cochlear implantation. Exploratory work in this area (Hutton, Politi and Seeger, 1995) indicates that paediatric implantation could be a cost-effective use of society's resources, if we consider long term educational and employment prospects. Davis, Fortnum and O'Donoghue (1995) recommend that the early rehabilitation factors for children, and the cost-effectiveness and educational benefits are researched urgently to facilitate future planning. The answers to these questions will only be available over a period of many years, and teachers and implant teams share the responsibility for ensuring that all children with implants are closely monitored. Teachers of the deaf must ensure that they have the skills and knowledge with which to fulfil this role, so that they can provide the best possible support for both the hearing aided and cochlear implanted children in their care.

Table 6.3 Programme costs and contents 1997–98: the Nottingham Paediatric Cochlear Implant Programme

Year 1: A minimum of eight full-day visits to Nottingham - £27,500

* Audiological assessment/ERA
* Medical assessment/CT scan
* Speech and language assessment involving visits to home and school.
* Preparation of child, family and local professionals by the implant team
* Surgical implantation
* Setting up and tuning of the device
* Medical checks
* Rehabilitation and monitoring of child's progress, and functioning of the device
* Monthly visits to home and school by members of the rehabilitation team
* Provision of an emergency service (spares/supplies/reasonable maintenance costs)

Years 2 and 3: A minimum of three full-day visits to Nottingham - £4,000

* Medical checks
* Tuning and monitoring of the device
* Rehabilitation and monitoring of child's progress, and functioning of the device
* Bi-monthly visits to home and school by members of the rehabilitation team
* Provision of an emergency service (spares/supplies/reasonable maintenance costs)

Annual maintenance: A minimum of one full-day visit to Nottingham - £2,300

* Audiological and medical checks and rehabilitation
* Annual visits to home and school by members of the rehabilitation team
* A replacement speech processor every six years as recommended by the manufacturer
* Provision of an emergency service (spares/supplies/reasonable maintenance costs)

References

Ajayi F, Garnham C, O'Donoghue EM (in press) Paediatric experience of the reliability of the Nucleus Mini 22 channel inplant, American Journal of Otology.

Archbold S (1992) The development of a paediatric cochlear implant programme; a case study British Journal of Teachers of the Deaf 16(1): 17-26.

Archbold S (1994a) Implementing a paediatric cochlear implant programme. In

McCormick B, Archbold S, Sheppard S (Eds) Cochlear Implants for Young Deaf Children. London:Whurr. pp 25-59.

Archbold S (1994b) Monitoring progress at the pre-verbal stage. In McCormick B, Archbold S, Sheppard S (Eds) Cochlear Implants for Young Deaf Children. London: Whurr. pp 197-213.

Archbold S, Tait M (1994) Rehabilitation: a practical approach. In McCormick B, Archbold S, Sheppard S (Eds) Cochlear Implants for Young Deaf Children. London: Whurr. pp 166-196

Archbold S, Robinson K (1997) Cochlear implantation, associated rehabilitation services and their educational implications: the UK and Europe. Journal British Association of Teachers of the Deaf 21: 34–41.

Archbold S, Robinson K (in press) A European perspective on paediatric cochlear implantation, rehabilitation services and their educational implications: the UK and Europe. American Journal of Otology.

Archbold S, Lutman M, Marshall D (1995) Categories of auditory performance. In Clark GM, Cowan RSC (Eds) Proceedings of the International Cochlear Implant, Speech and Hearing Symposium, Melbourne, 1994. Annals of Otology, Rhinolaryngology and Laryngology 104(9): 312-314.

BATOD (1995) Implant Centre Teachers of the Deaf: Guidelines for practice. Journal of the British Association of Teachers of the Deaf 19(5): 135-141. Teachers of the Deaf.

Beiter AL, Staller SJ, Dowell RC (1991) Evaluation and device programming in children. Ear and Hearing 12(4): 25S-33S.

Boothroyd A (1991) The assessment of speech perception capacity in profoundly deaf children. American Journal of Otology 12: 67S-72S.

British Deaf Association (1995) The BDA Policy on Cochlear Implants. Carlisle: BDA.

Chute PM (1993) Cochlear implants in adolescents. In Fraysse B, Deguine O (Eds) Cochlear Implants: New Perspectives. Basel: Karger. pp 210-215.

Clark GM (1997) Historical Perspectives. In Clark GM, Cowan RSC and Dowell RC (Eds) Cochlear Implantation in Infants and Children. San Diego: Singular Publishing Group Inc. pp 9-27

Clark GM, Cohen NL, Sheppard RK (1991) Surgical and safety considerations of multi-channel cochlear implants in children. Ear and Hearing 12: 15S-24S.

Clark GM, Cowan RSC, Dowell RC (1997) Cochlear implantation in Infants and Children. Singular Publishing Group Inc., San Diego: London.

Cohen NL, Waltzman SB, Fisher SG (1991) Prospective randomized clinical trial of advanced cochlear implants. Preliminary results of a department of veterans affairs cooperative study. Annals of Otology, Rhinolaryngology, Laryngology 100: 823-829.

Cohen NL, Waltzman SB, Fisher SG (1993) A prospective randomized study of cochlear implants. The New England Journal of Medicine 328: 233-237.

Cooper H (1991) Training and rehabilitation for cochlear implant users. In Cooper H (Ed) Cochlear Implants: A Practical Guide. London: Whurr.

Davis A, Fortnum H, O'Donoghue GM (1995) Children who could benefit from a cochlear implant: a European estimate of projected numbers, cost and relevant statistics. International Journal of Paediatric Otorhinolaryngology 31: 221-223.

Deguine O, Cormary X, Durrieu JP, Uziel AS, Fraysse B (1995) Comparison of human resources in adult and paediatric cochlear implant programme. In Uziel AS, Mondain M (Eds) Cochlear Implants in Children. Basel: Karger. pp195-201.

Dettman S, Dowell R, Barker E, Rance G, Hollow R, Cowan R, Galvin, Clark GM (1995) Results of multichannel cochlear implantation in very young children. Paper presented at the Third International Congress on Cochlear Implants, Paris, France.

Dewart H, Summers S (1988) Pragmatics Profile of Early Communication Skills. Windsor: NFER-Nelson.

Dyar D (1995) Assessing auditory and linguistic performances in low verbal implanted children. In Uziel AS, Mondain M (Eds) Cochlear Implants in Children. Basel: Karger. pp139-145.

Eisenburg LS (1985) Perceptual abilities with the cochlear implant: implications for aural rehabilitation. Ear and Hearing 6: 60S-69S.

Erber NP (1982) Auditory Training. Washington, DC: Alexander Graham Bell Association for the Deaf.

Fraser G (1991) The cochlear implant team. In Cooper H (Ed) Cochlear Implants: A Practical Guide. London:Whurr. pp 84-91.

Fryauf-Bertschy H (1992) Getting started at home. In Tye-Murray N (Ed) Cochlear Implants and Children: A Handbook for Parents and Teachers and Speech and Hearing Professionals. Washington DC: Alexander Graham Bell Association for the Deaf.

Geers AE, Moog JS (1989) Evaluating speech perception skills. In Owens E, Kesseler DK (Eds) Cochlear Implants in Young Deaf Children. Boston, MA: Little, Brown and Co. pp 227-256.

Geers AE, Moog JS (1991) Evaluating the benefits of cochlear implants in the educational setting. American Journal of Otology 12: 116-125.

Geers AE, Moog JS (1995) Impact of the cochlear implant on the educational setting. In Uziel AS, Mondain M (Eds) Cochlear Implants in Children. Basel: Karger. pp119-125.

Gibbin K, O'Donoghue GM (1994) Medical aspects of paediatric cochlear implantation. In McCormick B, Archbold S, Sheppard S (Eds) Cochlear Implants for Young Deaf Children. London:Whurr. pp 86-102.

Hellman SA, Chute PM, Krestchmer RE, Nevins ME, Parisier SC, Thurston LC (1991) The development of a children's implant profile. American Annals of the Deaf 136(2): 77-81.

House WF, Berliner KI (1991) Cochlear implants: from idea to clinical practice. In Cooper H (Ed) Cochlear Implants: A Practical Guide. London: Whurr. pp 9-33.

Hutton J, Politi C, Seeger T (1995) Cost-effectiveness of cochlear implantation of children. A preliminary model for the UK. In Uziel AS, Mondain M (Eds) Cochlear Implants in Children. Basel: Karger. pp 201-207.

Lane H (1994) The Cochlear implant controversy. World Federation of the Deaf News. No. 2-3.

Laurenzi C (1993) The bionic ear and the mythology of paediatric implants. British Journal of Audiology 27: 1-5.

Lesinski A, Hartrampf R, Dahm MC, Bertram B, Lenarz T (1995) Cochlear implantation in a population of multihandicapped children. In Clark GM, Cowan RSC (Eds) Proceedings of the International Cochlear Implant, Speech and Hearing Symposium, Melbourne, 1994. Annals of Otology, Rhinolaryngology and Laryngology 104(9): 332-334.

Lutman ME, Tait DM (1995) Early communicative behaviour in young children receiving cochlear implants:factor analysis of turn-taking and gaze orientation.

In Clark GM, Cowan RSC (Eds) Proceedings of the International Cochlear Implant, Speech and Hearing Symposium, Melbourne, 1994. Annals of Otology, Rhinolaryngology and Laryngology 104(9): 397-399.

Lutman ME, Archbold S, Gibbin KP, McCormick B, O'Donoghue GM (1996) Monitoring progress in young children with cochlear implants. In Allum-Mecklenburg DJ (Ed) Cochlear Implant Rehabilitation in Children and Adults. London: Whurr.

Mason SM (1994) Electrophysiological tests. In McCormick B, Archbold S, Sheppard S (Eds) Cochlear Implants for Young Children. London: Whurr. pp 103-139

Mason SM, Garnham CW, Sheppard S, O'Donoghue GM, Gibbin KP (1995) An intra-operative test protocol for objective assessment of the Nucleus 22-channel cochlear implant. In Uziel AS, Mondain M (Eds) Cochlear Implants in Children. Basel: Karger. pp 38-45.

McConkey Robbins A, Renshaw JJ, Berry SW (1991) Evaluating meaningful auditory integration in profoundly hearing-impaired children. American Journal of Otology 12: 144S-151S.

McCormick B (1977) The toy discrimination test: an aid for screening the hearing of children above the mental age of two years. Public Health (London) 91: 67-73.

McCormick B (1994) Suitability of implants for children under 5 years old. In McCormick B, Archbold S, Sheppard S (Eds) Cochlear Implants for Young Children. London: Whurr. pp 60-85.

McCormick B, Archbold S, Sheppard S (Eds) (1994) Cochlear Implants for Young Children. London: Whurr.

McKay C, McDermott H, Vandali A, Clark GM (1991) Preliminary results with a six spectral maxima sound processor for the University of Melbourne/Nucleus multiply electrode cochlear implant. Journal of the Otolaryngology Society of Australia 6(5): 354-359.

Mecklenburg DJ, Lehnhardt E (1991) The development of cochlear implants in Europe, Asia and Australia. In Cooper H (Ed) Cochlear Implants: A Practical Guide. London: Whurr. pp 34-58.

Miyamoto R, Robbins AM, Osberger MJ, Todd SL, Riley AI, Kirk KI (1995) Comparison of multichannel tactile aids and multichannel cochlear implants in children with profound hearing impairments. American Journal of Otology 16(1): 8-13.

Nevins ME, Chute PM (1995) The success of children with cochlear implants in mainstream settings. In Clark GM, Cowan RSC (Eds) Proceedings of the International Cochlear Implant, Speech and Hearing Symposium, Melbourne, 1994. Annals of Otology, Rhinolaryngology and Laryngology 104(9): 100-102.

Nevins ME, Chute PM (1995) Children with Cochlear Implants in Educational Settings. San Diego: Singular Publshing Group Inc.

Osberger MJ, Maso M, Sam LK (1993) Speech intelligibility of children with cochlear implants, tactile aids or hearing aids. Journal of Speech and Hearing Research 36: 186-203.

Osberger MJ, Miyamoto RT, Zimmerman-Phillips S, Kemink JL, Stoer BS, Firszt JB, Novak MA (1991a) Independent evaluation of speech production skills of children with the Nucleus 22-channel cochlear implant system. Ear and Hearing 12 (4): 66S-80S.

Osberger MJ, Robbins AM, Berry SW, Todd SL, Hesketh LJ, Sedey A (1991b) Analysis of the spontaneous speech samples of children with cochlear implants or tactile aids. American Journal of Otology 12: 151-164.

Parisier S, Chute PM, Popp AL (1995) Cochlear implant mechanical failures. Paper presented at the Third International Congress on Cochlear Implant, Paris, France.

Patrick JF, Clark GM (1991) The Nucleus 22-channel cochlear implant system. Ear and Hearing 12: 3S-9S.

Patrick JF, Seligman PM, Clark GM (1997) Engineering. In Clark GM, Cowan RSC, Dowell RC (Eds) Cochlear Implantation in Infants and Children. San Diego: Singular Publishing Group Inc. pp 125–145

Power DJ, Hyde MB (1992) The cochlear implant and the deaf community. Medical Journal of Australia 157: 421-422.

Quittner AL, Thompson Steck J, Rouiller RL (1991) Cochlear implants in children: a study of parental stress and adjustment. American Journal of Otology 12: 95-104.

Rance G and Dowell RC (1997) Speech processes. In Clark GM, Cowan RSC, Dowell RC (Eds) Cochlear Implantation in Infants and Children. San Diego: Singular Publishing Group Inc. pp 147–170

Roberts S (1991) Speech-processor fitting for cochlear implants. In Cooper H (Ed) Cochlear Implants: A Practical Guide. London: Whurr. pp 201-219.

Rose DE, Vernon M, Pool AF (1996) Cochlear Implants in Prelingually Deaf Children. American Ann Deaf 141: 3: 258–261.

Schindler RA, Kessler DK (1992) Preliminary results with the Clarion cochlear implant. Laryngoscope 102: 1006-1013.

Selmi A (1985) Monitoring and evaluating the educational effect of the cochlear implant. Ear and Hearing 6(3): 52S-59S.

Sheppard S (1994) Fitting and programming the external system. In McCormick B, Archbold S, Sheppard S (Eds) Cochlear Implants for Young Children. London:Whurr. pp 140-165.

Somers MN (1991) Effects of cochlear implantation in children; Implications for rehabilitation. In Cooper H (Ed) Cochlear Implants: A Practical Guide. London: Whurr.

Staller SJ, Beiter AL, Brimacombe JA, Mecklenburg DJ, Arnolt P (1991a) Paediatric performance with the Nucleus 22 channel cochlear implant system. American Journal of Otology 12: 126S-136S.

Staller SJ, Beiter AL, Brimacombe JA (1991b) Children and multichannel cochlear implants. In Cooper H (Ed) Cochlear Implants: A Practical Guide. London: Whurr. pp 283-321.

Summerfield AQ, Marshall DM (1995) Cochlear Implantation in the UK 1990-1994. London: HMSO.

Tait DM (1987) Making and monitoring progress in the pre-school years. Journal of the British Journal of Teachers of the Deaf 11(5): 143.

Tait DM, Lutman ME (1994) Comparison of early communicative behaviour in young children with cochlear implants and hearing aids. Ear and Hearing 15: 352-361.

Thelemeir MA (1984) Discrimination after Training. Los Angeles: House Ear Institute.

Tobey EA, Angelette S, Murchison C, Nicosia J, Sprague S, Staller S, Brimacombe JA, Beiter AL (1991) Speech production performance in children with multichannel cochlear implants. American Journal of Otology 12: 165S-173S.

Tye-Murray N (1993) Aural rehabilitation and patient management. In Tyler RS (Ed) Cochlear Implants: Audiological Foundations. London: Whurr. San Diego: Singular. pp 87-144.

Tyler R (1993) Cochlear implants and the deaf culture. American Journal of Audiology. March: 26-32.

Tyler RS, Tye-Murray N (1991) Cochlear implant signal-processing strategies and patient perception of speech and environmental sounds. In Cooper H (Ed) Cochlear Implants: A Practical Guide. London: Whurr. pp 58-83.

Tyler RS, Moore BCJ, Kuk FK (1989) Performance of some of the better cochlear-implant patients. Journal of Speech and Hearing Research 32: 887-911.

Vernon M, Alles CD (1994) Issues in the use of cochlear implants with prelingually deaf children. American Annals of the Deaf 139(5): 485-492.

Waltzman SB, Cohen NL, Shapiro WH (1992) Use of a multichannel cochlear implant in the congenital and prelingually deaf population. Laryngoscope 102: 395-399.

Waltzman SB, Cohen NL, Gomolin RH, Shapiro WH, Ozdamar SR, Hoffman RA (1994) Long-term results of early cochlear implantation in congenitally and prelingually deafened children. American Journal of Otology 15(2) 9-13.

Waltzman SB, Cohen NL, Gomolin RH, Shapiro WH, Ozdamar SR, Hoffman RA (1995) Effects of short-term deafness in young children implanted with the Nucleus cochlear prosthesis. In Clark GM, Cowan RSC (Eds) Proceedings of the International Cochlear Implant, Speech and Hearing Symposium, Melbourne, 1994. Annals of Otology, Rhinolaryngology and Laryngology 104(9): 341S-342S.

Webster A (1992) Images of deaf children as learners. In Cline T (Ed) The Assessment of Special Educational Needs: International Perspectives. London: Routledge.

Wilson B (1993) Signal processing. In Tyler RS (Ed) Cochlear Implants: Audiological Foundations. London: Whurr. San Diego: Singular. pp 35-86

Young NM, Johnson JC, Mets MB, Hain TC (1995) Cochlear implants in young children with Usher's syndrome. In Clark GM, Cowan RSC (Eds) Proceedings of the International Cochlear Implant, Speech and Hearing Symposium, Melbourne, 1994. Annals of Otology, Rhinolaryngology and Laryngology. 104(9): 342S-345S.

Chapter 7
Tactile Aids

W McCRACKEN

Introduction

For those involved in the education of deaf children, tactile perception of speech is not a new concept. Teachers of the deaf have historically used a variety of resonators to provide additional sensory information for profoundly deaf children. It was the pioneering work of Gault and his colleagues working in the 1920s, which led to the development of the first electrical device designed to deliver the speech signal to the skin. Research has, since then, been sporadic and many questions remain to be answered. The advent of cochlear implantation gave added impetus to tactile aid research as a non-invasive alternative for those with profound deafness. As knowledge of tactile perception, the physiology of the skin, and processing strategies increases, the range of alternatives also increases. Teachers of the deaf need to have an understanding of tactile aids, in respect of the processes involved, the device characteristics, research findings with pre-lingually deaf children, and training requirements. The ability of those professionals involved to deliver an educational programme, whatever the setting, will depend upon a clear understanding of the possible benefits and the constraints of employing tactile devices. This chapter will give consideration to the challenge of sensory substitution, the development of tactile aids and their characteristic features, candidacy, training needs and strategies and the research outcomes in relation to deaf children's utilisation of tactile aids.

Tactile aids provide information about:

- environmental and speech sounds,
- intensity,
- rhythm,
- duration,
- speed of delivery,
- spectral envelope, depending on the specific device,

- presence and absence of voicing,
- presence and absence of sibilant sounds.

(Smith, 1991)

At present tactile devices do not provide:

- sound localisation,
- access to environmental sounds where there is steady background noise,
- open set speech perception,
- spontaneous perception of spoken language in an unstructured speech environment.

(Perryman, 1992; Osberger et al., 1990)

A comparison between cochlear implants and tactile aids

Since the first child was implanted with a single-channel cochlear device in 1980, developments have been rapid. Both electrical and tactile devices aim to provide access to acoustic information that is unavailable via acoustic aids. Inevitably, comparisons concerning the efficacy of these devices are made. Whilst the decision concerning the most appropriate form of amplification will always involve a range of factors, some basic differences between cochlear implants and tactile aids should be noted:

- Tactile aids are non-invasive and carry no associated medical risk.
- Tactile aids use the skin and somatosensory system to perceive a processed auditory signal; this modality is comparatively restricted in its capacity to transduce auditory information. Cochlear implants make use of the auditory system, which is physiologically finely tuned for the perception of auditory information.
- Both types of device are body worn aids to hearing and are subject to the deleterious effect of background noise.
- Both types of device can be used in conjunction with an FM system. The cosmetic implications of employing an FM system with either device are considerable.
- There are formal protocols regarding the choice of candidates for implantation which involve a multi-disciplinary team (see Chapter 6). The situation regarding tactile aids is largely undefined.
- Cochlear implants replace other forms of amplification; tactile aids are used in conjunction with other forms of amplification.
- Cochlear implants are worn throughout a child's waking hours; tactile aids are often used only within a school setting. Experience of an alternative form of amplification is quantitatively different.

- In direct contrast to cochlear implants, tactile aids can provide access to suprasegmental and segmental aspects of speech, but do not provide open set recognition of words without speechreading.
- The cost of a tactile aid is approximately one tenth of a cochlear implant. It may well be that when the full costs of appropriate habilitation programmes are compared, the cost differential is far less.

Whilst the children who make use of electrical and tactile devices are audiologically similar, the devices used, the way in which candidates are identified, the type and level of support and the potential of such devices and their method of employment are markedly different.

Sensory substitution

Sensory substitution refers to a system where information normally received by one modality is transformed and received via another. The most familiar example of sensory substitution is Braille, where a code of raised dots is used to represent the written word. In this case touch is used as a substitute for vision. In the case of tactile hearing aids, touch is used in place of audition. The skin is used as a substitute for the cochlea to transduce vibrotactile information and to transmit electrical messages to the cortex. Touch has been described as "the variety of sensations evoked by stimulation of the skin resulting from mechanical, thermal, chemical or electrical events" (Cholewiak and Collins, 1991). Readers are referred to Cholewiak and Collins (1991) for detailed discussion of the mechanical and physiological characteristics of the skin. The cutaneous end organs thought to be responsible for transducing tactile stimuli into neural signals are illustrated in Figure 7.1.

The skin has a range of specialised receptors:

- Mechanoreceptors which respond to deformation of the receptor itself or an adjacent cell (for example, pressure on the surface of the skin causing a small indentation would result in the stimulation of these receptors).
- Thermoreceptors which respond to changes in temperature.
- Nociceptors which respond to physical or chemical damage to cell tissue ('noci' referring to noxious inputs).

Tactile aids may be either vibrotactile or electrotactile. Vibrotactile devices stimulate the sense receptors within the skin utilising a mechanical transducer. Electrotactile devices stimulate the underlying nerve fibres by means of an electrical current delivered to the skin surface. The skin itself acts as a low-pass band filter, being sensitive to a frequency range of 10–500 Hz (Keidel, 1974). A comparison between

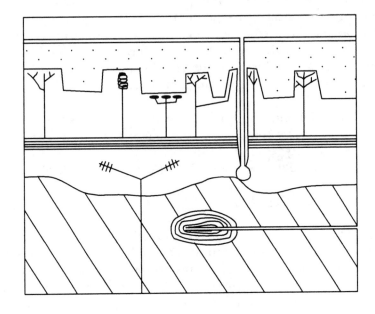

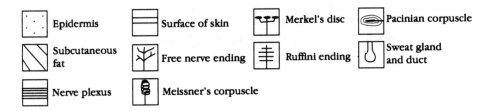

Figure 7.1 A simplified diagram of non-glaborous skin illustrating some of the sensory receptors thought to be responsible for tactile perception

auditory and tactile modalities in relation to the perception of auditory stimuli is given in Figure 7.2.

This illustrates the challenge presented to the effective design of tactile aids in seeking to substitute tactile perception for auditory perception. The ability of the tactile system to discriminate frequency, temporal cues and intensity cues in relation to the auditory system is very limited. The decision on how to present an auditory signal via a tactile device to ensure that the wearer obtains optimum benefit is controversial. While tactile aids supplement acoustic information provided through hearing aids, as well as visual information, they are not a substitute for other modes of sensory information. Tactile aids do provide access to information that may otherwise be inaudible or non-visible.

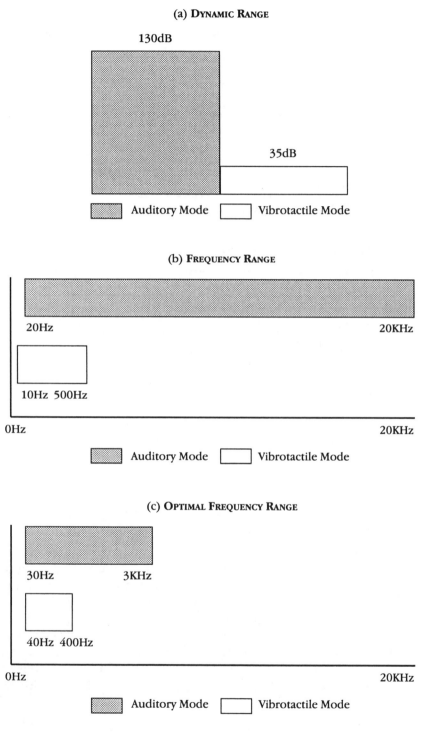

Figure 7.2 A comparison of auditory and tactile senses in relation to the perception of acoustic variables

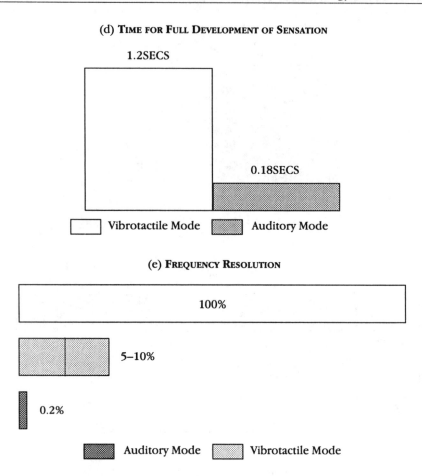

Figure 7.2 (continued) A comparison of auditory and tactile senses in relation to the perception of acoustic variables

Device design

The Teletactor designed by Gault (1926, 1934) employed a high quality microphone with an amplifier and a receiver in the form of a vibrator unit to deliver a speech signal to the skin. Despite the restrictions of the skin in resolving information above 300 Hz, the results of studies were promising. Gault suggested that the tactile channel had the potential to provide beneficial information to aid deaf learners in accessing the speech signal. Carhart (1935) reports on a group of eight deaf children who were followed for a study period of three years. A desk-top device was employed. The extended experience of tactile information is reported to have resulted in:

- an improvement in the children's ability to lip read,
- an increased awareness within a range of sounds,

- an ability to monitor their own voice,
- an improvement in aspects of voice production.

(Goodfellow, 1934)

At this time relatively little was known about the physiology of the skin. Despite the gross nature of the signal delivered to the skin, Gault was able to demonstrate that tactile information could be used to enhance speechreading ability. In developing tactile devices to aid in speech reception, researchers have considered the features of speech that would be most appropriately extracted from the auditory signal and presented via the tactile channel. This is an area in which there is no consensus, and research continues to seek to identify the aspects of the speech signal which it is most beneficial to extract and recode into tactile information. Bernstein notes that "In theory, for a tactile aid to be as effective as an auditory signal, not only must the signal processing preserve the critical speech information, but the tactile psycho-physical display must be designed to convey this information to the skin". A hierarchy of listening tasks illustrating finer and finer degrees of analysis of the input stimulus is described by Weisenberger and Miller (1987). In the case of tactile perception of sound, the poor ability of this system to transduce an acoustic signal would appear to be a major stumbling block. Research and experience in this area suggest that, as a supplement to visual information, tactile information can play a major role in enhancing comprehension of spoken discourse. The interested reader is referred to Soderlund, 1995.

Coding approaches

Two approaches are employed in delivering the acoustic signal to the skin: direct and processing. In the case of the direct approach, the acoustic signal is delivered to the skin and the problem of extracting useful information is left to the sense of touch. The relatively poor information transfer afforded by the skin presents some problems to this approach. All high frequency information will be lost because the skin is unable to transmit information above 500Hz. In the processing approach, specific features of the acoustic signal are selected as being of importance in the perception of speech. These features are extracted, coded and presented to the skin. This strategy aims to ensure that the most salient features of the speech signal are presented to the skin. There are a variety of coding approaches, and the interested reader is referred to Summers, 1992.

Single, dual and multi-channel devices

Tactile devices vary in the number of channels that are used to present acoustic information to the skin. Single-channel aids convey information via a single transducer, dual-channel aids utilise two transducers and multi-channel aids employ a number of channels; seven – sixteen or more, depending on the specific device. Acoustic information is received from the immediate environment and filtered into a number of channels. Each channel transmits a signal to the skin. In dual and multi-channel devices, frequency differences are signalled by place of stimulation. Intensity within the acoustic signal is signalled by a corresponding change in channel intensity. It may initially appear obvious that multi-channel devices offer more information and would therefore have greater potential in delivering information about an acoustic signal. The research is not conclusive on this matter (Carney, 1988; Plant, 1989; Kishon-Rabin, Hanin and Boothroyd, 1990). Controversially, some research suggests that there is no clear benefit from multi-channel aids in the perception of connected speech (Spens, 1995). It appears that an increase in the number of channels may result in masking effects which diminish the gains that might have otherwise been expected from additional channels (Huss and Spens, 1996).

User controls

Tactile aids incorporate a range of features and user controls. The microphone may be built into the speech processor or may operate as a satellite microphone. Satellite microphones offer the opportunity for an effective voice-to-tactile-signal link. In the case of Tactaid systems, the microphone is powered by a battery separate from the speech processor. The processor frequently incorporates a rechargeable Ni-Cad battery that will recharge overnight. Devices frequently employ automatic noise suppression circuitry and the majority additionally have automatic gain control circuitry. User controls allow for individual setting of a number of features. The intensity control is set to determine the strongest vibration generated by the transducers. The sensitivity control sets the threshold for the quietest sound to be delivered to the unit and determines the level at which background noise is introduced.

The following user controls are found on tactile aids:

M	microphone setting for normal use
T	to allow for use with induction based devices, e.g., loops, telephones
MT	to allow for signals to be received from the M and T settings simultaneously.
ON/OFF	switch
Indicators	Several systems use light emitting diodes (LED) to indicate when the aid is in use, and to provide other status indications.

In the case of Tactaid 7, an LED display situated on top of the processor provides visual representation of the pattern of stimulation being delivered to the seven transducers, and also allows faulty transducers to be identified and appropriate remedial action taken. An eighth LED indicates when the battery is functioning below the optimum level. The auxiliary input jack can be used to connect the device to a satellite microphone, FM system or tape recorder. The skin transducer will be attached to the device via the output jack and an appropriate lead. In the case of single and dual-channel aids, the transducer/s are attached to the skin by a strap. In the case of Tactaid 7, the vibrator array is housed in a cloth sleeve which is then held in place by a harness. It is important to ensure close contact of the transducers with the skin. The microphone and transducers should be physically separated to avoid the possibility of feedback problems, indicated by a buzzing noise. Similar problems of feedback may occur if the transducers are in close contact with a hard surface. Dual and multi-channel aids should always be worn with the transducers in the same position, for example, the Tactaid 7 array should always be worn in the same orientation – low vibrator on the left, high frequency vibrator on the right. All devices should include clear trouble-shooting guidelines, and the audiologist and teacher of the deaf should feel confident in their management of tactile devices. As with any form of amplification, there should be a range of spares readily available to ensure continuity of sensory experience.

Single-channel	Dual-channel	Multi-channel
TAM	TACTAID 11 +	TACTAID 7
Input signal modulated @ 190 Hz Input sensitivity control External mic. jack Internal omnidirectional mic. LED signal indicator Telecoil Rechargeable battery or disposable GMS types PX625N	Channel 1 100–1800 Hz] AM Channel 2 1500–100000 Hz] Input signal modulated @ 250 Hz Input sensitivity control Output sensitivity control Automatic gain control Automatic noise suppression Ext. output jack – satellite mic FM, tape. Rechargeable battery	Channel 1: 200–400 Hz Channel 2: 400–600 Hz F1 Channel 3: 600–800 Hz Channel 4: 800–1200 Hz Channel 5: 1200–1600 Hz Channel 6: 1600–3000 Hz F2 Channel 7: 3000–7000 Hz AM: input signal modulated @ 250 Hz Automatic gain control Automatic noise suppression internal mic
MINIVIB 4	TRILL	

Input signal modulated @ 220 Hz
Input sensitivity control
Noise suppression circuitry
for continuous noise
Mic can be used for isolation or
Telecoil and mic.
AA battery or rechargeable
	Mode 2: Channel 1 <2500 Hz] AM
	          Channel 2 > 2500 Hz]
	input encoded @ 250 Hz
	
	Mode 3: Channel 1 <2500 Hz
	@ 150 Hz; >2500 Hz @ 250 Hz
	          Channel 2 – all
	          frequencies unmodulated
	Automatic gain control
	Automatic noise suppression
	ext output jack for satellite mic
	FM, tape
	Rechargeable battery
		LED display verifying signal
		Ext output jack for
		Satellite mic, FM, tape
		Rechargeable battery

Figure 7.3 Examples of single, dual and multi-channel tactile device characteristics

Information available via a tactile device

Early vibrotactile devices aimed to provide information on time and intensity cues, as they were known, to enhance speechreading performance. More recent developments aim to provide access to some of the spectral cues of speech (Osberger et al., 1990).

Candidates for tactile aids

There are two contrasting approaches to the use of tactile devices with children. The National Acoustic Laboratories (NAL) in Australia considered that tactile devices should be available to all those children who showed little benefit from conventional acoustic amplification. In the period 1986-1990, 18.8% of all profoundly deaf children in three states in Australia were recommended for fitting (Plant, 1992) (see Tables 7.1 and 7.2).

Table 7.1 Audiometric test results for 149 children recommended for tactile aids by NAL audiologists*

	Test Frequency (kHz)				
	0.25	0.5	1	2	4
Number of responses	104	86	40	12	3
Mean (dBSPL)	95.1	108.4	113.2	111.2	95.0
Range (dBSPL)	75-110	90-120	95-120	80-120	70-110

*the thresholds given are for each child's better ear.

Table 7.2 Aided thresholds for 148 children recommended for tactile aids by NAL audiologists*

	Test Frequency (kHz)				
	0.25	0.5	1	2	4
Number of responses	91	69	44	14	3
Mean (dBSPL)	72.75	70.4	63.5	65.0	55.0
Range (dBSPL)	60-105	45-110	45-85	50-80	50-60

*the thresholds given are for each child's better ear.

Recommended (G Plant):-	250Hz	500Hz	1kHz	2kHz
aided threshold levels>	70 dBSPL	65 dBSPL	60 dBSPL	55 dBSPL

Tactile aids were always used as a supplement to conventional amplification. Specific 'at risk' criteria were established in identifying candidates who would potentially benefit from tactile devices:

- Audiometric data, responses within the vibrotactile range.
- Aided thresholds greater than 70 dBSPL @ 250 Hz, 65 dBSPL @ 500 Hz, 60 dBSPL @ 1 kHz, 55 dBSPL @ 2 kHz.
- Speech test results, typically able to detect vowels and voiced consonants, but not voiceless fricatives, difficulty with identifying syllable number, able to discriminate long versus short vowels but unable to discriminate contrasts on higher level tasks.
- Aided and unaided lip reading, the lack of appropriate test materials for younger deaf children restricted assessment in this area.
- Subjective reports from parents and family members – the need to follow a structured training programme makes it essential that parents, teachers and therapists understand the implications for supporting the use of tactile devices.

(Plant, 1992).

The NAL approach contrasts sharply with that of the Mailman Center in Florida. This programme encourages all the severely and profoundly deaf children in their project to utilise tactual vocoders to supplement information gained from conventional acoustic aids. For those children who are deemed unsuitable for implantation, tactile aids offer an alternative avenue of learning.

Additionally it is important that children who are waiting for consideration by a cochlear implant team are provided with access to the acoustic environment and ongoing support. A tactile aid can be used to bridge the gap between acoustic aids and cochlear implants. Not only does this allow a child to develop skills in attending to auditory stimuli, but it also encourages the use of a body worn device and sets the scene for ongoing habilitation sessions.

For children who are learning in a sign language environment, the ultimate goal is one of competent bilingualism, allowing individuals to move along the communication continuum. In communicating with non-signing individuals, tactile aids offer access to aspects of the spoken word that are visually unavailable. In addition, tactile aids provide access to the immediate acoustic environment, alerting individuals to changes that may otherwise be missed. For those with a profound hearing loss, tactile aids may offer a feeling of 'connectedness' to the world (Weisenberger, 1992).

There is a small, but nevertheless important, group of deaf children who offer a major challenge to the field of audiology. These children have a range of complex learning needs compounded by a hearing loss. Identification of auditory status may be very difficult. Proving appropriate amplification is similarly challenging. Within this group, some children will find the insertion of an earmould distressing and may show prolonged and determined resistance. Any form of amplification should be seen as an aid to communication. An aid which causes disengagement is failing in this basic role. For this group of children, a tactile aid offers the chance of engaging in simple awareness and detection work whilst working on a desensitisation programme.

The ability to offer sensory input at a distance can be used to focus the child away from themselves and allow contact with the outside world. The danger of exceeding comfortable listening levels with acoustic hearing aids is also overcome. Whilst the aim would always be to establish appropriate amplification, it is essential that time is not lost. The communication channels for children who face the greatest challenges in making sense of their learning environment are of critical importance. The longer this is delayed the greater the task that faces both the child and the professionals responsible for ensuring an optimum learning environment.

Training approaches for tactile aids

Research suggests that an appropriate training programme is essential if children are to gain maximum benefit from tactile aids (Plant, 1995). In the case of a blind child learning Braille, the need for training would be obvious; there appears to be some confusion in the case of tactile 'hearing' aids. The financial implications of cochlear implantation include the cost of the provision of a rehabilitation programme. For children fitted with tactile devices, who are within the same audiological category as those receiving implants, the provision of a teacher or therapist who is responsible for training seldom appears to be seen as essential. This group of children are employing sensory substitution to access the acoustic environment. The responsibility for ensuring an individual programme is developed for each child lies with the audiologist, teacher of the deaf, and speech and language therapist.

Structured tactile training programmes

A number of structured programmes (Plant, 1989; Franklin, 1989; McConkey Robbins et al., 1993; Vergara and Miskiel, 1994) have been developed. Programmes are developed either in relation to the use of a specific device to take advantage of device design, or to provide a comprehensive developmental curriculum in relation to the use of acoustic, electronic and tactile aids (Vergara and Miskiel, 1994).

The **Tactaid II training programme** (Plant, 1989) was designed specifically for use with children using the Tactaid II, a dual-channel vibrotactile device, now superseded by the Tactaid II + (Figure 7.4). The programme covers four areas:

- Sound detection exercises.
- Tactile pattern perception exercises.
- Word syllable number and type exercises.
- High frequency detection exercises.

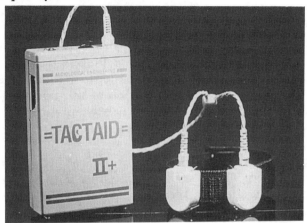

Figure 7.4 Tactaid II+, an example of a dual-channel vibrotactile device (reproduced with permission of Audiological Engineering)

The programme follows an analytical approach. It includes record sheets and a suggested developmental sequence. Plant suggests that 10 minutes' individual work per day should be available for specific training, but that children should wear the devices throughout the day.

The **Tactaid reference guide and orientation (TARGO)** was developed by McConkey Robbins et al. (1993) to support the use of the Tactaid 7 vibrotactile device. This provides a comprehensive guide to the use, care, maintenance and management of the Tactaid 7. Information relating to the in-service training required by teachers and other therapists and to management approaches with reluctant users are discussed. The training programme is divided by age into four groups: 0–3 years, 3–6 years, 6–9 years, and 9–12 years. The programme details learning goals, device related goals and parent–teacher goals at each level and for each age group. The programme includes:

- exposure, 0–6 years only,
- detection, all groups,
- beginning pattern perception, all groups,
- advanced pattern perception, all groups,
- segmental pattern perception, all groups.

The activity sequence key section provides a range of teaching suggestions for parents and teachers to use with the Tactaid 7.

The **Miami cochlear implant, auditory and tactile skills curriculum (CHATS)** (Vergara and Miskiel, 1994) presents an alternative approach by providing a comprehensive training manual for use with children utilising a range of sensory aids to assist in the development of speech perception and production. The programme focuses on the need to ensure that information offered to children is accessible. In order to make effective use of tactile information, it is important that individuals are able to synthesise a variety of inputs. A simple analogy of this is when a film sound track is out of synchronisation with the visual lip pattern – even a slight mismatch will be perceived by the viewer and temporarily disrupt the flow of information. For children employing tactile aids, the extra sensory information should add to that already available, rather than compete with it. The Miami programme initially uses a multi-modal approach, including auditory, visual and tactile channels. The programme develops awareness of specific sensory channels by employing uni-modal tasks, i.e., where only one of the senses is employed. This is complemented by training in dual sense tasks, for example auditory/tactile, tactile/visual.

A specific goal of the programme is to encourage multi-modal perception, where supplementary sensory information is integrated and enhances a child's learning. An interesting feature of the Miami project is the incorporation of sign language. Sign is not presented simultaneously with speech. For specific parts of each day, children are taught in sign language. The use of sign alone allows for fast efficient communication incorporating the full range of sign language structures, including non-manual markers. "Speech success is spurred on by rapid growth of sign language knowledge, and hinges on a curriculum designed accurately to predict the sequence of progress that can be expected for deaf children through various speech communication skills" (Oller et al., 1995).The programme actively encourages teachers to develop complementary activities that relate to the specific interests of individual children. Tasks are divided into receptive and expressive areas and are hierarchical in nature:

- Receptive: awareness, discrimination, recognition and comprehension.
- Expressive: imitation, initiative.

The programme aims to establish phonological foundations that characterise early vocal play and then to move on to training suprasegmental features and segmental training. A developmental approach is followed in order to decide the sequence in which sounds are taught (Ingram, 1976; Oller and Eilers, 1981; Locke, 1983, cited in Oller et al., 1995). As children develop their skills in utilising tactile information within specific tasks, the programme moves on to generalisation in a broader communicative framework. A full range of activities, progress charts, evaluation procedures, and a parents/infants supplement are included. The interested reader is referred to Oller et al., 1995.

Learning outcomes

Proctor (1995) provides an excellent overview in a summary of the research that has been undertaken in relation to the use of tactile aids with deaf children. Benefits are considered under five headings:

- Sound perception.
- Sound discrimination.
- Speechreading.
- Speech production.
- Communication.

Learning outcomes with single-channel aids:

- Increased awareness of sound, suprasegmental aspects of speech and discrimination of vowels (Sheehy and Hansen, 1983), developed awareness of own speech and speech of others (Geers, 1986).
- Ability to distinguish syllabic patterns and voicing (Boothroyd, 1972).
- Enhanced speechreading performance (Plant, 1979; Goldstein, Jr. and Proctor, 1985; Geers, 1986).
- Improved suprasegmental qualities of speech (Neate, 1972; Sheehy and Hansen, 1983; Geers, 1986).
- Rapid rate of lexical acquisition (Goldstein, Jr. and Proctor, 1983).
- Improved rate of language acquisition (Proctor and Goldstein, Jr., 1983; Geers, 1986).

Learning outcomes with dual-channel tactile aids:

- Awareness of environmental sounds and own voice.
- Discrimination of the suprasegmental aspects of speech and syllabic patterns, discrimination scores comparable with those obtained by subjects with single and 22 channel cochlear implant (Osberger et. al., 1990).
- Enhanced speechreading performance (Lynch et al., 1989).
- Increased levels of vocalisation (Smith, 1991), increased intelligibility (Osberger et al., 1990).

Learning outcomes with multi-channel tactile aids:

- Ability to discriminate a range of environmental sounds (Scilley, 1980), improved feature perception (Brooks et al., 1987; Alcantra et al., 1990).
- Ability to achieve fine speech discrimination (Engleman and Rosov, 1975).
- Enhanced visual reception of isolated words and connected discourse (Scilley, 1980; Kozma-Spytek and Weisenberger, 1987).

- Increased speech intelligibility (Franklin and Saunders, 1981; Oller et al., 1986), increased amounts of vocalisation (Goldstein and Stark, 1976).
- Improvement in perception of conversational skills, syntax and semantics (Friel-Patti and Roeser, 1983).

Placement of tactile aids

A number of body sites have been investigated in order to ascertain the optimum location for the delivering information that will help in the perception of speech. These include the hand, wrist, forearm, neck, back and abdomen. A recent study involving the use of a multi-channel tactile device confirmed the findings of earlier studies in identifying the fingertips as being the most sensitive. The neck, forearm, back and abdomen follow in order of reduction in sensitivity (Connelly et al., 1995). There are a range of factors that may influence the effectiveness of a tactile device, in relation to placement, cited in this study:

- the degree of innervation,
- the amount of fatty tissue,
- the ability to stimulate bone rather than muscle,
- comfort and acceptability.

Ergonomically and ethically there are constraints on the placement of tactile transducers. Whilst the fingers are the most sensitive area, making use of this sensitivity is impractical. Children are actively involved in exploring their immediate environment in a range of activities including painting, water play, building and writing; this compromises the use of the most sensitive area and forces a more pragmatic approach to transducer placement. The practical problems faced by children in making effective use of cumbersome equipment should not be underestimated. Children working within a specialised school facility may accept relatively bulky equipment. However, within the UK, the vast majority of children with severe and profound hearing losses are educated within the mainstream of education. Placement of a tactile array on the chest or abdomen may present a considerable problem in this situation.

Discussion

Since the early work of Gault (1926), tactile aids have been recognised as an important adjunct to conventional acoustic aids for children with profound deafness. Many challenges yet remain if children are to be provided with a miniaturised tactile device which gives access to the fine spectral aspects of the speech signal. Indeed, what portion of the speech signal should be made available through tactile perception, to aid in the development of communication skills, remains a subject of research. Tactile aids can, however, function as extremely effective supplements to learning for severely and profoundly deaf children. In the early stages of establishing vocal play, in developing awareness of voice quality and enhancing the perception of speech, tactile aids can support the development of listening skills. Later, in enhancing speechreading performance and encouraging expressive skills, tactile devices offer support in providing a complementary route to communication. The challenges which remain are considerable. It is inappropriate to view tactile aids as the 'end of the line' when all other amplification options have been exhausted. There is sufficient research to support the early use of tactile aids with deaf children, as a supplement to acoustic aids. There is a pressing need for the habilitation needs of children using tactile aids to be recognised, agreed and implemented. In the face of such a challenge there is a need to establish the rights of this group of children to the support of a comprehensive, multi-disciplinary team over an extended period. Training for all those concerned in the use of tactile aids as a supplement to learning is essential.

The efficient use of tactile aids will be heavily dependent on the audiologist and teacher of the deaf in ensuring that an appropriate programme of training is implemented. A growing body of research demonstrates the benefits of utilising tactile devices within education programmes for deaf children. It is essential that the professionals involved ensure multi-disciplinary research continues and that knowledge is shared to enhance the learning opportunities offered to pre-lingually deaf children.

References

Alcantra JI, Blamey PJ, Cowan RSC, Clarke GM(1990) Speech feature recognition by profoundly hearing impaired children using a multiple-channel electrotactile speech processor and aid residual hearing. Journal of Acoustical Society of America 88:1260-1273.

Boothroyd A (1972) Sensory aids research project at the Clarke school for the deaf. In Fant G (Ed) Speech Communication Ability and Profound Deafness. Washington, DC: AG Bell Association. pp 367-377.

Brooks PL, Frost BJ, Mason JL, Gibson JJ (1987) Word and feature identification by profoundly deaf teenagers using the Queen's University tactile vocoder. Journal of Speech and Hearing Research 30: 137-141.

Carhart R (1935) A method of using the Gault-Teletactor. American Annals of the Deaf 80: 260-263.

Carney AE (1988). Vibrotactile perception of suprasegmental features of speech: A comparison of single and multichannel instruments. Journal of Speech and Hearing Research 31: 348-448.

Cholewiak RW, Collins AA (1991). Sensory and physiological bases of touch. In Heller MA, Schiff WR (Eds) The Psychology of Touch. Hillsdale, NJ: Lawrence Erblaum Associates. pp 23-60.

Connelly K, Addison MA, Sentelik MS (1995) Assessment of body sites for the optimum placement of multichannel tactile aids for the deaf. Paper presented at the 18th International Congress on the Education of the Deaf, Tel Aviv, Israel.

Engleman S, Rosov R (1975) Tactual hearing experiments with deaf and hearing subjects. Exceptional Child 41: 243-253.

Franklin B (1989) A Tactaid II Training Program for Deaf Blind Children. San Francisco: San Francisco State University.

Franklin B, Saunders FA (1981) The use of tactile aids with the deaf. Paper presented at the American Speech-Language-Hearing Association, Los Angeles, CA, USA.

Friel-Patti S, Roeser RJ (1983) Evaluating changes in the communication skills of deaf children using vibrotactile stimulation. Ear and Hearing 4: 31-40.

Gault RH (1926) Touch as a substitute for hearing in the interpretations and control of speech. Archives of Otolaryngology 3: 121-135.

Gault RH (1934) An interpretation of vibrotactile phenomena. Journal of the Acoustical Society of America 5: 252-254.

Geers AE (1986) Vibrotactile stimulation: Case study with a profoundly deaf child. Journal of Rehabilitation Research and Development 1: 111-117.

Goldstein MH Jr, Proctor A (1985) Tactile aids for profoundly deaf children. Journal of the Acoustical Society of America 77: 258-265.

Goldstein MH, Stark RE (1976) Modifications of vocalizations of pre-school deaf children by vibrotactile and visual displays. Journal of the Acoustical Society of America 59: 282-286.

Goodfellow LD (1934) Experiments on senses of touch and vibration. Journal of the Acoustical Society of America 6: 45-50.

Huss C, Spens K-E (1996) Radial and tangential tactile stimulation; some masking aspects. Paper presented at the International Sensory Aid Conference, Sint-Michielsgestel, The Netherlands.

Ingram D (1976) Phonological Disability in Children. New York: Elsevier.

Keidel WD (1974) The cochlear model in skin stimulation. In Geldard FA (Ed) Cutaneous Communication Systems and Devices. Austin,TX: Psychonomic Society. pp 676-673.

Kishon-Rabin L, Hanin L, Boothroyd A (1990) Lipreading enhancement by a spatial tactile display of fundamental frequency. Paper presented at the International Conference on Tactile Aids, Hearing Aids and Cochlear Implants, Sydney, Australia.

Kozma-Spytek L, Weisenberger JM (1987) Evaluation of a multichannel electrotactile aid for the hearing impaired: A case study. Paper presented at the Meeting of the Acoustical Society of America, November, Miami,Fl. Journal of the Acoustical Society of America 82: 523.

Locke JL (1983) Phonological Acquisition and Change. New York:Academic Communication Options. San Diego:College Hill Press.

Lynch MP, Eilers RE, Oller DK, Cobo-Lewis AB (1989) Multisensory speech perception by profoundly hearing impaired children. Journal of Speech and Hearing Disorders 54: 57-67.

McConkey Robbins A, Hesketh LJ, Bivins C (1993) Tactaid 7 Reference Guide and Orientation (TARGO). Somerville, MA: Audiological Engineering Corporation.

Neate DM (1972) The use of tactile aids in the teaching of speech to profoundly deaf children. The Teacher of the Deaf 70:137-146.

Oller DK, Eilers RE (1981) A pragmatic approach to phonological systems of deaf speakers. In Lass N (Ed) Speech and Language Advances in Research and Practice. New York:Academic Press 6: 103-141.

Oller DK, Eilers RE, Vergara KC, LaVoie EF (1986) Tactual vocoders in a multisensory program training speech production and reception.Volta Review 88: 21-36.

Oller DK, Vergara K, Eilers RE (1995) Education of deaf children with tactual aids:the Miami Experience. In Plant G, Spens K-E (Eds) Profound Deafness and Speech Communication. London: Whurr. pp 89-110.

Osberger MJ, Miyamoto RT, Robbins AM, Renshaw JJ, Berry SW, Myers WA, Kessler K, Pope ML (1990) Performance of deaf children with cochlear implants and vibro-tactile aids. Journal of American Academy of Audiology 1: 7-10.

Perryman PR (1992) Tactile Sensory Aids for Hearing Impaired Children in New Zealand. A resource guide for parents, educators, speech/language therapists, advisers on deaf children and audiologists. Christchurch, NZ: Van Asch College.

Plant G (1979) The use of tactile supplements in the rehabilitation of the deafened: A case study. Australian Journal of Audiology 1: 76-82.

Plant G (1989) Tactaid II Training Program. Sydney: National Acoustic Laboratories.

Plant G (1992) The selection and training of tactile aid users. In Summers IR (Ed) Tactile Aids for the Hearing Impaired. London: Whurr. pp 146-166.

Plant G (1995) Training approaches with tactile aids. Seminars in Hearing 16(4): 394-403.

Proctor A (1995) Tactile aid usage in young deaf children. In Plant G, Spens K-E (Eds) Profound Deafness and Speech Communication. London: Whurr. pp 111-146.

Proctor A, Goldstein MH Jnr (1983) Development of lexical comprehension in a pro-foundly deaf child using a wearable vibrotactile communication aid. Language Speech and Hearing Services in Schools, 14: 138-149.

Scilley PL (1980) Evaluation of a vibrotactile auditory prosthetic device for the pro-foundly deaf. Unpublished master's thesis, Queen's University, Kingston, Canada.

Sheehy P, Hansen SA (1983) The use of vibrotactile aids with preschool hearing impaired children: Case studies.Volta Review 85: 14-26.

Smith DL (1991) The use of vibrotactile aids with young profoundly deaf children. Proceedings of the National Conference on Pediatric Amplification, Boys Town, Omaha. pp 163-172.

Soderlund G (1995) Tactiling and tactile aids: a user's point of view. In: Plant G, Spens K-E. (Eds.) Profound Deafness and Speech Communication. London: Whurr.

Spens K-E (1995) Evaluation of speech tracking results: some considerations and examples. In Plant G, Spens K-E (Eds) Profound Deafness and Speech Communication. London: Whurr.

Summers IR (Ed) (1992) Tactile Aids for the Hearing Impaired. London: Whurr.

Vergara KC, Miskiel LW (1994) Miami Cochlear Implant, Tactile and Auditory Curriculum (CHATS). San Diego: Singular Press.

Weisenberger JM (1992) Communication of the acoustic environment via tactile stim-uli. In Summers I (Ed.) Tactile Aids for the Hearing Impaired. London: Whurr.

Weisenberger JM, Miller JD (1987) The role of tactile aids in providing information about acoustic stimuli. Journal Acoustical Society of America 82(3): 906-916.

Section C:
Knowledge and Practice

Introduction

A clear understanding of the implications of all aspects of audiology as
they relate to the deaf child and his/her environment has now been
established. The teacher of the deaf has the responsibility to set child-
centred goals that will lead to the optimum development of listening,
language and learning. A prerequisite to this is the need to establish
baseline information which lays the foundation for continual assessment
and evaluation. This will lead to the establishment of programmes that
are individually tailored to the needs of each child, whatever the educational setting. It means that the teacher of the deaf can share valuable
information with professionals who see the child in a clinical setting on
an infrequent basis. This kind of positive interdisciplinary interaction
will ensure that the child has the opportunity of reaching his/her
optimum potential. Preventative and interventional strategies which are
carefully thought out will provide security for parents and children.

The listening/learning environment of a child changes dramatically in
the course of a single day. The soundscape will be varied and dynamic
ranging from hostile to acoustically friendly. An overview of current
technological aids can only be meaningful when viewed within the
context of the listening environment. This will never replicate the
acoustically controlled clinical setting.

The following chapters describe how the deaf child can be provided
with good management which will involve the co-operation of parents and
families, educational audiologists as well as classroom teachers and head
teachers. They will establish criteria for providing the deaf child with
the opportunity to compete within an appropriate listening/learning
environment.

Chapter 8
Management

S LEWIS and D LYON

Photographs by K Wilbraham

Introduction

The practical benefit that children derive from hearing aids and other amplification equipment depends upon a number of factors. Clearly the aids must be suitable for the child in terms of dealing with both the characteristics of the hearing loss, and the environments and conditions in which he/she will need to use them. In essence, the aid must provide appropriate amplification.

Effective use of residual hearing, however, is not just a question of finding the right hearing aid and amplification system for the right context, although this is undoubtedly the starting point. Effective amplification also involves the provision of consistently high quality sound experience via such systems. Such quality is not simply a case of whether the aid is functioning according to the manufacturer's specifications or not; it is also a function of the opportunities for, and the quality of, the listening experience provided, the regular monitoring of the child's hearing status both with and without hearing aids, and the careful monitoring of the acoustic characteristics of the environments in which the child is both learning to listen and has to apply his or her burgeoning listening skills.

However effective the hearing aid fitting, whatever the range of amplifications options made available to the child, however good the input data going into the hearing aids, the effectiveness of the provision will break down unless procedures are in place for the practical management of such aids – in terms both of their everyday use and their functioning. Since children do not work and play in clinical contexts these procedures must be ones which allow the aids' effectiveness to be tested and evaluated in everyday contexts by those who are working on a day-to-day basis with the children – parents, teachers of the deaf, mainstream teachers, support assistants and of course the children themselves.

This chapter is particularly concerned with the systems and procedures that are in place to ensure that the hearing aid and other amplification systems worn by the child are functioning and continue to function as intended, so that the child does have the opportunity to derive maximal benefit from them. Specifically, it will review the evidence as to those aspects of hearing aid functioning and use that teachers, parents and indeed hearing-impaired children themselves need pay particular attention to on a day-to-day basis. It will then describe the routine procedures that should be in place at home and in school for the testing of hearing aids and other amplification equipment, including those using hearing aid analysers (electro-acoustic tests) and more subjective listening and visual checks and procedures (psycho-acoustic tests). It will also provide examples of the record keeping, literature and equipment that parents, services and schools should keep, to allow for the short and long term evaluation of an aid's functioning, and effective trouble shooting procedures and back-up provision that should be in place.

Effective and consistent amplification

Effective hearing aid management is characterised by a number of essential aspects:

1 Daily subjective listening tests and battery checks.
2 Regular electro-acoustic tests (at least once a month).
3 Ongoing assessment of aided thresholds.
4 Regular impedance checks.
5 Attention to detail in earmould acoustics and plumbing.
6 A good acoustic environment.
7 Provision of high quality input to the hearing aid.

The first two of these are particularly within the scope of this chapter, but all are central to the smooth audiological management of the child once the initial fitting of hearing aids and/or other amplification has been carried out. The fitting of aids to children is never final. As children mature and they provide more evidence of their hearing/listening levels, as they move from context to context and their listening needs vary, then the process becomes one of constant evaluation, assessment and adjustment. The aim is clearly to provide such children with the most effective auditory support possible for their learning and interaction with people and the world, and all evidence gathered by clinicians, teachers, parents and others contributes to this process. Much of these data will be observational evidence based on children's everyday use of amplification, the evidence of their functional use of hearing and their emergent listening skills.

It is difficult, however, to evaluate the adequacy of a child's current hearing aid fitting for learning and for everyday life, if the reliability of the aids in terms of their ability to deliver the optimum signal has been compromised in some way. Hearing aids are not robust instruments; they have a number of small intricate parts and connections, and delicate electronic and electro-acoustic components. They are fitted on the premise that the earmould by means of which the aid is attached to the wearer fits properly and does not radically change the amplification configuration, unless specifically designed to do so. Any support amplification attached to, or worn with, the hearing aid is provided to enhance the listening/ hearing opportunity, and should not intervene to the detriment of the quality of sound and amplification configuration originally prescribed.

Potential problems

In any hearing aid use situation, there are many potentialities for problems. This is particularly so when the hearing aid wearers are young children who are developmentally young listeners, and cannot therefore themselves monitor the functioning and performance of their own hearing aids. Thus, although pupils should be encouraged to be increasingly responsible for the management and functioning of their own amplification equipment, the responsibility for monitoring its on going performance and use falls heavily on teachers, parents and other adults who work with the child, i.e., those who are in day-to-day contact with the child.

Such monitoring cannot be done at a distance. In the United Kingdom, health authorities retain the ultimate responsibility for the prescription, provision and maintenance of hearing aids, but most readily acknowledge the importance of co-operation with the educational services for hearing-impaired children in the evaluation of the child's use of amplification, the monitoring of hearing aid performance and its appropriateness for the range of contexts in which the child operates. Often teachers of the deaf are supplied with spares for the most common hearing aids in use – tone hooks, leads, receivers and batteries and such like – so that the child's listening experience is disrupted as little as possible should an aid or component malfunction. Parents are provided with spares for their child's individual hearing aids and/or FM system. Such practice recognises that early identification of faults, loan facilities during repair times, rapid turn around of faulty aids, are all essential components of an effective management programme. It recognises that all who are involved with the child therefore must be convinced of the central nature of the sound experience for the child, and the need to support its quality. All must be capable of recognising a breakdown in the system, have a sense of urgency in responding to such a breakdown, and must have swift access to spare equipment so that the disruption to the child's listening programme and to his/her quality of life and education is minimised.

There are few educational management programmes for hearing-impaired children currently in operation that do not have the goal of maximising and supporting hearing-impaired children's use of residual hearing as a major priority. Teachers cannot support and deliver this component of an individual child's programme if there is not an effective system in place that ensures children are receiving consistently high quality signals through their ears. Special school, peripatetic and resource based teachers of the deaf should be routinely carrying out subjective and electro-acoustic tests on pupils' hearing aids and FM systems, and be reporting back regularly to their colleague educational audiologists and to health authority personnel, audiology departments and ear, nose and throat consultants, on the aids' functioning and on earmould problems as well as on pupils' current hearing status, use of amplification and amplification needs.

Integration

In the United Kingdom there has been a minor revolution over the last 20 years in terms of the management patterns of hearing-impaired children, and particularly in relation to the education of severely and profoundly deaf children. Whereas the majority of such pupils were to be found previously in special schools for the deaf or segregated units attached to mainstream schools, the majority are now educated in mainstream schools or resource bases, and quite often within their local neighbourhood school. Although the reasons for this are complex and very much linked to the general climate and thinking as regards the education of all pupils with special educational needs, there is no doubt that within deaf education the movement towards inclusion of hearing-impaired children within mainstream education has been facilitated by the support technology available – a wider range and type of hearing aid, the availability of radio aids and the support technology associated with them. Such amplification options not only support the child's language acquisition and access to experience in general, they also support and maintain access to curriculum. Many older pupils will openly voice their difficulties in accessing mainstream lessons should their equipment break down or be inappropriately managed by the class teacher. Younger pupils, however, are not always mature enough listeners to recognise an equipment fault, and are left in these instances not only under-supported, but often confused by inconsistent and distorted sound messages.

Resources

Systems in place for checking hearing aid and FM system functioning must take account of this. Put quite simply, early identification, sophisticated hearing aid and earmould technology and other advances in the field are of little benefit unless children are wearing equipment that works. In every school that has a hearing aid wearer enrolled, there needs therefore to be at least one adult who both knows how to check the functioning of that child's systems, and has been trained to recognise the indicators of system breakdown.

Research demonstrates quite clearly the propensity of the new born infant, the child and the adult to try and impose order, to classify, to seriate and to make sense of the world (Siegler, 1991). However, "Perceptual development requires reliable sense organs. Only with a consistent and predictable relationship between physical and neural messages can the child learn to interpret the information received from the environment. Periodic fluctuations cause a lowering of priority for the modality concerned." (Boothroyd, 1982, p.192). The implications of this are quite clear. Boothroyd does not set fully intact sense organs as a prerequisite, but rather stresses the consistency and predictability of the messages and of the organs' functioning.

Although factors such as the involvement of a middle ear condition, and instability of the hearing loss, can result in such a lessening of priority in respect of listening, poor establishment of hearing aids, the wearing of malfunctioning hearing aids and/or of badly fitting earmoulds will result in a similar effect, i.e., for children who already have a hearing difficulty, inconsistent and inadequate amplification will not only render the whole auditory discrimination/processing/learning process more difficult, but also, for some, may well lead them actively to 'switch off' in listening terms and never realise their full potential as listeners. Such inadequate and inconsistent sound experiences will influence children's and indeed parents' views of, and attitudes towards, the hearing aids and FM systems they wear. It may lead to some pupils being wrongly classified as 'poor' listeners, when in effect they have been provided with an impoverished base from which to develop their listening skills.

Consistency

Consistent and effective amplification provides the essential support for pupils' emergent listening skills and for movement towards higher levels of auditory processing. Consistent and high quality sound is a product of the aids' quality itself, of the current appropriateness of the aid fitting, and of the efforts that are taken to maintain and monitor their functioning within the manufacturer's specifications and in relation to the desired amplification configuration for the child.

Research

Problems with hearing aid malfunction are common in educational settings. Smith (1994) reviews a number of these surveys, many of which present a gloomy picture of the effectiveness for children of hearing aids in routine use. More than thirty years ago, Gaeth and Lounsbury (1966) reported that 50% of a sample of 134 hearing aids worn by children in school were malfunctioning. Similar levels of malfunction were reported by Zinck (1972), Bess (1977), Hoverstein (1981) and Skinner (1988). Cracked cases, cracked receivers, broken cords, faulty connections and low battery voltage were the most common problems reported. Studies of classroom FM systems have reported similar levels of problems. Bess, Sinclair and Riggs (1984) reported that 50% of student receivers and teacher transmitters they investigated were not working properly. For FM systems such faults fall into two main areas – those faults connected with a malfunction and wearing of the system itself, and those faults that result from an inappropriate balancing of the system with the hearing aid. In the latter case, the hearing aids and FM system may have interacted in such a way that the amplification configuration delivered to the child was no longer that prescribed as optimal, in terms of either frequency response or amplitude, and/or may have introduced unacceptable levels of harmonic distortion. More recent studies (Lyon and Swain, 1989; Maxon, Bruckett and van den Berg, 1991; Thibodeau, McCaffrey and Abrahamsan, 1988) confirm such high levels of malfunction in both hearing aids and FM systems.

Two recent surveys in England and Canada confirm the persistent and widespread nature of such problems, but also point the way forward in terms of preventative approaches to them. Smith (1994) reported on a sample of 89 school-aged children, including matched groups within different educational settings (an auditory-oral special school, total communication special schools, and auditory-oral mainstream schools). All pupils' audiological management was overseen by a trained audiologist as well as by teachers of the deaf. Regular electro-acoustic testing and hearing aid evaluation was a part of all pupils' audiological management. Scrutiny of aids as worn by the children, using both subjective and electro-acoustic tests, revealed however only 34% of the total sample to be wearing aids without faults or without evidence of misuse (e.g., switched off!). This improved to 64% once earmould and tubing faults were eliminated, but still represents a figure of faulty aids as large as that reported by Gaeth and Lounsbury (1966) thirty years ago. A simple observational routine and a more rigorous battery checking regime would have identified most of the faults – damaged casing, switches and ear hooks, flat batteries, split earmoulds, problems with earmould tubing and so on.

Electro-acoustic testing of the hearing aids revealed that most aids were performing broadly in line with manufacturers' specifications, although the match between hearing aid functioning and such specifications was less secure for those pupils within the total communication special school contexts.

The existence of a regular programme of electro-acoustic testing was clearly a strength for all environments; it may be however that this very strength may have diverted some teachers and parents away from the simple yet frequent observational and listening procedures that should be in place to check the efficacy of the whole system as it is worn by the child, including earmoulds. Hearing aid and FM faults may develop at any point, and parents, teachers and children need to be alert to the tell-tale signs that signify an aid is not functioning properly, and to the factors such as poor earmould condition that may contribute to this. Both subjective tests and electro-acoustic tests are essential components of an effective audiological management programme. Neither is sufficient alone.

A recent study in two Canadian provinces, Nova Scotia and New Brunswick, illustrates the large number of repairs carried out to children's aids. During the 1994–1995 school year, when hearing aid and FM support was being co-ordinated for approximately 600 children, 650 repairs were carried out on personal hearing aids either on-site or by the manufacturer. 1200 repairs were carried out on FM systems, the bulk of them related to FM transmitters or receivers, although FM charger faults were also a common occurrence. Clearly, this high incidence of repairs indicates that the problems have been identified at least in these aids. Other studies, such as Smith's 1994 study, centre on the high incidence of non-identified faults. Smith offers evidence that poor monitoring of the condition and functioning of hearing aids and their appropriateness as worn may be more a feature of particular educational regimes than others.

Exchange of information

Parents, teachers and audiologists must recognise the benefits of hearing aid provision for severely and profoundly hearing-impaired pupils if they are to carry out management programmes with conviction. They also need appropriate information from audiologists, in order to optimally support the child's wearing of the aids. At minimum this should comprise:

- The make and type of hearing aid, including the serial number.
- The internal settings of the aid. When aids are repaired these settings are often adjusted and it is imperative that all involved check the aid settings are appropriate before putting it back on the child. The teacher of the deaf or audiologist will also need to adjust the settings of any replacement aid loaned to produce a similar amplification configuration to the child's own aid.
- The volume level required.
- The type of battery necessary, how often it should be changed.

- The type of ear hook (tone hook) e.g., Mini, filtered.
- The type of receiver, cord (for BW aids).
- The date of manufacture of the most recent earmould, and any specific details (tubing diameter, bore size and venting).
- Copies of the print-out from the hearing aid analyser at user setting, against which current aid performance can be compared.

If the child is using an FM system a similar range of information is required including:

- The type of FM system and its serial number.
- The environmental and FM 'volume' or balance wheel control settings. Sometimes these have to be in diagrammatic form. Usually there will also be a print-out from the hearing aid analyser that demonstrates clearly the output at user setting of the combined systems via the child's hearing aid.
- The type of battery, recharging arrangements and the amount of FM use that this will support.
- The type of direct input shoe and leads/cords.
- The type of button receiver and cords (for Type 1 systems).

Such information provides the background against which hearing aid and FM functioning can be monitored and maintained.

Some (Allard and Cordry-Golden, 1991; Thibodeau et al., 1988) have suggested that there is a lack of teacher confidence and/or expertise in hearing aid management, particularly given the range and complexity of amplification systems now available. There are, however, a number of fairly simple routine procedures that both teachers and parents can carry out on a regular basis to check the functioning of aids, trouble-shoot for common problems and guide remedial action. Indeed, Smith (1994) refers to several studies wherein the introduction of more detailed checking procedures for hearing aids and FM systems produced a significant improvement in the identification of faults and the state of children's aids.

Subjective tests: looking and listening checks

Smith's study is a timely reminder to us that, although more objective testing of hearing aids through electro-acoustic tests should be part of every child's hearing aid management programme, such procedures must be supported by a much more regular programme of looking and listening checks by parents, teachers, support workers and the child himself. In stressing the role and involvement of adults in monitoring the functioning of the child's hearing aids and other amplification equipment, one should not be diverted from the responsibility that children must be encouraged to take on, from the very beginning of their amplification experience, for monitoring the quality of the sound that they are experiencing and the condition of the various components of their equipment. In the earliest stages, this is prepared for when parents and teachers involve the child in some aspects of the checking routine – drawing the child's attention to casing damage, clean or dirty earmoulds, blocked or damaged tubing, dead batteries and so on. Indeed there are a whole host of opportunities for adults to signal to the child that their involvement in hearing aid maintenance and their evaluation of an aid's functioning is critical and that such an involvement is expected. Some parents do need careful support in encouraging such a responsibility in their children – both in terms of the child's ability to set and wear the aid appropriately, and to indicate that the sound they are experiencing is not as it should be. The foundations for this are laid by teachers and parents who comment not only on faults when found, but also reinforce the fact that an aid is working and is clean, that an earmould does fit well. When an aid is switched on they may well ask the child "Is it working properly?"; they may momentarily put a malfunctioning aid back in the child's ear before correcting the fault or replacing the aid so that the child can experience the difference between poor sound and good sound quality, sound and no sound and so on.

Many schools and teachers routinely train not just parents, but also pupils, to re-tube earmoulds; many also involve older pupils in the test box procedures for balancing FM systems with hearing aids, and for testing hearing aids themselves. The temptation is for the testing and general management procedures to be carried out by adults because it is less time consuming; it is however ultimately less cost effective in terms of the child's own hearing aid and FM management and use.

Starting points

Equipment

A certain amount of basic equipment and of course basic training must be provided for parents and teachers, in order that they can both check children's aids efficiently and respond to any apparent faults quickly and accurately. Stetosets or stetoclips with acoustic dampers/attenuators should be used to establish hearing aid performance in subjective listening tests. A variety of dampers are now available for this purpose, varying in attenuation according to the requirements of the tester and the potential output of the aid in question. If acoustic dampers are not used then adults must of necessity listen-in to aids at relatively low levels of amplification, i.e., not at the child's user setting. Clearly an aid may well be functioning appropriately at low volume, but be distorting badly or be under-powered at higher volumes, or there may be a 'dead spot' in the volume range or similar problems. Although this can be clarified by the use of a hearing aid analyser or test box, access to such equipment may be limited. The use of attenuators and stetoclips allows the listener to evaluate the hearing aid's response at the child's prescribed setting, without being in danger of damaging their own hearing.

The range of other equipment necessary to test an aid and support its use will depend on the type of aid and FM system that the child has been provided with. For BTE aids, parents and teachers will need to have spare tone hooks (including mini hooks where appropriate), batteries and tubing, spare 'huggie' bands and/or toupee tape, as necessary. In the case of BW aids and Type 1 FM systems, spare leads and button receivers will also need to be made available. For cochlear implanted children, spare leads and if possible microphones need to be provided; prompt access to a spare processor is necessary in the event of breakdown.

An air blower should be available to pupils and adults so that condensation does not build up in either tubing or tone hook. The impact of such condensation on the quality of sound received by the child should not be underestimated. Figure 8.1 represents the impact of a large amount of condensation in the tubing on the output and frequency response of one particular aid at user setting. The effect is predominantly in the high frequency areas, but note also the increased distortion and reduced output that is present at both mid and low frequencies. In this case, the hearing aid itself is working perfectly in terms of manufacturer's specifications and its output and gain at user settings, but the whole system fails to deliver an amplification configuration appropriate to the child's needs because of the condensation problem. The use of an air blower and re-tubing of the earmould with tubing specifically designed to minimise the problem (such as 'Stay Dri' tubing) vastly ameliorates the problem and restores the integrity of the system. Many parents and teachers do not recognise that moisture in tubing can have such a dramatic effect on the amplification configuration that a child is receiving, and may negate the very good work that has been done in establishing and providing for optimum listening levels to be delivered to the child.

Battery tester

A battery tester will enable the voltage and drain of the battery to be quickly and easily tested. However, the use of a battery tester is usually supported by a regular battery changing schedule for young children or older, as yet less reliable, listeners, i.e., parents and children are encouraged to change batteries routinely at least once a week, twice a week or as required by a particular aid's known parameters, rather than risk a deteriorating or dead battery being in a child's aid for any length of time.

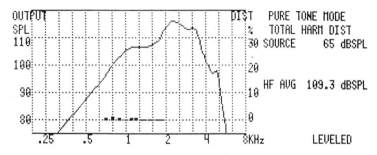

Aid set to user setting (vol. 3), output measured through earmould.

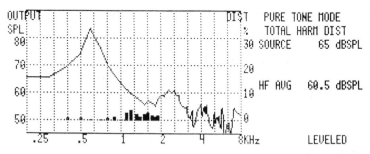

Same aid, same setting but with considerable amount of condensation in the tubing.

Figure 8.1 Effect of condensation in earmould tubing on hearing aid output

Although the newer FM systems can now be powered for up to 40 hours by their power source, usually rechargeable nickel cadmium (Ni-Cad) or nickel metal hydride batteries (NiMH), which means that most systems do not now require overnight charging every night, there is still the possibility of a battery failing in an FM system whilst the child is wearing it. Teachers and parents need to be aware of the limitations of rechargeable Ni-Cad batteries and their progressive loss of ability to hold their charge. Most FM systems now incorporate a 'low battery' light to alert the users to this problem; remedial action requires of course that there are spare charged batteries readily accessible to the child. If the child is based in a resourced unit or a school for the deaf then the school or unit carries adequate fully charged spares. For the child who is individually integrated and using an FM system, then a six-battery system is to be preferred – two batteries being used by the child, two fully charged and two being charged.

Battery chargers

Rechargeable batteries do not have an indefinite life. Most teachers now clearly identify a battery according to the date that it was first brought into service, so that a systematic replacement and checking procedure is possible. Most rechargeable batteries have a charging cycle of 14 to 16 hours. In practical terms, a full night's charge will give a full school day's usage for older type FM systems, and 40 hours or so usage for the latest generation of radio aids. Care must be taken, however, that parents, teachers and children fully understand the particular type of battery charger with which they have been supplied. The newer full-cycle chargers work on the principle of discharging a still partially charged battery to an optimum level before beginning the charge phase. This process has been shown to prolong battery life in comparison with the frequent topping up of partially charged batteries. It should be noted, however, that if the power supply is interrupted during the charging phase,whereas a basic charger would simply resume charging when the power supply is restored, a full cycle charger will begin the whole discharge/charge process again. Alternative chargers should be used in those contexts in which the power supply is erratic or the charger is likely to be unplugged during its recharging cycle. Children may well arrive in school with an undercharged battery because someone has unplugged the charger to make an early morning cup of tea and then plugged it in again!

Kits: cleaning

For all aids, cleaning and sterilising kits will be necessary, and wax guards may also be required for ITE aids. All such items may be important components of the trouble-shooting repair and spares kit that is located with individual children to support their use and management of their aids. Educational services for hearing-impaired children and/or local health authority audiology departments will often jointly supply a kit containing the basic items mentioned above to individual parents and schools. In the United Kingdom The National Deaf Children's Society through their Technical and Information Centre have basic testing kits available for purchase by parents and professionals, and some local branches will fund the provision of such a kit to the parents of newly diagnosed children. Most teachers of the deaf, however, require a much more extensive kit, that they carry with them for the routine maintenance of aids and support of hearing aid wearers. A typical kit might consist of the following items:

- WD-40 cleaning spray (penetrating oil)
- Earmould disinfectant cleaner
- ITE aid cleaner
- 'Super seals'
- 'Dri-Aid' kit
- Earmould blower
- Earmould tubing and cement
- Reamer

- Brush
- Battery tester
- Stetoclip
- Alcohol swabs
- Watchmaking screwdrivers
- Wax pick and brush
- 'Huggie' band
- Pointed pliers
- Scissors
- Earmould tubing expander
- 'Ad-Hear' wax guards

Kits: spares

A classroom spares kit is necessary to support both hearing aid and FM use. The exact contents of such a kit will vary according to the type of hearing aid worn by the child and the FM type and particular system used, but will include battery chargers and testers, spare microphones, direct input leads and shoes, aerials, modules or oscillators as appropriate. A much fuller kit including direct input leads or cords of varying length, type and thickness, direct input shoes, neck loops, a range of button receivers, FM system batteries, battery chargers, spare microphones, oscillators, modules and aerials, as well as the spares detailed above for hearing aids, should be carried by the teacher of the deaf.

Once a fault is diagnosed in a hearing aid or FM system itself, access to a spare system or aid becomes critical. In the United Kingdom, hearing aids are supplied free of charge via the local district health authority. Some local authorities will provide three hearing aids to newly diagnosed children, so that they always have available a working spare aid of the same type as their own; this can be fitted immediately to the child if one aid is malfunctioning or indeed suspect. If such provision is not available, then parents and schools will need to have immediate access to spare hearing aids of a similar type to the child's own; they need to know who to contact and where. This is particularly important during weekends and school holidays as well as during school terms. Children will also need access to a spare FM system. Such provision and urgency recognises two principles – that time spent without a working hearing aid is wasted listening time, and that replacement aids need to be capable of maintaining the quality and consistency of auditory experience that the child's own hearing aids provide.

Visual checks

The importance of the initial visual check within the test battery either for a hearing aid or an FM system should not be underestimated. A careful observational routine which systematically examined earmoulds, microphones, tubing, tone hooks, battery compartments, switches, button receivers, and the condition of the hearing aid casing itself would have eliminated a very high percentage of barriers to aids working effectively within Smith's study. In the case of BW hearing aids and FM systems, detailed examination of earmoulds, button receivers or direct input shoes, leads, sockets, battery compartments, microphones, switches and hearing aids is the starting point.

Many services for hearing-impaired children do produce leaflets and guidelines for parents to guide such a check and resultant action. Appendix C is an example of a protocol for checking BTE hearing aids, and takes the parent and user through a careful observation of the hearing aid before moving on to the listening check and basic troubleshooting procedures. Appendix C provides a further example of procedures for checking BW hearing aids. The fact that such a percentage of problems existed in Smith's and other studies, however, points to such checks either not taking place, or to the potential significance of such faults as discoloured tubing, cracked and damaged earmoulds, damaged switches and casing not being recognised, or, as Markides (1988) suggests, of a pattern of less detailed attention to such things as children get older.

Tubing

Some, but not all, schools, services and parents do recognise the potential weakness in relation to earmoulds and tubing and institute a routine replacement regime (at least every 6 weeks) for tubing to minimise the risk of discoloured, damaged or twisted tubing going unnoticed for any length of time. Many also either ask for earmoulds to be routinely tubed with high quality wide bore, thick walled tubing, or will re-tube even new moulds with such tubing themselves. They also have a regular programme for replacement of earmoulds that requires new earmoulds to be made at least every 6 weeks or whenever there is no longer spare capacity in the current mould. They do not wait until the earmould is so poor that the aid has to be turned down, which would compromise the child's input, but take further impressions when a child is wearing the aid at recommended user settings, although there is no reserve.

Earmoulds

Although all those involved in the audiological management of hearing-impaired children acknowledge the potential weakness of the earmould in the system, it is clear that for many pupils the quality of the earmould is still a major determining factor in respect of both the quality and level of amplification that they receive. Earlier writers (Gaeth and Lounsbury,

1966) commented on the then common practice of hearing aid gain controls and listening levels being set according to when acoustic feedback occurred. Smith (1994) did not compare aids worn by pupils with their recommended user settings. He does however report a situation in which the deafest of the three groups (the total communication special school group) used "significantly less gain in both absolute (user gain) and relative terms (functional gain)" than the two auditory oral groups.

Nearly a quarter of this group had poorly fitting earmoulds even for gain used. Only four children in the TCS group were wearing their aids at levels and settings that would provide any access to the speech signal. On the whole, this was not a function of the hearing aid provided, since some of the most high powered aids were being used with least gain; these pupils for varying reasons, such as earmould inadequacies, habit, the 'lack of priority' warned of by Boothroyd above, were not able to make use of the potentialities within the amplification systems provided. Clearly for some pupils, 'within child' factors might be operating. As teachers advising parents and supporting children, however, we must be careful that we do not confuse a lack of support for delivery of the signal – as in the case of children who repeatedly have problems with poorly fitting earmoulds or malfunctioning aids – with the child's ability to benefit from it.

Leads

Leads are also potentially weak components of BW or pocket hearing aids and of FM systems. It is important therefore that the visual examination takes particular note of the condition of any leads, checking for signs of fraying, splitting or stress around connecting joints (microphone leads, leads to button receivers or to FM direct input shoes), as well as monitoring the condition of the jack plugs and input sockets.

It is clearly not possible to carry out electro-acoustic testing or listening checks on cochlear implants or indeed vibro-tactile aids and bone anchored hearing aids. For these aids, the importance of the visual check cannot be overestimated. Like all other aids, they need checking (in so far as they can be) every day to ensure that they are working. Although older pupils may be able to indicate that there is a fault, young children and those who have just received their aids or implant devices will be dependent on their teachers and parents for an effective management programme. Appendix C provides an example of a check list for parents and teachers for checking the speech processor and microphone of a cochlear implant. Most implant centres, and indeed manuals relating to specific implant systems, provide such a checking procedure. All stress the importance of visually checking the processor, microphone and leads and then systematically changing batteries, leads and microphone if the system appears to be less responsive than usual. Similar proformas exist for checking bone anchored aids and vibro tactile aids, although there are of course only limited components that can be replaced with these. Ultimately, with such systems and cochlear implants, the back-up provision that exists in terms of access to spare processors or aids (as applicable), and access to clinics for reappraisal of the system, is critical.

Listening checks

Daily subjective listening tests are the cornerstone of any hearing aid monitoring programme. Within such a programme, parents and teachers will quickly become accustomed to the quality of sound produced by a particular hearing aid, and are alerted to any variations from usual in the signal. A systematic test routine which involves listening-in to the aid with a stetoclip in similar acoustic conditions, and uses similar test inputs, facilitates this and ensures that intermittent faults as well as persistent ones are picked up. Intermittent faults in particular are not always identified by a test box.

Some indication of the integrity of the frequency response of the hearing aid and the level of distortion it is delivering can be gained by using the Ling (1976) five-sound test supplemented by /m/ (/m/ /oo/ /ee/ /ah/ /sh/ /s/). When attenuators are used, this will enable these to be checked at user setting, and judgements to be made as to the output of the aids in comparison with their usual output, frequency response, clarity and other operating parameters.

Internal noise

Every aid produces some noise from the amplifier, which may manifest itself as a quiet buzz. If internal noise is too loud then this will interfere with the listener's ability to attend to and discriminate the external inputs such as speech. The internal noise generated by the aid can be monitored using the stetoclip either at low levels of amplification or at the child's own setting if a stetoclip with an attenuator is available. Checking internal noise must be done in quiet conditions. The aid is attached to the stetoclip, turned to a low to mid volume setting and held in the hand. The level of buzzing is monitored in the signal, compared with when the aid was new.

The provision of a written protocol by health and education authorities, such as those reproduced in the appendices, supports effective hearing aid management, particularly by inexperienced adults. A number of commercially published booklets and videos also exist for this purpose. Examples include the Ewing Foundation's videotape *Are Their Hearing Aids Working?* (Ewing Foundation,

1995) which illustrates the checking procedures for BTE and BW hearing aids and FM systems, and *The Hearing Aid Handbook* (Waynor, 1990). Most FM system manufacturers and cochlear implant programmes also provide clear and well illustrated testing and user guides for their systems (see for example *The CRM 220 Handbook*, Connevans, 1995).

Fault finding and adjustment

Systematic substitution of one component of a hearing aid system or an FM system with a new one is the most logical way to approach an aid that sounds faulty. For all aids, changing first the battery and then moving on to changing other components is the sensible starting point. For BW aids, this means replacing leads and then receivers by ones that are known to be perfect. For BTE hearing aids there is the tone hook to be considered and for cochlear implants the lead and microphone. Fault finding and testing procedures are covered in Appendix C.

Faults in FM systems

The list of potential components to replace becomes much longer when dealing with FM systems, particularly Type II systems. Appendix C shows an example of a checking procedure for radio aids used with parents. The starting point for checking such a radio aid system is always to establish that the hearing aid itself is working. Then, after following the visual check for the radio aid (FM) receiver and transmitter, it is possible to listen-in to, and check, the radio aid's functioning. A number of FM manufacturers provide a specific listening stick for this purpose. In listening-in to the FM receiver, it is important that sufficient distance be placed between the FM transmitter microphone and the receiver that the transmitter range is checked. The range checked should of course be equivalent to the most extensive range that the child is likely to use the aid in – for example the hall for assembly or the far end of the class room for group work.

Most teachers and parents ask the child or a sibling to wear the transmitter elsewhere in the room, or will use a distant radio or television input to support the testing of the FM system. Near-testing of an FM system, i.e., placement of a transmitter in close proximity to a receiver – or even around the tester's neck so that they themselves can speak in to it – is not to be recommended, as a number of systems will appear to be functioning when close to the speaker, but will in fact have transmitter or receiver faults. If a fault is indicated at this stage, then systematic substitution of transmitter microphone, aerials, receiver microphone, oscillators, and finally replacement of the transmitter or receiver unit itself, is carried out until the fault is eliminated.

Balancing FM systems

Once the efficacy of both hearing and radio aid have separately been established, then any ensuing problems once the systems are linked must be a product of their interaction. This can result from two main causes – either an inappropriate balancing of the aid and the FM system or faults with the leads, input shoes and induction links between the systems. Although subjective balancing of radio aid systems with hearing aids is possible, its accuracy is only as skilled as its listener's ears. Figure 8.2 illustrates the effects of inappropriate and appropriate balancing of FM and hearing aid systems on the frequency response, output and distortion levels of hearing aids. The FM system is illustrated correctly balanced using a test box; the two other inputs demonstrate the problems of subjective balancing of radio aids when test boxes are not used, and unacceptable levels of distortion and indeed output are introduced.

FM systems and hearing aids are most effectively balanced by electro-acoustic methods; poorly balanced systems compromise the integrity of the listening experience prescribed for the child, and instead of facilitating

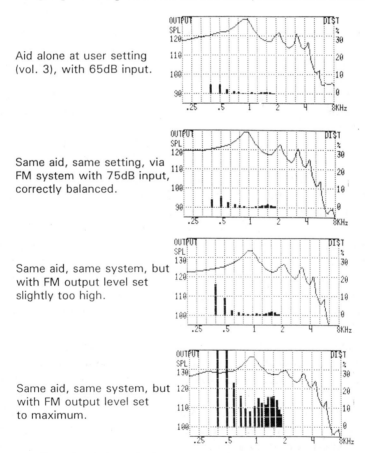

Aid alone at user setting (vol. 3), with 65dB input.

Same aid, same setting, via FM system with 75dB input, correctly balanced.

Same aid, same system, but with FM output level set slightly too high.

Same aid, same system, but with FM output level set to maximum.

Figure 8.2 Effect of maladjusted radio system on hearing aid output

access to the curriculum, may actually impede it. The procedures for testing hearing aids and fitting and balancing radio aids in hearing aid analysers are described later in this chapter.

Aids will need to be re-balanced whenever there has been any adjustment to hearing aid setting, or if a spare aid or a replacement radio aid transmitter/receiver is being used. Most services routinely check that the radio and hearing aid listening levels are still well matched, whenever hearing aids are run through the test box. This should happen at least once per month, and more often for pre-school hearing-impaired children and those who are very delayed listeners. Such young listeners are also more at risk if the balance or volume wheel of a radio aid cannot be locked once balanced with the hearing aids, or are part of the on/off switch system of the radio aid. The fixed screw-type balance wheel has much to recommend it when using radio aids with young children. Where this is not possible, then a locking device, or simple indication marks (using, for example, nail varnish) showing exactly where the volume or 'balancing' wheel should be turned to, will help prevent inappropriate settings being used.

The balancing of radio aids with cochlear implants and titanium implant bone conduction aids is problematic. It is clearly not possible to measure the output of the implants or of the combined FM/implant systems through electro-acoustic means, or even subjectively, except in the broadest terms by comparing pupil responsiveness. As a result, FM systems tend not to be used with such systems until the pupils themselves are able to make a listening judgement about the equivalence in quality and output of the combined systems compared with the implants, and about the contexts in which the FM genuinely offers support for listening and learning. There have been particular problems in the United Kingdom with the provision of appropriate FM cables and operating frequencies in relation to implants. Cochlear UK does now supply an attenuated FM cable and recommends an operating frequency for FM systems around 174 MHz. Different FM systems show different performance in conjunction with cochlear implants, and careful selection in order to find the best system for an individual is critical. Leads and an audio adapter are also now available for use with bone anchored hearing aids to allow connection to a range of audio equipment as well as to FM systems. The cochlear implant and bone anchored hearing aid manufacturers provide guidance on both fitting and checking procedures.

FM systems are used by some pupils in conjunction with bone conduction aids, and again balancing and checking the interaction of such systems is problematic, given that most services do not readily have access to an artificial mastoid. A very creative use of the bone conduction facility on a portable audiometer to support subjective balancing was seen by one author recently. The tester first matched the output of the audiometer bone conductor with the output on the hearing aid through tactile means on the fingers, or by listening with the bone conductor placed on the forehead. This was then compared with the target gain for the child for accuracy. A radio aid input of 75 dBSPL was then transmitted via the FM receiver to the bone conduction aid. The resultant output in bone conduction form was compared with that of the audiometer bone conductor, and matched as closely as possible. The comfort level and appropriateness of the fitting was then confirmed or adjusted, following observation and basic speech discrimination checks with the child.

Microphone faults

Microphone faults are common, particularly where lapel microphones are used. Figure 8.3 illustrates the impact on the hearing aid output of a faulty 'crackly' microphone, and a situation in which the interaction of the FM system and the hearing aid had a major impact on the output, frequency range and response curve of the hearing aid.

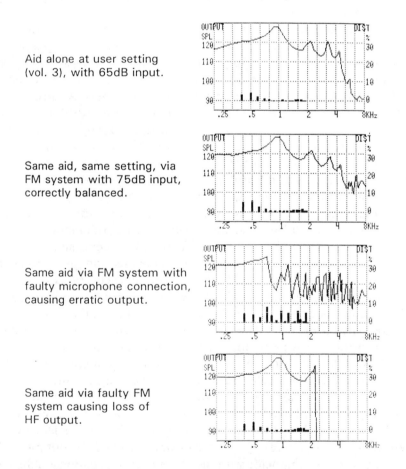

Aid alone at user setting (vol. 3), with 65dB input.

Same aid, same setting, via FM system with 75dB input, correctly balanced.

Same aid via FM system with faulty microphone connection, causing erratic output.

Same aid via faulty FM system causing loss of HF output.

Figure 8.3 Effect of faulty radio system on hearing aid output

Listening checks of the system as worn will reveal weaknesses and problems in the links between the FM system and the hearing aids. Some of these are system-specific, others are more general. Again, a systematic substitution of components with new ones should reveal the source of the problem, and in most cases, given that both parts of the system have already been identified as functioning appropriately, will ameliorate it. Problems will relate to shoes, leads, the neck loop, the direct input contacts on the aid, a faulty telecoil in the aid, switching systems or inappropriate balancing. The new type of transparent shoes are particularly useful for checking that children really have matched shoes and contacts appropriately. Careful listening checks must be carried out, however, to ensure that the hearing aid and FM system are jointly able to deliver all the functions for which they are designed. Thus for example, aids which offer both an audio input alone, and an audio input in conjunction with the environmental microphone of the hearing aid, must be checked in both positions. If direct input shoes which provide a similar listening opportunity (microphone on-off shoes) or shoes with attenuators are used, then the effectiveness and impact of such a facility must be checked both by listening and using electro-acoustic means. Many children benefit from the provision of such options, but they and the adults supporting them need training in the effective use of the facility and in the use of the switches to optimum advantage in varying listening conditions. This is also true for Type 1 FM systems, which must be checked in hearing aid alone, FM alone and FM/hearing aid microphone positions and comparisons made in respect of functioning, output, gain and frequency response for all three settings.

Problems with neck loops

Listening checks on neck loops can be particularly revealing. Fewer and fewer children are now being issued with these systems. This is for a number of reasons, but in particular is related to the weaknesses of this method of transferring the signal from the radio receiver to the personal aid. Figure 8.4 demonstrates the problem quite explicitly – the addition of the FM system with direct input reproduces the aid's output accurately and introduces minimal additional distortion; the addition of an FM system coupled by a neck loop however, even though as in Figure 8.4 balanced (i.e., with the aid worn at ear level and the loop round the neck), affects the frequency response and introduces high levels of distortion. The nature of the exact interaction between an aid, FM system and neck loop will vary from hearing aid to hearing aid and according to type of neck loop worn. In addition, the strength of the signal received by the aid is dependent on its distance from the neck loop and its relative angle to the loop. Therefore as the head moves, both of these variables are constantly changing, and the aid's output with them.

T position

The frequency response curve of the aid when used on the 'T' position may also be different from the frequency response of the aid when used in the microphone position. This clearly can negate all the good work done in establishing optimum listening levels and amplification configuration for a particular child. These two characteristics of neck loops – the potential instability of the signal and the effect of selecting the T position on the aid on the frequency response curve of the aid – make them options that should only rarely be considered for use with children. Although some older children do manage the orientation problem effectively, the majority of hearing-impaired children benefit most from a direct audio input system that is effectively maintained and properly balanced. In such circumstances they are reluctant to be without it in classroom contexts.

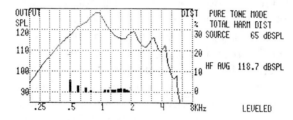

Aid only, at user setting (vol, 3), with 65dB input.

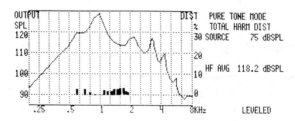

Same aid, same setting, via FM system using direct input.

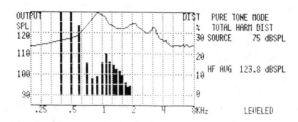

Same aid, same setting, via FM system using neck loop.

Figure 8.4 Comparison of hearing aid outputs using direct input and inductive coupling from radio system

Auto-muting

Some radio aids have an auto-muting facility which many teachers and indeed pupils value both for the priority it gives to the transmitter voice, and also because it alerts the child to the need to listen and watch for key information. However auto-muting does not function with all hearing aids, and any aid that has attenuation in the shoe should be treated with caution in this respect. The light on the receiver that indicates that voice priority is active may be on, but this is not confirmation that the muting is actually taking place. A practical listening test is necessary. Similar difficulties have also been experienced by some ITE users with these systems.

The point at which such priority systems 'switch in' is dependent in part upon the setting of the microphone sensitivity control on the transmitter. Any adjustment of the microphone sensitivity means that the whole system will need to be re-balanced. If this type of FM system is being used in isolation then it is possible to adjust the microphone sensitivity for optimum performance in the circumstances in which it is being used, i.e., according to teacher voice level and background noise variables. Difficulties may be encountered, however, in those contexts in which there is more than one transmitter in use, and the child moves from teacher to teacher, changing frequencies and transmitters, but not receivers. Although this is part of the flexibility of the system, it is also a potential weakness. Ideally, listening checks and balancing should be checked against all possible transmitters. Often transmitters end up set to very similar microphone sensitivity levels to facilitate this. In being so, however, part of the very flexibility of the system to respond to perceived need is lost – the ability to respond to varying teacher inputs and classroom noise conditions.

Extra care needs to be taken with these auto-muting systems, that the transmitter user switches off the transmitter when not communicating with the receiver wearer either individually or in a group. Although this is true of any radio aid, it is particularly so when the auto-muting facility is being used, since inappropriate use not only results in the child receiving irrelevant information but also reduces access to more relevant information by shutting down the environmental microphones on his or her hearing aid. Young children are particularly at risk from such poor management and, although many older children appear to like the auto-muting facility, a number of teachers of the deaf have reservations as to its use with children in the early stages of listening.

Other amplification systems

Free-field or sound field FM systems

Free-field FM systems as shown in Figure 8.5 consist of an FM teacher microphone, an FM receiver with antenna and an arrangement of loudspeakers. The sound signal is transmitted in the same way as the personal FM system, but instead of these being a personal receiver, the loudspeakers direct the sound to the students. The speakers are placed at strategic positions in the classroom, enabling the teacher's voice to be heard clearly by all children. Free-field systems are usually installed by manufacturers and daily trouble-shooting should not be an issue, although clearly the weak parts are the microphone, the speaker cables, the antenna and the batteries. Visual checks of these components as well as listening checks to the system are necessary as for other amplification systems.

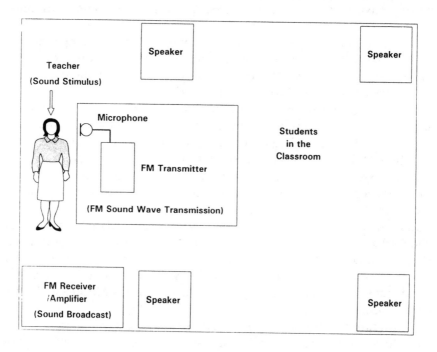

Figure 8.5 Sound field or free-field FM systems

Auditory trainer units (ATUs) and hard wire systems

It is surprising, given the well documented difficulties that exist in the provision of effective amplification for severely and profoundly hearing-impaired children, that more use is not made of single or linked auditory training units. An effective management programme for such children would involve the use of a number of amplification options with a child. There are many situations both in schools and at home where the use of headphone listening would be appropriate and would deliver a signal of higher quality than is available via current hearing aids, with or without an FM system. ATUs do not suffer from the drawbacks associated with delivery via earmoulds and offer a more wide-band listening experience. Their effective use of course is dependent on parents' and teachers' ability to operate them effectively, and a checking routine that allows for child and adult microphones, child headphones and auditory trainer output to be checked separately. It also requires that recommended settings are known and that child responsiveness is monitored. There is much evidence (Markides et al., 1980; Smith and Richards, 1990) of the merits of such systems when used in schools and homes. Although some manufacturers will supply varying sizes of headphones for these systems, there are not as yet truly lightweight high powered headphone-based systems available for use with severely and profoundly hearing-impaired children.

Appendix C explores a procedure for balancing FM systems with hearing aids, and Figures 8.6 and 8.7 demonstrate the procedure being carried out for direct input and neck loop systems respectively, although the exact procedure will vary according to the specific test box in use, and the decision taken as to recommended input levels by a particular service for hearing-impaired children. Most services operate on an input to the radio aid transmitter of 10 dB more than that used when testing a BTE aid by itself. Thus if an input signal of 65 dBSPL is used to test aids at user setting, then one of 75 dBSPL input is used when balancing the radio and hearing aid. However, a signal of 60 dBSPL is used with a BW aid then 75 dBSPL will be used when adjusting the FM system for use with the hearing aid.

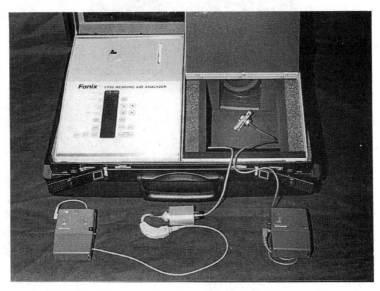

Figure 8.6 Using a test box to balance a hearing aid and an FM system: direct input

Not all aids and FM systems will be balanced using the inputs suggested above, however, and there is currently a great deal of interest in the use of composite, more speech-like signals when balancing FM systems for use with hearing aids (Rowson and Bamford, 1995). Certainly there is some concern that, given the very real problems with and variations in signal to noise ratio in some mainstream schools, there is not a more flexible response to the balancing problem, i.e., that although matching the output curves at user setting with the 65/75 dBSPL input is the starting point, for some children in some environments, a balancing 'up' in terms of measured hearing aid or FM output might be necessary, provided that unacceptable levels of distortion are not introduced and uncomfortable listening levels are not exceeded.

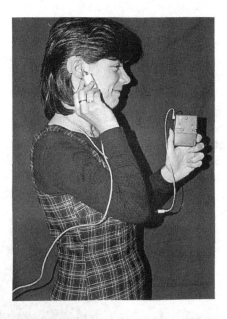

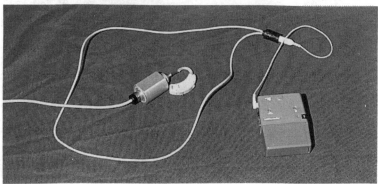

Figure 8.7 Using a test box to balance an FM system and a hearing aid with a neck loop

Electro-acoustic testing of hearing aids

Most teachers when training as teachers of the deaf will spend some time studying the principles and gaining the practical skills both of using electro-acoustic test boxes and analysing and interpreting their results. Hearing aid test boxes or analysers allow the electro-acoustic characteristics of hearing aids and FM systems to be measured accurately, both for comparison with the manufacturer's specifications and/or to determine how well an aid is performing at the setting at which the wearer is currently wearing it.

There is a variety of such equipment currently available, some designed as portable test boxes for the field, others being much more complex and highly sophisticated laboratory models. All however have three essential parts – a sound generator, an acoustic (anechoic) chamber and a measurement system. Figure 8.8 shows such a system in diagrammatic form. The sound generator produces a signal, the frequency and amplitude characteristics of which the user can control. The acoustic chamber provides a controlled environment within which the sounds can be made. Hearing aids, and indeed other amplification equipment, are connected to a coupler within the acoustic chamber which in turn is linked to the sound level measuring equipment. Different types of coupler are available according to the equipment to be tested, but for hearing aid and FM purposes the coupler used is generally a 2cc coupler (IEC 126), which is considered to be approximately equal to the volume of the human ear canal plus the equivalent volume of the middle ear. The output and configuration of the sounds coming from the hearing aid can be compared with the original input signal and its adequacy assessed. By varying the input

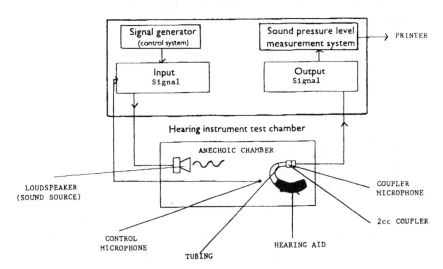

Figure 8.8 Basic hearing aid test box in diagrammatic form (Adapted from and reproduced by permission of Phonat Ltd.)

signal to the hearing aid and the hearing aid settings themselves (see below), the test box user is able to verify whether the hearing aid still functions according to manufacturer's specification, and is working optimally at user setting. The user can also monitor the aid's performance over a time. An example of such a commercial test box system can be seen in Figure 8.6. A protocol for testing hearing aids using a test box system is given in Appendix C.

Hearing aids are manufactured and tested according to standardised specifications as prescribed by national standards institutes. Those most commonly used include:

HAIC (Hearing Aid Industry Conference)
ANSI (American National Standards Institute)
BSI (British Standards Institute)
IEC (International Electrotechnical Commission)

Currently, hearing aid performance should always be quoted in terms of the requirements of IEC 118 and the coupler specified in IEC 711, even if other measurements are cited for comparison in manufacturers' literature.

There are clearly a very large number of individual aids and FM systems in use, and the generic descriptions and protocols provided here will not apply to all hearing aids and all systems. Teachers should have access to manufacturers' information on all aids they have to deal with, and should follow manufacturers' specific instructions as regards inputs and internal settings to be used when comparing individual aids with manufacturers' specifications.

Most services for hearing-impaired children use a test routine which compares the child's aids directly with the original test box print-out for that aid when new and working optimally. Usually the measures taken will include all or some of the following:

* Maximum gain
* Maximum output
* Frequency response
* Random noise
* Harmonic distortion
* User setting information in particular gain, random noise and harmonic distortion.

When an aid is new and performing optimally the print-out of such parameters is often made into an acetate sheet or overlay, which then functions as the target performance for that aid. This permits a direct comparison with current functioning, including tolerances for each of the measures above.

Maximum gain

The maximum gain of a hearing aid is usually checked with all output limitation controls switched off or set to minimum limitation, and tone controls set to normal; volume controls and internal gain controls are usually set to maximum. Maximum gain at any frequency is the highest possible gain at that frequency, although maximum gain is often specified for 1 kHz. The recommended input for calculating and checking maximum gain is either 50 or 60 dBSPL. For most hearing aids tested using portable test boxes, an input of 60 dBSPL is advantageous because of the problem of ambient noise. However, aids which have automatic gain control or compression circuitry (AGC), and some of the more powerful aids which have very high gain, must be tested using an input of 50 dBSPL and their manufacturers' data will reflect this.

Maximum output

Maximum output or SSPL (saturated sound pressure level) is almost always tested using an input signal of 90 dBSPL. Volume controls and internal gain controls are full on and all other controls are set to 'normal' or as indicated within manufacturer's specifications.

Frequency response

The basic frequency curve of an aid is usually checked with a 60 dBSPL input and by adjusting the volume control of the aid such that 40 dB of gain is delivered at 1 kHz, i.e., the output figure on the test box screen for 1 kHz is 100 dBSPL. All controls are set to normal and all output limitations are normally off. The gain at each frequency is calculated and plotted on a frequency response curve; the frequency range may also be quoted from this curve.

Internal noise

It is also possible to measure in the test box the background or internal noise produced by the amplifier. This is usually expressed as 'equivalent input noise', i.e., the equivalent signal needed to produce that amount of signal in the output (output – gain = input equivalent). The level of equivalent input noise should obviously be considerably less than average speech levels (60 to 70 dBSPL) if it is not to interfere in speech discrimination.

Harmonic distortion

It is important to get an accurate measure of harmonic distortion because as teachers we are concerned that the signal reaching a child's ears should be the most high fidelity signal possible. Harmonic distortion can however be expressed and presented in a number of ways, according to the standards used. All hearing aids produce some form of distortion, particularly when they operate at near maximum gain or where specific output limitations such as AGC are employed to meet listeners' sensitivity needs. Most manufacturers use an input of 70 dBSPL, with the gain of the aid in reference test position (see manufacturers' data to clarify this) to present harmonic distortion. However the frequencies that are used to exemplify harmonic distortion will vary, and specification sheets must be examined carefully to ensure distortion levels are being checked along similar dimensions.

Most teachers of the deaf, however, primarily want to know whether there is an acceptable amount of distortion in the hearing aid output at user settings for normal speech inputs. The comparisons that they tend to use for this measure are the aid's current functioning at user settings – in terms of total harmonic distortion (THD) across a range of frequencies – compared with that when the aid was new and functioning optimally. The quality of the current generation of high powered hearing aids is such that most have minimal distortion figures even when operating at near saturation level. The aids that are particularly at risk in terms of THD, however, are those catering for children with severe or profound hearing losses, and who utilise practically all of an aid's gain, i.e. are wearing the aids on maximum or near maximum volume levels, with all gain controls and output controls set to maximum. Although Lindblad (1982) measured the average just detectable harmonic distortion as being around 19% for hearing-impaired people, this does not mean that such levels of distortion are acceptable. Quite the opposite, it reinforces the notion that adults must be checking aids and FM systems in terms of distortion levels, since pupils themselves will not necessarily identify such distortion until it has reached unacceptable levels and is rendering the speech processing and discrimination task more problematic than it needs to be. Small increases in distortion levels or frequency-specific increases, such as those often seen emerging at 500 Hz in some of the low frequency emphasis aids, are difficult to pick up by listening checks alone until the distortion has become quite pronounced. Frequent electro-acoustic testing of children's aids allows THD to be monitored and any significant increase in distortion levels to be tracked and responded to.

Testing at user setting

Such a use of test box measurements to examine and monitor an aid's functioning at user settings is one of the most common uses of hearing aid analysers by teachers of the deaf. Two measures in particular tend to be taken – output at user setting and THD for comparison with an earlier baseline or 'standard' print-out taken when the aid was first fitted. Most teachers wish to consider the output of an aid when a conversational speech level input is used (60–70 dBSPL) and so each service or school will settle on the recommended input for these purposes, usually 65 or 60 dBSPL. Some services choose to differentiate between the input to be provided for BW aids (60 dBSPL) and that provided to BTE and ITE aids (65 dBSPL) to take account of their different wearing positions.

According to the model of test box used, the graph on the visual display screen and/or the current print-out for the aid set to user settings is compared with the past 'ideal' print out within defined tolerance levels – usually +3 dB. Distortion levels are similarly compared, but with the proviso that distortion levels of 10% or more are generally unacceptable whatever the starting point. Similarly, for an aid that originally exhibited no distortion at a particular frequency at user setting, an increase to 6 or 7% might indicate that a component is beginning to malfunction and the aid needs further investigation. Figure 8.9 represents one way in which such information is recorded. In addition, most services keep a log in relation to individual aids and FM systems which records when they were last put through the test box, and the result. This enables the functioning of individual aids to be carefully monitored on both a short and long term basis. 'Rogue' aids and FM systems that are repeatedly being returned for repair and are proving very expensive to maintain can thus be identified for replacement.

Hearing aid and earmould

It is important that, when a child has new earmoulds, some measure is taken of the impact of the earmould on the amplification configuration of the aid. Most services include the electro-acoustic testing of aids, with and without earmoulds, as part of their regular testing programme. Chapter 5 has explored fully opportunities that are available via the earmould for both supporting and enhancing the signal delivered by the aid to meet children's needs more effectively. There is also the risk of their detracting from the signal either because of poor fitting (and nothing illustrates more graphically the impact of an ill-fitting earmould on the sound the child receives than a print-out of the level at which the child is currently listening), or because the mould has features that enhance or reduce relative gain at particular frequencies in ways not prescribed for the child.

Test setting

The procedure for running hearing aids through portable test boxes is explored in Appendix C, but is not just a question of deciding on inputs and parameters. In particular, it is important that the surroundings in which the testing is to take place are taken into account. One of the

problems of portable test box use is that the sound chamber itself is not
sealed and this can sometimes dramatically affect the stability of the
figures obtained. Care must be taken to test in conditions as quiet as
possible; the portable test box should be optimally located on a surface
that is not too hard (some teachers carry a small foam mat or a cloth

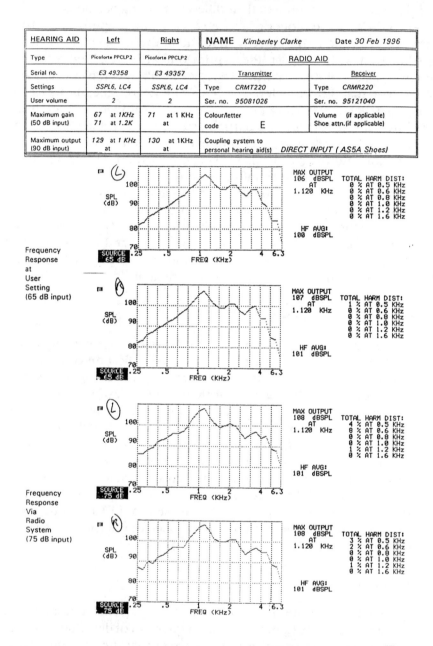

HEARING AID	Left	Right	NAME Kimberley Clarke		Date 30 Feb 1996
Type	Picoforte PPCLP2	Picoforte PPCLP2	RADIO AID		
Serial no.	E3 49358	E3 49357	Transmitter		Receiver
Settings	SSPL6, LC4	SSPL6, LC4	Type CRMT220		Type CRMR220
User volume	2	2	Ser. no. 95081026		Ser. no. 95121040
Maximum gain (50 dB input)	67 at 1KHz 71 at 1.2K	71 at 1 KHz at	Colour/letter code	E	Volume (if applicable) Shoe attn.(if applicable)
Maximum output (90 dB input)	129 at 1 KHz at	130 at 1KHz at	Coupling system to personal hearing aid(s)	DIRECT INPUT (AS5A Shoes)	

Figure 8.9 Frequency responses of a hearing aid recorded using a test box

with them for this purpose). Results that give rise for concern should always be replicated to check that they are not being influenced by some transient environmental condition. Many services always re-check print-outs of suspect aids in a more static test box, or at least in a more stable acoustic environment than the average school or home can provide, before sending an aid away for repair.

Limitations of test boxes

It must be remembered that hearing aid test boxes help us to balance FM systems and hearing aids, monitor the functioning of aids and to identify faulty aids. They do not of course indicate the source of the problem. The authors have watched both student and qualified teachers of the deaf waste many hours of precious time trying to balance up radio aids with hearing aids in test boxes, without first listening-in to the aids or checking the battery condition. It is usual to use a fresh battery when testing aids at user settings. It also helps if the listening and visual checks have already eliminated basic and intermittent faults.

Summary

All involved in the prescription, provision, management and use of hearing aids systems for children must be convinced of the urgency with which faults should be responded to and of the value of the listening experience for the child. Such urgency is reflected to varying degrees in current support programmes offered to hearing-impaired children and their families. For hearing-impaired children to make effective use of their residual hearing they must have appropriate hearing aids, but they must also be wearing working hearing aids at the levels at which they need to wear them – that is the bottom line.

References

Allard BJ, Cordry-Golden D (1991) Educational audiology: a comparison of service delivery systems utilised by Missouri schools. Language, Speech and Hearing Services in Schools 22: 5-11.

Bess FH (1977) Conditions of hearing aids worn by children in a public school setting. In HEW Pub. No. (OE) 77-05002 The Condition of Hearing Aids Worn by Children in a Public School Program. Washington, DC: Government Printing Office.

Bess FH, Sinclair JS, Riggs DE (1981) The condition of classroom amplification in a public school program (Grant Project No. 6007902254). In Bess FH, Freeman BA, Sinclair SJ (Eds) Amplification in Education. Washington, DC: A.G. Bell Association Press. pp 373-379.

Boothroyd A (1982) Hearing Impairments in Young Children. Englewood Cliffs: Prentice Hall Inc.

Connevans (1995) The CRM 220 Radio Microphone Aid 2nd Ed. Connevans Ltd, Reigate, Surry UK.

Ewing Foundation (1995) Are Their Hearing Aids Working? (video tape) Ewing Foundation, Centre for Audiology, Education of the Deaf and Speech Pathology, University of Manchester.

Gaeth J, Lounsbury E (1966) Hearing aids and children in elementary schools. Journal of Speech and Hearing Disorders 31: 283-289.

Hoverstein GH (1981) A public school audiology program: Amplification maintenance, auditory management and in-service education. In Bess FH, Freeman BA, Sinclair SJ (Eds) Amplification in Education. Washington, DC: A.G. Bell Association Press. pp 224-227.

Lindblad AC (1982) Detection of non linear distortion on speech signals by hearing-impaired listeners. Karolinska Institute, Stockholm: Report TA105.

Ling D (1976) Speech and the Hearing-impaired Child: Theory and Practice. Washington DC: The Alexander Graham Bell Association for the Deaf.

Lyon DJ, Swain G (1989) Battery voltage drop in frequency modulated amplification systems. Journal of the Association of Canadian Educators of the Deaf 15: 73-80.

Markides A (1988) Speech intelligibility: Auditory oral approach vs. total communication. Journal of the British Association of Teachers of the Deaf 12: 6.

Markides A, Huntingdon A, Kettley A (1980) Comparative speech discrimination of hearing impaired children achieved through infra-red, radio and conventional hearing aids. Journal of British Association of Teachers of the Deaf 4(1): 5.

Maxon AB, Bruckett D, van den Berg SA (1991) Classroom amplification use: A national long-term study. Language, Speech and Hearing Services in Schools 22: 242-253.

Rowson VJ, Bamford JM (1995) Selecting the gain for radio aid microphone (FM) systems: Theoretical considerations and practical limitations. British Journal of Audiology 3: 161-171.

Siegler RS (1991) Children's Thinking. Englewood Cliffs: Prentice Hall Inc.

Sinclair JS, Freeman B, Riggs D (1981) The use of the hearing-aid test box to assess the performance of the FM auditory training units. In Bess FH, Freeman BA, Sinclair JS (Eds.) Amplification in Education. Washington DS: AG Bell Association.

Skinner MW (1988) Hearing Aid Evaluation. Englewood Cliffs: Prentice Hall Inc.

Smith MS (1994) Children's Use of Hearing Aids. Unpublished Ph.D. dissertation, University of Manchester.

Smith MS, Richards SE (1990) Some essential aspects of an effective audiological management programme for school age hearing impaired children. Journal of the British Association of Teachers of the Deaf 14: 4.

Thibodeau LM (1992) Physical components and features of FM transmission systems. In Ross M (Ed) FM Auditory Training Systems, Characteristics, Selection and Use. Maryland: York Press.

Thibodeau LM, McCaffrey H, Abrahamsan J (1988) Effects of coupling hearing aids to FM systems via neck loops. Journal of the Academy of Rehabilitative Audiology 21: 49-56.

Waynor DS (1990) The Hearing Aid Handbook: User's Guide for Children

Zinck GD (1972) Hearing aids children wear: A longitudinal study of performance. The Volta Review 74: 40-41.

Chapter 9
Selection and Assessment of Classroom Amplification

D E LEWIS

Introduction

Given the variety of amplification systems that are available, how do we select the one that will be most appropriate for a given student in his/her educational environment, and how do we assess the system's performance? To begin the process, we must start with its end. That is, what are the goals of amplification in an educational setting? Firstly, we want the student to be able to hear and understand the main speaker (usually the teacher, but often another student or a television or cassette player). For this to occur, the talker's voice must reach the student's ear(s) at a loudness level which is above the background noise in the environment. The reader is referred to Chapter 10 for a discussion of issues related to noise in the classroom listening environment. Secondly, we want the student to monitor his/her own voice. Self-monitoring will help the student control the volume, as well as the clarity, of what he/she is saying. Thirdly, we want the student to hear and understand talkers other than the primary speaker, who may be at differing distances from the student, during discussions or question/answer periods.

It is important to keep these three goals in mind when selecting amplification systems for students. However, constraints related to the amplification system, the student, and the educational environment itself may affect the ability to achieve all of these goals with any single amplification system. Compromise often is necessary, and decisions must be made about which goal is given priority. In a lecture setting, for example, the priority will be to hear the main speaker, because the student may spend little or no time speaking or listening to others. In contrast, if the student is required to read aloud, the priority becomes the monitoring of his/her own voice.

The assessment of amplification begins before the individual is fitted with a device and testing is performed. It begins by considering the persons who will be using the system (both student and teacher) and the student's varied listening needs, and selecting amplification options that best meet those needs. The next section will address issues that should be considered when pre-selecting a classroom amplification system.

A hearing aid can be coupled to another amplification system for use in the classroom, but its performance will need to be assessed to ensure an appropriate fit. A number of studies have shown that the response of a hearing aid may change when it is coupled to another amplification system such as an FM system (Van Tasell and Landin, 1980; Hawkins and Van Tasell, 1982; Hawkins and Schum, 1985; Thibodeau, McCaffrey and Abrahamson, 1988; Thibodeau, 1990; Lewis, 1991; Lewis, 1994). If the amplification system is not assessed as it will be used in the classroom, the student may receive inappropriate amplification and reject the system.

Educational environment

Potential sources of interference within the student's educational environment must also be considered in the pre-selection of any amplification system using a remote transmitter. The cause of interference will vary depending on the mode of transmission. Infrared systems may be affected by natural light and do not transmit well around barriers. FM systems may be affected by other, more powerful FM transmissions within the area, such as FM radio stations, and beepers/pagers. An FM transmitter may also interfere with other FM systems in the same school if used too close to them. Inductive systems may be affected by electromagnetic interference from any device within close proximity that emits electromagnetic energy, including fluorescent lights, computer video display terminals, and electrical wiring in the walls. If large-area inductive loop systems are being used, the signal from one area may 'bleed over' into another if they are in close proximity. In addition, hearing aids with remote controls that use ultrasonic transmission technology may be affected by some ultrasonic devices such as motion detectors.

Background noise, both outside and inside classrooms, should be evaluated during the selection of amplification systems. Even when classroom amplification devices intended to improve the S/N ratio are being considered for a student, noise reduction strategies such as those discussed in Chapter 10 are important for enhancing the learning environment. In many amplification systems, the environmental microphone and the teacher's microphone are active simultaneously. The environmental microphone will amplify noise in the classroom, the student's own voice and the voices of others. Because all of the students within the classroom are a source of background noise (Blair, 1977), it will also be helpful for them to understand the noise they make, what effects it has on understanding, and how it can be reduced.

Individual user characteristics

The student who will be using the amplification system should be considered in the selection process. Taking user characteristics into consideration in the selection process will improve the chances of a successful fitting.

One characteristic to be considered is the age and physical size of the student. It is important to determine if the system being examined will fit the student comfortably. For very small children, the size of some body worn devices may make them cumbersome and uncomfortable. Selecting a smaller body worn or ear level device, or using a sound field amplification system may greatly improve adjustment. In many cases, simply keeping the components of the system stabilised can be a challenge. The use of accessories designed for children, such as shorter cords, paediatric-sized neck loops and kiddie tone hooks can be helpful in keeping the system situated. Other ways to keep the system in place can be as simple as using toupee tape to keep a behind the ear (BTE) receiver from flopping, or using eyeglass holders or ribbons to hold binaural BTE receivers in place. Sweat bands can be used to hold button receivers and earmoulds in the ear or to hold a bone-conduction transducer in place. Vests with pockets or waist packs may be more comfortable for holding a BW receiver than the more traditional chest worn placement. If chosen, however, the environmental microphone of the system should be placed at ear level so that amplification of the student's own voice and the voices of others is not compromised.

A child's behaviour is another aspect that should be considered in the selection process. If a child is easily distracted by the cords or switches on a BW receiver, he/she may pay more attention to them than to the teacher and may adjust the controls inappropriately. In these cases, it may be necessary to place the receiver unit on the child's back (if the system has ear level environmental microphones), to select a neck loop coupling that could be placed under clothing, or to use covers over the volume control and switches. Alternatively, a large-area induction loop that requires the child to wear only his/her own hearing aid or a sound field amplification system that requires no device on the child may be considered. An ear level FM receiver would also be an option, if the child is able to wear it without distraction.

Especially with older students, cosmetic concerns play a role in the selection process. Even those who willingly wore a particular amplification system when they were younger, may reject it as they get older. For these students, the perceived benefit of the amplification device may be outweighed by concerns about appearing different from their peers. Options to consider when cosmetic concerns are an issue include a neck loop coupling that can be worn under clothing, or a large-area induction system, if the student is willing to wear his/her hearing aid. An ear level

FM system may be more acceptable than a body worn receiver unit. A system that is coupled to the ear via headphones might be acceptable because of the popularity of 'Walkman-style' radios, cassettes and compact disc players. A sound field system will be the least obtrusive because the student is not required to wear any type of receiver. However, for students who change classes throughout the day, this option requires sound field systems in each classroom.

Finally, physical limitations will play a role in the selection process. Chronic ear drainage, for example, may require a non-occluding coupling option such as open earmoulds, lightweight headphones, or earbuds. Cranio-facial anomalies may preclude fitting a traditional earmould coupling to the ear. Use of a bone-conduction transducer if the hearing loss is conductive, or headphones, may be considered as alternatives. A sound field system may also be an appropriate option. For individuals with dexterity problems, a body worn receiver, with its larger volume control and switches, may improve the student's independence when small systems would be too difficult to manipulate.

It is important that the audiologist, educational personnel, the student, and his/her family work closely together to select device options that will be beneficial and acceptable. Time spent in the pre-selection process will be time saved in the next phase of the evaluation, the assessment of aided performance.

Assessment of aided performance

As with the entire process of selection, the assessment of aided performance must begin with the goal. That is, what benefit do we want the user to obtain from the amplification device? If the primary goal is to improve audibility of speech, whose speech do we mean (the teacher, other students, the student using the system) and how do we know when we have achieved our goal?

Numerous approaches for selecting amplification targets have been developed for adult hearing aid users (Skinner et al., 1982; McCandless and Lyregaard, 1983; Berger, Hagberg, and Rane, 1984; Byrne and Dillon, 1986; Cox, 1988). Although these methods are often used in the selection of amplification systems for children, there are a number of concerns that must first be addressed.

Firstly, in determining appropriate amplification for children, it is important to remember that they are not simply 'little adults'. Test techniques and habilitation needs will be different for children. Children are just learning speech and language, while the adult with acquired hearing loss requires amplification of something he/she already knows. As a result, amplification appropriate for an adult may not be appropriate for a child with a very similar hearing loss. Children lack the world knowledge that often allows adults to 'fill in' parts of a message they are unable to hear.

Secondly, when fitting children with amplification, we often have less audiological information than we would have with an adult. Especially with younger children, threshold information may be limited, test reliability may vary from good at one visit to very poor at the next, and word recognition information may be limited or non-existent. In addition, middle ear pathology may cause frequent changes in the degree and configuration of the hearing loss.

Thirdly, children may be unable or unwilling to communicate problems that arise with amplification. If the child rejects the device or we are not seeing the anticipated benefit, we may not always know why. They may not communicate that the device is not working, that the signal is distorted, that it does not sound the same today as it usually does, or a host of other minor or major difficulties that can occur on a daily basis. This problem is illustrated in a study by Bess, Sinclair, and Riggs (1984). They examined FM systems in classrooms for students with hearing loss. Results indicated that 53% of the student receivers and 50% of the teacher transmitter/microphones failed at least one category on their checklist for physical defects. Clearly, involvement of parents, caregivers and educational personnel is critical to acceptance, adjustment and maintenance of classroom amplification systems.

Selecting amplification targets

When evaluating performance with amplification, many of the subjective measures that currently are used with adult patients are not appropriate for children. Therefore, selection of instruments is often based on a target or goal for amount of amplification at different frequencies relative to degree and shape of hearing loss. Using target based or formula approaches with children is problematic because most of these formulas were based on information obtained for adults with hearing loss. As a result, many of the factors discussed above were not considered in the design. Of equal importance, children have ear canals that are much smaller than those of adults (Feigin et al., 1989). Targets that produce appropriate sound levels for adults result in much louder sounds for a small child.

Two approaches designed specifically to select amplification targets for children will be addressed in this section; the first employs guidelines for aided thresholds versus unaided thresholds (functional gain) and the second is the desired sensation level approach (Seewald, Ross, and Spiro, 1985; Seewald, Ross, and Stelmachowicz, 1987; Seewald, 1988; Seewald et al., 1991; Seewald et al., 1993).

Functional gain

Matkin (1987) provided recommendations for aided thresholds for young children with moderate to severe hearing losses (Table 9.1), to provide optimal audibility of average conversational speech. These guidelines were not intended for use with profound hearing losses where the amplification goal may be just detection of sound. In setting the maximum output of the hearing aid, Matkin used Cox's (1986) recommendation that the SSPL90 (i.e., the maximum output of the system in a 2cc coupler) equals 100 dBSPL plus one quarter of the average hearing loss. He recommended that this level be further reduced by 5 dB for pre-schoolers and 10 dB for infants and toddlers. For example, for a 4 year old child with a hearing loss of 60 dB, the recommended SSPL90 would equal 100 dB + 15 ($^1/_4$ of the hearing loss) – 5 dB (for a pre-schooler) or 110 dBSPL.

Table 9.1 Optimal aided thresholds for young children as recommended by Matkin (1987)

Frequency	250 Hz	500 Hz	1000 Hz	2000 Hz	4000 Hz
Threshold	30 dBHL	30 dBHL	25 dBHL	20 dBHL	20 dBHL

Desired sensation level approach

The desired sensation level (DSL) approach is a formula based procedure, based on the assumption that hearing aid selection for children differs in important ways from hearing aid selection for adults. The goal of this approach is "to provide the child with amplified speech that is consistently audible, comfortable and undistorted across the broadest relevant frequency range possible" (Seewald et al., 1991). Using hearing threshold data that can be gathered in a variety of ways, targets are developed for 2cc coupler, sound field functional gain or probe-tube microphone measures of amplification for both average conversational speech and maximum output of the hearing aid(s).

Both Matkin's functional gain guidelines and the DSL methods assume that variations from the target will occur in the final fitting, when based on information that is particular to an individual child. In addition, both methods assume that the speech being amplified is average conversational speech at approximately 3 feet from the listener. Neither method accounts for differences that occur when the speaker is further away (e.g., in a lecture hall or gym) or closer (e.g., when a remote microphone is placed close to the speaker's mouth or when the speech being amplified is the user's own voice). For this reason, they must be considered 'guidelines' – a starting point for measurements of amplified speech – which will be modified as needed to account for the variety of listening situations that are encountered throughout the day.

Evaluation

Functional gain measures

When an amplification system has been selected and amplification targets have been developed, the next step is to measure the performance of the system and verify that it meets our goals for the student. Aided performance can be assessed in a number of ways. One of the most common methods utilises behavioural testing in a sound booth. First, unaided thresholds are obtained for each ear, if possible. Then the amplification system is placed on the ear to be evaluated and threshold measures are repeated in the sound field (the signal coming from a loudspeaker). The difference between the two thresholds is the functional gain with the hearing instrument. For example, if a child's unaided threshold is 50 dBHL and his/her aided threshold is 20 dBHL, the hearing instrument is said to provide 30 dB of functional gain.

The test method by which unaided and aided thresholds are obtained will vary depending on the age of the child. Test methods are presented in detail in Chapter 1 and therefore will be addressed only briefly here. Children approximately 5–6 months to 2 years of age are most often tested using visual reinforcement audiometry (VRA) (Suzuki and Ogiba, 1961; Liden and Kankkunen, 1969; Moore, Wilson, and Thompson, 1977).

Children of 2–4 years of age can be tested using play audiometry tasks (Thompson and Weber, 1974). By 5 years of age, most children can respond using a hand-raising task. If the test session is long, however, younger children may become bored and it is often helpful to use play tasks to maintain their interest and attention.

The physical arrangement of the test room also will vary, depending on the amplification system that is being evaluated. When the system's microphone is worn by the child (e.g., personal hearing aid), he/she is placed in the appropriate position in the sound booth and signals are presented via the loudspeaker (Figure 9.1). If the amplification system uses a remote microphone (e.g., FM microphone/transmitter), it is placed in the spot in the booth where the child would have been, and the child, wearing the receiver, is placed some distance away.

Once the functional gain measures have been completed, they are compared with the level of unamplified speech to determine if speech will be audible. Figure 9.2 shows an example of an aided audiogram. The Xs represent unaided thresholds for the left ear and the As represent aided thresholds for that ear. The shaded region represents the levels of conversational speech. Any area where the shaded region is below (i.e., louder than) the As would be expected to be audible. In this example, results suggest that average conversational speech, as well as the peaks and valleys of speech, would be audible with the exception of softer components of speech at 250 Hz and 4 kHz.

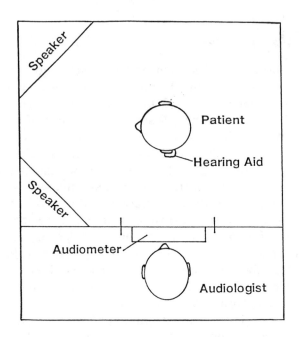

Figure 9.1 Physical arrangement for sound field functional gain testing of a hearing aid

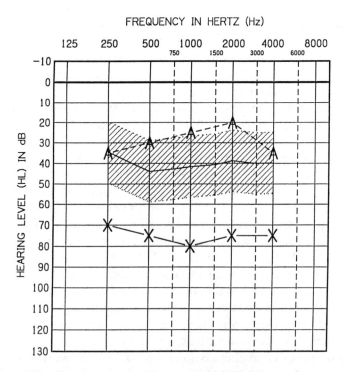

Figure 9.2 Aided audiogram obtained using sound field functional gain measures. Xs represent unaided thresholds and As represent aided thresholds for the left ear. The shaded area represents the levels of conversational speech

Benefits

Functional gain testing uses procedures that typically are familiar to the child, family and audiologist and requires test equipment that is available in most audiology practices. Functional gain measures also provide information about the lowest sound level that can be detected with an amplification system.

Limitations

Functional gain measures do not evaluate the system at input levels that are comparable to the level at which speech, typically, will reach the microphone of the system. As a result, functional gain measures can overestimate the amount of amplification the system will provide in real-life situations. Figure 9.3 illustrates this problem. The curves show gain produced at different sound input levels for three hypothetical hearing aids. Note that at low input levels (10–40 dBSPL) comparable to those that would be used in functional gain measures, the gain of the three hearing aids is the same. At inputs above 40 dBSPL, hearing aid C begins to deviate from the other two, with lower gain across the remaining input levels. At inputs above 60 dBSPL, hearing aid B begins to deviate from hearing aid A. If only low input levels were used to test these instruments, one might conclude that the three hearing aids would respond similarly in the classroom. However, at higher inputs (comparable to the level of speech at the hearing aid microphone) the responses are very different. This discrepancy between the response of the amplification system using functional gain measures and the response of the system in actual use would also be a problem for any amplification system that uses a remote microphone close to the talker's mouth. For these systems, the typical input to the microphone would be much higher

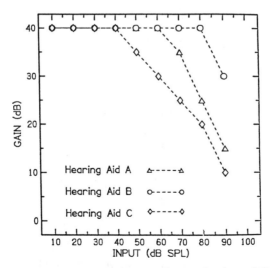

Figure 9.3 Gain (dB) as a function of input (dBSPL) for three different hearing aids

than the inputs used for functional gain measures (e.g., 80–85 dBSPL for a chest level microphone). Functional gain measures also do not provide information about the maximum output of the system, an issue that is especially important when fitting young children to prevent discomfort, rejection and possible further hearing loss.

Furthermore, evaluation by functional gain measures is limited because it cannot provide information about the amount of amplification provided by a system in regions of normal hearing. In addition, when there are significant differences in hearing thresholds between ears, the better ear must be masked in order to test the poorer ear. Many younger children have difficulty ignoring the masking noise while trying to listen for the signal being tested. Functional gain measures also may require co-operation from the child for extended periods of time, especially if different amplification systems or settings are being evaluated.

Probe-tube microphone measures

Aided performance may also be assessed with probe-tube microphone measures. Probe-tube microphone measures assess amplification provided by the device in the ear canal of a user. For these measures, a small flexible tube is attached to a microphone and placed in the ear canal at an appropriate depth (Stelmachowicz and Seewald, 1991; Hawkins and Mueller, 1992). A signal is generated from a loudspeaker and a measurement is made in the unoccluded ear canal (Figure 9.4).

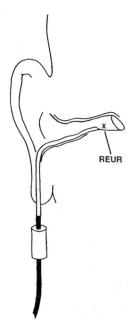

Figure 9.4 Measurement of the real ear unaided response (REUR) in an unoccluded ear canal using a probe-tube microphone

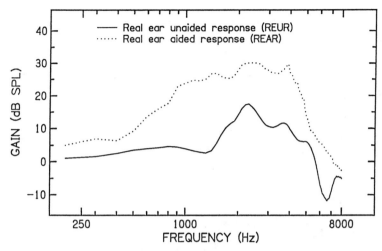

Figure 9.5 Real ear unaided response (REUR) (solid line) and real ear aided response (REAR) (dotted line) as a function of frequency as measured in the ear canal using a probe-tube microphone system

This measurement, which represents the natural amplification effects of the external ear, is termed the real ear unaided response (REUR) (Figure 9.5 – solid line).

Next, the amplification device is placed on the ear, turned on, and the measurement is repeated (Figure 9.5 • • • dotted line). This measurement, representing the gain or output of an amplification device in the ear canal, is termed the real ear aided response (REAR) (Figure 9.6). The

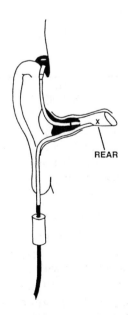

Figure 9.6 Measurement of the real ear aided response (REAR) with the amplification device coupled to an earmould and placed in the ear canal

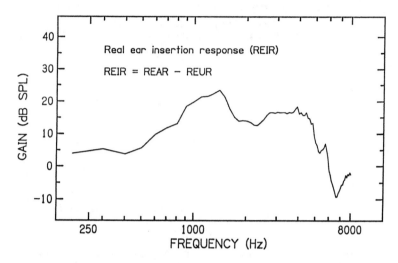

Figure 9.7 Real ear insertion response (REIR) as a function of frequency

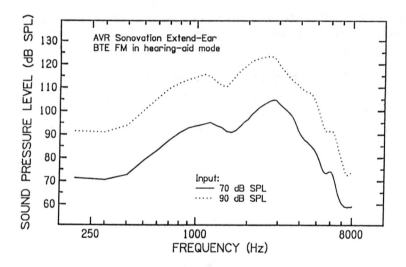

Figure 9.8 Real ear output sound pressure level as a function of frequency for an AVR Sonovation Extend-Ear BTE FM system in the hearing aid mode. The solid line represents output with a 70 dBSPL speech-weighted noise input and the dotted line represents output with a 90 dBSPL swept pure-tone input

difference between the REAR and REUR is termed the real ear insertion response (REIR) (Figure 9.7). When describing the REIR at a specific frequency, the term real ear insertion gain (REIG) is used. The sound level used for these measurements will differ depending on the information needed. For example, the audiologist may use a 70 dB, 75 dB, or 60 dBSPL input signal to assess how much amplification is provided to the student for average, loud or soft conversation, respectively. The audiologist may want to use an 80 dBSPL signal to assess how much amplification the student receives with a system where the microphone is worn very close to the mouth (e.g., lapel or head worn microphone). In addition, the maximum output of the device may be assessed with high input levels (usually 90 dBSPL). This measurement is termed the real ear saturation response (RESR).

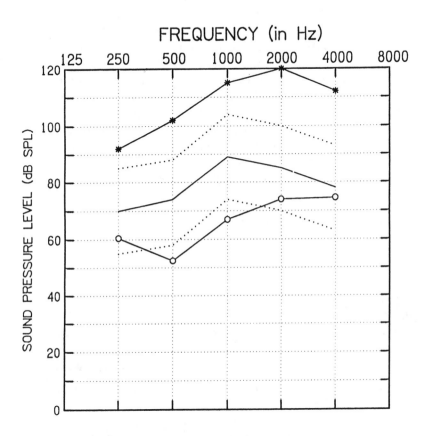

Figure 9.9 Real ear amplified long term average speech spectrum (LTASS) using outputs shown in Fig. 9.8. Os represent unaided thresholds for the right ear; solid line represents the LTASS; dotted lines represent the +15/–15 range of speech; asterisks represent the maximum output of the amplification system

Figure 9.8 illustrates results from probe-tube microphone measures using a behind the ear FM system in the hearing aid mode of operation. The solid line shows sound output from an amplification system when a 70 dBSPL noise input is used (REAR). The dotted line shows output of the same system with a 90 dBSPL input (RESR). In Figure 9.9, these results are used to plot the level to which speech is amplified with the amplification system. The Os represent unaided thresholds for the right ear, the solid line represents the level to which average conversational speech is amplified with the system, and the dotted lines on either side represent the peaks and valleys of amplified speech. The asterisks represent the maximum output of the amplification system. On this graph, any parts of speech that are above threshold (Os) and below maximum output (asterisks) would be audible. Therefore, in this example, average conversational speech, as well as the peaks of speech, would be audible across the frequency range 250 Hz to 4kHz. Some of the softer components of conversational speech would not be audible at 250 Hz, 2 kHz and 4 kHz.

The physical set-up used for probe-tube microphone measures depends on the particular measurement equipment being used and the amplification system being assessed. Figure 9.10 is an example of the equipment array for assessing an FM system. The probe microphone assembly is in place in the ear and the student is wearing an FM receiver. The FM microphone/transmitter is placed at an appropriate distance from the probe-microphone loudspeaker for the particular measurement equipment. Measurements representative of the amplification received from the FM system when the teacher is wearing the transmitter and the student is wearing the receiver in a typical classroom setting are made.

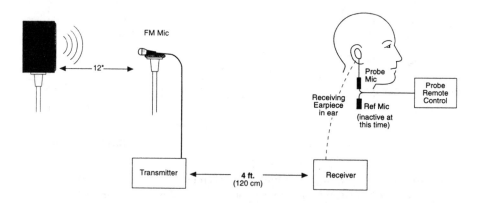

Figure 9.10 Example of physical arrangement for probe-tube microphone evaluation of an FM system for the FM-only mode of operation (from American Speech-Language-Hearing Association, 1994. Used with permission)

Benefits

Assessment with probe-tube microphone measures can resolve many of the limitations posed by functional gain measures. One important benefit, which was discussed above, is the ability to evaluate the student's amplification system with sound levels he/she would typically encounter in the classroom. In addition, probe-tube microphone measures provide information about the maximum output of the system to ensure safety, comfort, and adequate amplification of speech, and can evaluate amplification provided in regions of normal hearing. Probe-tube microphone measures are typically faster than functional gain measures, requiring co-operation for a shorter period of time. They also are able to define the frequency response of the amplification system more completely than is possible with functional gain measures and allow relatively easy evaluation of each ear independently, even when there are significant differences in thresholds between ears.

Limitations

Probe-tube microphone measures do require specialised equipment. However, the availability of probe-tube microphone equipment is increasing as companies develop systems that can be used with current audiological equipment. Also, measurement equipment is portable so that a single system can be used in multiple locations.

Probe-tube microphone measures are limited by the requirement that the user be co-operative, still and have ear canals free of cerumen. With young children, especially, it may be difficult to achieve these goals on all occasions. However, there are general guidelines to help improve success with these measures when evaluating young children (Stelmachowicz and Seewald, 1991; Moodie, Seewald, and Sinclair, 1994). Probe-tube microphone measures cannot be used when there is drainage from the ear canal or in cases of ear canal atresia. In addition, they should not be used when it is suspected that the user's thresholds are vibrotactile rather than auditory.

Coupler or test box measures

A third method of assessing a student's aided performance is with coupler measures. For these measures, the receiver of an amplification system is attached to a standard coupler (usually 2cc) and the micro-phone of the system is placed in the sound chamber of a hearing aid test box. In instances where the microphone is in the same case as the receiver, the entire receiver is placed in the sound chamber. A signal is presented to the microphone from a loudspeaker in the sound chamber and the hearing aid analyser records the amount of amplification across frequencies. Figure 9.11 illustrates an example of the set-up for analysing an FM system using coupler measures. In this case, the micro-phone of the FM system has been placed in the test box and the receiver, which is outside the test box, is attached to the coupler. The hearing aid analyser then records the amplification the system provides for the particular input signal.

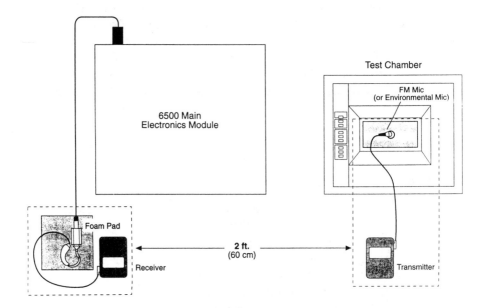

Figure 9.11 Physical arrangement for 2cc coupler measurements of an FM system in the FM-only mode of operation (from American Speech-Language-Hearing Association, 1994. Used with permission)

Benefits

As with probe-tube microphone measures, coupler measures can evaluate amplification at input levels comparable to those experienced during actual use. Coupler measures also provide information concerning maximum output of the system and harmonic distortion, both at use and full-on volume settings. Coupler measures are able to delineate the frequency response of the system more completely than functional gain measures and, unlike functional gain and probe-tube microphone measures, they do not require the user to be present. In addition, use of a standard coupler allows comparison to manufacturer's specifications.

Limitations

Coupler measures do require an analysis equipment system. However, these systems are available in most audiological practices. Care must be taken when using coupler measures for evaluating the amount of amplification received by the student because the size of the coupler may vary considerably from the size of the child's own ear canal. As stated earlier,

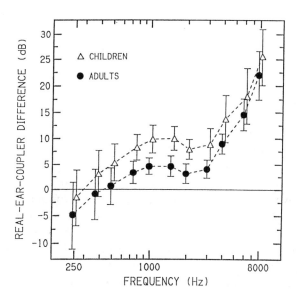

Figure 9.12 Real-ear-to-coupler difference (in dB) as a function of frequency (in Hz) for children (open triangles) and adults (filled circles). Error bars represent +/– 1 standard deviation from the mean (from Feigin et al., 1989. Used with permission)

the size of the ear canal will have an effect on the actual sound pressure levels that the individual hears with the amplification system. The smaller the canal, the higher the output in that canal in relation to the standard coupler. Figure 9.12, from Feigin et al. (1989), illustrates this point. The graph shows differences between measurements made in the ear canal and in a 2cc coupler for children aged 4 weeks to 5 years (open triangles) and adults (filled circles). For both groups, the differences between the actual ear canal and coupler measures increase with frequency. However, across the entire range, the differences are larger for the children. In addition, the standard deviations suggest that use of average correction values may not adequately reflect the actual difference between the coupler and a particular individual's ear. If no corrections are made to compensate for these differences when evaluating the amplification system, an inappropriate fitting may result. Therefore, corrections must be used to predict how the amplification will perform in the child's ear. Detailed information on average correction factors, as well as methods of measuring the difference between the coupler and real ear on an individual basis, can be found elsewhere (Bentler and Pavlovic, 1989).

As stated earlier in this chapter, no method of assessing aided performance is useful unless it is used with some goal in mind for determining if the amount of amplification provided by the system will make the desired signal audible to the user. In addition, the amount of amplification needed will vary depending on the signal(s) the user must be able to hear.

Speech recognition measures

When audibility has been assured (to the best of our ability given the hearing loss, amplification system, signal level, etc.), the battle is partly won. However, ensuring audibility does not always ensure that the signal can be understood. The next step of the evaluation process, therefore, is to assess speech recognition with the amplification system of choice. Again, the goal must be kept in mind when selecting both the test materials and test environment. The results of speech recognition testing will be affected not only by the degree and shape, but also by the distortion that may result from the hearing loss. Consequently, improvement in speech recognition resulting from use of an amplification

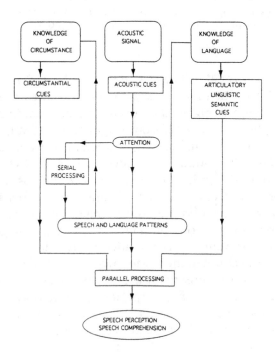

Figure 9.13 Simplified model of speech perception (from Smaldino, 1995. Used with permission)

system can only be determined when compared with unaided test results. Therefore, whenever possible, speech recognition should first be assessed without amplification.

There are a number of standardised tests that are available for assessing children's speech recognition. In addition to hearing loss, the test selection, and, therefore, the results obtained, will be affected by age, world knowledge, language and cognitive level, and the information the tester is seeking. Figure 9.13, from Smaldino (1995), provides a simple model of speech perception. As can be seen in this model, the ability to perceive and, more importantly, to comprehend speech is not a simple task.

In general, speech recognition tests range from those which measure only awareness of sound, to those which require identification of phonemes, words or sentences. It is important to select tests that are within the range of a child's capabilities to ensure that results reflect auditory skills and are not limited by other factors such as language delay. For example, tests may simply require children to point to pictures or words, or may require them to write or repeat what has been heard. A test that requires a child to respond by selecting among a group of printed alternatives will be affected by reading skills and phonological and vocabulary knowledge. Open ended tests usually will be more difficult than those which use a limited set of possible responses.

Educational personnel are an important asset to audiologists selecting speech recognition tests as a part of an audiological test battery. Because these individuals work with the student on a day-to-day basis, they have a more comprehensive knowledge of that student's skills than the audiologist, who may only see the student infrequently. Developmental and educational advances (or the lack thereof) since the last time the child was evaluated may require different tests from those originally planned to ensure, again, that auditory skills are being assessed rather than language, vocabulary, reading level, etc. Conversely, the results of appropriately selected speech recognition tests will be helpful to educational staff as they plan activities and goals for individual students in their classrooms. For example, tests have been designed to assess speechreading ability as well as to compare performance on tasks in auditory only, visual only, or auditory plus visual modes of presentation. A student who scores significantly higher on a task in the auditory plus visual mode than in the auditory only mode may function better in a classroom setting where the talker's face is visible during educational activities than one where the talker often is in a position where his/her face is not visible. During activities when the talker's face cannot be seen, such as a film whose talkers are often off-camera, additional assistance may be needed, such as closed captioning, a written transcript of dialogue, or an interpreter.

Although a complete discussion of available speech recognition tests is not possible in the context of this chapter, Appendix B2, from the Pediatric Working Group of the Conference on Amplification for

Children with Auditory Deficits (1996), provides an extensive list of materials that are available in the English language. Again, note that degree of hearing loss, age, response task, and response format are factors to be considered in test selection. Further information regarding speech recognition testing is available in Chapter 1.

The Pediatric Working Group of the Conference on Amplification for Children with Auditory Deficits (1996) indicates that "measures of aided performance are not to be used for the purpose of changing hearing aid settings unless there is an obvious behavioural indicator to the contrary. These include loudness tolerance problems or an inability to perceive particular speech cues that should be audible in the aided condition" (page 56). The Group further recommends that "performance measures be obtained in a binaural presentation mode unless one's intent is to document asymmetry in aided auditory performance" (page 56).

The physical arrangement for testing may depend on the information that is needed. For example, if the goal is to determine the child's speech recognition under ideal conditions, testing may be completed in a quiet environment (such as a sound suite) with the amplification system in place. If the effects of background noise are to be assessed, multi-talker babble or speech noise may be added to the test environment at a level that would approximate to that of the classroom.

Distance effects can be simulated in a sound suite by varying the level at which the signal is presented. For example, Figure 9.14a illustrates speech recognition testing in noise with a monaural hearing aid. The hearing aid is placed on the left ear and the student is seated in the appropriate spot in the sound booth. Speech is presented from the left loudspeaker at 55 dBHL and noise is presented from the right loudspeaker at 50 dBHL (a +5 S/N ratio). Speech recognition testing is completed. Figure 9.14b illus-

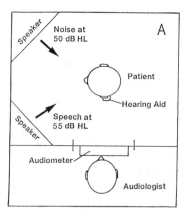
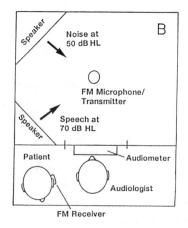

Figure 9.14 Display of speech recognition testing in a sound booth for both hearing aids (Panel A) and FM systems (Panel B) to simulate actual classroom conditions. A +5 dB S/N ratio is used for speech perception testing with hearing aids and a +20 dB S/N ratio with FM systems (from Lewis et al., 1991. Used with permission)

trates testing in the sound suite with the same noise level (50 dBHL), but using an FM system in place of the hearing aid. The FM microphone, not the student, is placed in the appropriate spot in the sound booth. The level of speech from the left loudspeaker has been increased to 70 dBHL to simulate the level of speech at a lapel microphone. The child, wearing the FM receiver on an FM-only setting, has been moved outside the sound booth to ensure that the signal being tested is from the FM microphone only. Speech recognition testing is repeated and the score can be compared to that with the hearing aid alone.

As stated previously, it may also be helpful to assess speech recognition ability with auditory input alone, visual input alone and auditory and visual input combined. This information can be helpful to classroom instructors as they assess teaching style and consider possible adaptations for students with hearing loss.

Although testing in a sound suite can simulate the educational environment, it may be helpful to do some informal testing in the actual educational setting(s) the student will encounter. Comparisons can be made at varying distances and with different amplification systems in the types of environments the student will experience throughout the day. For example, the teacher could present a list of words or sentences in a typical voice in the classroom while the students are seated at their desks. The students' responses can be compared for unaided, hearing aid, individual FM system, and/or sound field FM system conditions. Responses also could be compared for a particular amplification system or in the presence of noise sources (e.g., fans, classroom equipment, open windows) while the teacher and student are at different distances from each other. These comparisons can be helpful in selecting the system that will provide the most flexibility for the student and teachers.

Follow-up

Even when the initial evaluation and assessment have been completed and the student has been fitted with appropriate classroom amplification, the fitting process should not be considered complete. It is important that everyone who will be using the system be trained in its use, care and maintenance, as well as in the benefits and limitations of the selected system. Appropriate expectations can be very important to the student's success with the amplification system. As educational personnel change, ongoing training will be necessary. In addition, changes in the student's educational environment, hearing loss or personal amplification system may necessitate re-evaluation of the original choices that were made. Educational personnel play a very important role throughout evaluation and follow-up because they will be using the system on a daily basis and are often the first to note changes in the performance of the system and/or in the student's use of the system. Close contact among the audiologist, educational personnel, student and the student's family will help to ensure that the best benefit possible is achieved with classroom amplification systems.

Conclusion

The evaluation and assessment of classroom amplification cannot be confined to a single visit with an audiologist. Pre-selection issues must be addressed to ensure that appropriate options are selected for evaluation. The testing itself must be appropriate, both for the developmental level of the student and for the equipment that is being evaluated. Once an initial selection has been made, evaluation in the educational environment and close follow-up are important to the successful use of the system. When all aspects of evaluation and assessment are addressed, the student is most likely to receive amplification that will meet his/her particular needs.

References

American Speech-Language-Hearing Association (1994) Guidelines for fitting and monitoring FM Systems. ASHA 36(12): 1-9.

Bench J, Koval A, Bamford J (1979) The BKB (Bamford-Koval-Bench) sentence lists for partially-hearing children. British Journal of Audiology 13: 108-112.

Bentler RA, Pavlovic CV (1989) Transfer functions and corrections factors used in hearing aid evaluation and research. Ear and Hearing 10: 58-63.

Berger KW, Hagberg EN, Rane RL (1984) Prescription Hearing Aids: Rationale, Procedures, and Results (4th Edition). Kent: Herald Press.

Bess F, Sinclair JS, Riggs D (1984) Group amplification in schools for the hearing impaired. Ear and Hearing 5: 138-144.

Blair J (1977) Effects of amplification, speech reading, and classroom environments on reception of speech. Volta Review, Dec.: 443-449.

Boothroyd A (1968) Developments of speech audiometry. Sound 2: 3-10.

Boothroyd A (1995) Speech perception tests and hearing-impaired children. In Plant G, Spens CE (Eds) Speech Communication and Profound Deafness. London: Whurr Publishers.

Boothroyd A (1996) Speech perception and production in hearing-impaired children. In Bess FH, Gravel JS, Tharpe AM (Eds) Amplification for Children with Auditory Deficits. Nashville, TN: Bill Wilkerson Center Press.

Byrne D, Dillon H (1986) The National Acoustic Laboratories' (NAL) new procedure for selection of the gain and frequency response of a hearing aid. Ear and Hearing 7: 257-265.

Cox RM (1986) Hearing aids and aural rehabilitation: A structured approach to hearing aid selection. Ear and Hearing 7: 226-239.

Cox RM (1988) Distribution of short-term RMS levels in conversational speech. Journal of the Acoustical Society of America 84: 1100-1104.

Erber NP (1974) Pure-tone thresholds and word-recognition abilities of hearing-impaired children. Journal of Speech and Hearing Research 17: 194-202.

Erber N (1980) Use of the auditory numbers test to evaluate speech perception abilities of hearing-impaired children. Journal of Speech and Hearing Disorders 45: 527-532.

Erber NP (1982) Auditory Training. Washington, D.C.: Alexander Graham Bell Association for the Deaf.

Feigin JA, Kopun JK, Stelmachowicz PG, Gorga MP (1989) Probe-microphone measures of ear-canal sound pressure levels in infants and children. Ear and Hearing 10: 254-258.

Finitzo-Hieber T, Gerlin IJ, Matkin N, Cherow-Skalka E (1980) A sound effects recognition test for the pediatric audiological evaluation. Ear and Hearing 1: 271-276.

Haskins H (1949) A phonetically balanced test of speech discrimination for children (unpublished Master's thesis). Northwestern University.

Hawkins D, Schum D (1985) Some effects of FM-system coupling on hearing aid characteristics. Journal of Speech and Hearing Disorders 50: 132-141.

Hawkins D, Van Tasell D (1982) Electroacoustic characteristics of personal FM systems. Journal of Speech and Hearing Disorders 47: 355-362.

Hawkins DB, Mueller HG (1992) Procedural considerations in probe-tube microphone measurements. In Mueller HG, Hawkins DB, Hawkins JL, Probe Microphone Measurements: Hearing Aid Selection and Assessment. San Diego, CA: Singular Publishing Group. pp 67-90.

Hirsch IJ, Davis H, Silverman SR, Reynolds EG, Eldert E, Benson RW (1952) Development of materials for speech audiometry. Journal of Speech and Hearing Disorders 17: 321-337.

Jerger S, Lewis S, Hawkins J, Jerger J (1980) Pediatric speech intelligibility test: I - Generation of test materials. International Journal of Pediatric Otorhinolaryngology 2: 217-230.

Katz D, Elliott L (1978) Development of a new children's speech discrimination test. Paper presented at American Speech and Hearing Association Convention.

Levitt H, Resnick SB (1978) Speech reception by the hearing impaired: Methods of testing and the development of new test. Scandinavian Audiology 6, 107S-130S.

Lewis D (1991) FM systems and assistive devices: Selection and evaluation. In Feigin JA, Stelmachowicz PG (Eds) Pediatric Amplification: Proceedings of the 1991 National Conference. Omaha, NE: BTNRH. pp 115-138.

Lewis D (1994) Assistive devices for classroom listening: FM systems. American Journal of Audiology 3: 70-83.

Lewis D, Feigin J, Karasek A, Stelmachowicz P (1991) Evaluation and assessment of FM systems. Ear and Hearing 12: 268-280.

Liden G, Kankkunen A (1969) Visual reinforcement audiometry. Acta Otolaryngology 67: 281-292.

Ling D (1978) Auditory coding and reading: An analysis of training procedures for hearing impaired children. In Ross M, Giolas TG (Eds) Auditory Management of Hearing-Impaired Children. Baltimore, MD: University Park Press. pp 181-218.

Ling D (1989) Foundations of Spoken Language for Hearing-Impaired Children. Washington, D.C.: Alexander Graham Bell Association for the Deaf.

Matkin ND (1987) Hearing instruments for children: Premises for selecting and fitting. Hearing Instruments 38: 14-16.

McCandless GA, Lyregaard PE (1983) Prescription of gain/output (POGO) for hearing aids. Hearing Instruments 34: 16-21.

Moodie KS, Seewald RC, Sinclair ST (1994) Procedure for predicting real-ear hearing aid performance in young children. American Journal of Audiology 3: 23-31.

Moore J, Wilson J, Thompson G (1977) Visual reinforcement of head-turn responses in infants under twelve months of age. Journal of Speech and Hearing Disorders 42: 328-334.

Mueller HG (1992) Terminology and procedures. In Mueller HG, Hawkins DB, and

Northern JL, Probe Microphone Measurements: Hearing Aid Selection and Assessment. San Diego: Singular Publishing Group. pp 41-66.

Pediatric Working Group of the Conference on Amplification for Children with Auditory Deficits (1996) Amplification for infants and children with hearing loss. American Journal of Audiology 5(1): 53-68.

Renshaw J, Robbins AM, Miyamoto R, Osberger MJ, Pope M (1988) Hoosier Auditory Visual Enhancement Test (HAVE). Indianapolis, IN: Indiana University School of Medicine, Department of Otolaryngology-Head and Neck Surgery.

Robbins AM, Renshaw J, Miyamoto R, Osberger MJ, Pope M (1988) Minimal Pairs Test. Indianapolis, IN: Indiana University School of Medicine, Department of Otolaryngology-Head and Neck Surgery.

Ross M, Lerman J (1970) A picture identification test for hearing-impaired children. Journal of Speech and Hearing Research 13: 61-66.

Schweitzer HC, Sullivan FF, Beck LB, Cole WA (1990) Developing a consensus for "real ear" hearing instrument terms. Hearing Instruments 41: 28, 46.

Seewald RC (1988) The desired sensation level approach for children: Selection and verification. Hearing Instruments 39: 18-22.

Seewald RC, Ramji KV, Sinclair ST, Moodie KS, Jamieson DG (1993) DSL 3.1: User's Manual. London, Ontario: Hearing Health Care Research Unit, The University of Western Ontario.

Seewald RC, Ross M, Spiro MK (1985) Selecting amplification characteristics for young hearing-impaired children. Ear and Hearing 6: 48-53.

Seewald RC, Ross M, Stelmachowicz PG (1987) Selecting and verifying hearing aid performance characteristics for young children. Journal of the Academy of Rehabilitative Audiology 20: 25-37.

Seewald RC, Zelisko DL, Ramji KV, Jamieson DG (1991) DSL 3.0: User's Manual. London, Ontario: Hearing Health Care Research Unit, The University of Western Ontario.

Siegenthaler B, Haspiel B (1966) Development of two standardized measures of hearing for speech by children. Co-operative Research Program, Project No. 2372, United States Office of Education, Washington, DC.

Skinner MW, Pascoe DP, Miller JD, Popelka GR (1982) Measurements to determine the optimal placement of speech energy within the listener's auditory area: A basis for selection of amplification characteristics. In Studebaker GA, Bess FH (Eds) The Vanderbilt Hearing Aid Report: State of the Art Research Needs. Upper Darby, PA: Monographs in Contemporary Audiology.

Smaldino JJ (1995) Speech perception processes in children. In Crandell CC, Smaldino JJ, Flexer C (Eds) Sound-Field FM Amplification: Theory and Practical Applications. San Diego: Singular Publishing Group, Inc. pp 17-28.

Stelmachowicz PG, Seewald RC (1991) Probe-tube microphone measures in children. Seminars in Hearing 12: 67-72.

Suzuki T, Ogiba Y (1961) Conditioned orientation reflex audiometry. Archives of Otolaryngology 74: 192-198.

Thibodeau L (1990) Electroacoustic performance of direct-input hearing aids with FM amplification systems. Language, Speech and Hearing Services in Schools 21: 49-56.

Thibodeau L, McCaffrey H, Abrahamson J (1988) Effects of coupling hearing aids to FM systems via neckloops. Journal of the Academy of Rehabilitative Audiology 21: 49-56.

Thompson G, Weber B (1974) Responses of infants and young children to behavioral observation audiometry (BOA). Journal of Speech and Hearing Research 39: 140-147.

Tillman TW, Carhart R (1966) An expanded test for speech discrimination utilizing CNC monosyllabic words: Northwestern University Auditory Test No. 6. Technical report no. SAM-TR-66-55. USAF School of Aerospace Medicine, Brooks Air Force Base, TX.

Van Tasell D, Landin D (1980) Frequency response characteristics of FM mini-loop auditory trainers. Journal of Speech and Hearing Disorders 45: 247-258.

Chapter 10
Optimum Listening and Learning Environments

F S BERG

Schools and homes include acoustically hostile environments for children's listening and learning. This chapter describes acoustical problems in schools and homes as well as their acoustical solutions. Discussion is organised under three headings: acoustical problems, noise control, and signal control.

Acoustical problems

Introduction

Teachers of the deaf should initially become aware of acoustical problems and related phenomena in schools and homes that affect speech intelligibility. The problems include speech energy loss; room modal interference; echoes; reverberation; and noise. They degrade speech intelligibility, which is the percentage or ratio of the speech of the talker understood by one or more listeners.

Speech energy loss

In an enclosed space, speech energy is transmitted from teacher to students through a combination of direct and reflected sound. Direct sound is sound that travels outward from its source before or without being reflected. Reflected sound is sound after it has struck one or more objects or surfaces in a room. Direct sound energy predominates close to the teacher and reflected sound energy predominates away from the teacher (Figure 10.1). Speech energy reaching the student through direct and reflected sound waves is more intense than when only direct sound waves reach a listener (Davis and Jones, 1989). In a room the distance from the sound source to places where the direct sound level and the reflected sound level are equal is called the critical distance. At this distance, the total sound level is 3 dB higher than either the direct sound or the reflected sound.

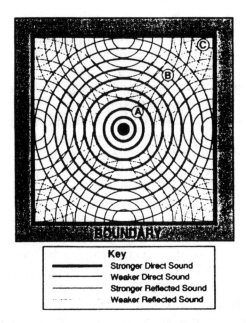

Key
Stronger Direct Sound
Weaker Direct Sound
Stronger Reflected Sound
Weaker Reflected Sound

Figure 10.1 Direct and reflected sound field in an enclosed acoustic environment. (A) Direct sound field near sound source. (B) Room location where intensity of direct sound equals that of reflected sound. (C) Room location where reflected sound is predominant. From *Sound Reinforcement Handbook* (p.58) by G. Davis and R. Jones, 1989. Milwaukee: Hal Leonard. Copyright 1989 by Yamaha Corporation of American and Gary Davis & Associates. Reprinted by permission

Sound in air travels at a speed of 1100 feet per second. As sound is propagated from its original source, it spherically expands so that for each doubling of distance, the sound energy is distributed to four times the area. This means that a student seated 6 feet from the teacher receives only a quarter as much direct sound as a student seated 3 feet from the teacher. The decrease in direct sound pressure level for each doubling of distance is 6 dB (inverse square law). For example, if the direct sound pressure level of propagated voice is 57 dB at 3 feet, it will decrease to 51 dB at 6 feet, 45 dB at 12 feet, and 39 dB at 25 feet (Berg, 1993). Remember we are talking about direct sound and not total sound, which is a combination of direct and reflected sound.

The fall-off of total sound energy with doubling of distance between teacher and student is not 6 dB. If room surfaces are completely reflective, there is no (or 0 dB) fall-off. It is only when room surfaces are completely absorptive that the fall-off is 6 dB. In a typical classroom, the fall-off may be about 3 dB between 3 and 6 feet, 2 dB between 6 feet and 12 feet, and 1 dB between 12 feet and 25 feet (Waterhouse and Harris, 1979).

The teacher's vocal effort also determines the sound energy heard by students. If the sound pressure level of the teacher's voice is 57 dB at

3 feet with normal vocal effort, it diminishes to about 52 dB with casual vocal effort. If raised voice, loud voice, or a shout is used, the sound pressure level at 3 feet increases to about 63 dB, 71 dB, and 80 dB, respectively (Brook and Uzzle, 1987).

The sound energy of the teacher's voice is also diminished when the teacher does not face the students. High speech frequencies, particularly important for speech intelligibility, are especially affected. Sound levels for high and low speech frequencies are most intense in front. Sound levels of high speech frequencies are diminished by about 6 dB at the sides and 20 dB at the rear. Sound levels of low speech frequencies are diminished very little at the sides and 8 dB at the rear (Egan, 1988). This directional problem applies especially when students are relatively close to the teacher or when room surfaces reflect little or no sound.

Sound energy intended for distant students can be diminished further by sound absorption, reflection, or diffraction from nearby students. Absorption of sound energy by nearby students transfers it to heat energy, reflection causes it to bounce back, and diffraction causes it to bend or change direction. Any one, or a combination, of these phenomena can happen when a teacher is seated (Brook, 1991). When the teacher is standing, most sound energy from his or her voice passes over the heads of nearby seated students (Berg, 1993).

Sound energy within a room is also diminished by absorptive treatment of its surfaces, which attenuates reflection. Absorption is the most familiar acoustic treatment employed by architects and builders. The least expensive and most used forms of absorbent material in school classrooms are acoustic ceiling tile and carpet on foam rubber padding. A special problem with these materials is that they absorb high frequency speech sounds much better than low frequency speech sounds. As a result, consonant sounds, which contain primarily high frequency energies, are not transmitted well as sound reflections. This is a problem because controlled transmission of high frequency sound is especially important to speech intelligibility (D'Antonio, 1989).

The dB level of a teacher's voice is directly related to the percentage of speech recognised by students. The S-shaped curve of Figure 10.2 shows this relationship in quiet and with a 40 dBA background noise level. A dBA level is a decibel measure with a sound level meter switched to a weighting in order to filter out low frequency noise and compensate for less sensitive human hearing at low audio frequencies. A nearly straight line relationship exists when speech levels are between 20 dB and 60 dB in quiet and between 30 dB and 80 dB in 40 dBA background noise, which is still relatively quiet. As speech levels decrease within these ranges, syllable recognition correspondingly decreases from about 95% to 5–10%. These data are based on studies of listeners with normal hearing in mid-life years, when their listening and language skills are optimum (Brook and Uzzle, 1987). The speech level for children with

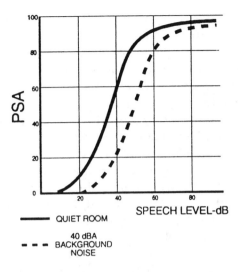

QUIET ROOM

40 dBA
BACKGROUND
NOISE

Figure 10.2 Relation of speech level to percentage of syllables repeated correctly. Adapted from "Rooms for Speech, Music, and Cinema" by R. Brook and T. Uzzel in *Handbook for Sound Engineers* (p.160) edited by G. Ballou, 1987, Carmel, IN: Howard W. Sams. Copyright 1987 by Howard W. Sams. Reprinted by permission

bilateral hearing impairments must be higher than for adults with normal hearing to reach the same level of speech intelligibility.

In a typical school classroom, speech intelligibility is depressed somewhat for nearby students and more so for distant students. Leavitt and Flexer (1991) measured the distance over which a speech signal could be transmitted faithfully in a college classroom by using a rapid speech transmission index (RASTI) measurement system. They found that perfect transmission (score of 1.0) could be obtained 6 inches from the transmitter and that the signal in the back of the room was degraded (0.60) when compared with that in the front of the room (0.80). They concluded that it is only when a student is very near a teacher that the student has no difficulty with speech recognition. Crandell (1990) measured the speech recognition scores of twenty 5–7 year old children with normal hearing at 6, 12 and 25 feet speaker–listener distances. The stimuli were simple sentences with key words. The mean scores of the subjects were 82%, 55% and 36% at 6, 12 and 25 feet, respectively.

Room modal interference

Modes or standing waves with 'dead' and 'live' spots in specific locations can also occur within rooms. This is a resonance condition that degrades speech within the 80 to 300 Hz frequency range. The resulting modal interference occurs when the wavelengths of speech or noise fit the room dimensions. Each room has its unique set of resonant frequencies at which it will vibrate and produce standing waves if stimulated with sound containing these specific frequencies. When room dimensions are multiples of a wavelength such as 10 feet, 20 feet and 30 feet, more modal phenomena occur. There are three types of modes: axial, tangential, and oblique (Figure 10.3). Each axial mode results from standing waves produced when two sound waves travel past each other in opposite directions between two room surfaces. Each tangential mode results from standing waves produced when travelling waves reflect from four room surfaces. Each oblique mode results from standing waves produced when travelling waves reflect from all six surfaces of a room: ceiling, floor, and four walls. The speech signal and noise background include frequencies with relatively high intensities that coincide with axial, tangential and oblique modes (Everest, 1989).

Room modes particularly degrade speech intelligibility when most or all surfaces in a room are hard. Sound then bounces around like billiard balls, creating modes that are more intense than if room surfaces are softer. Sound energies at these modal frequencies also decay more slowly in hard rooms. Even when acoustic ceiling tile or

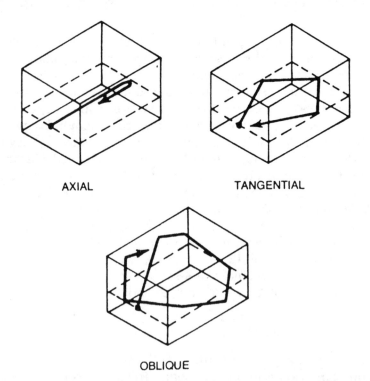

AXIAL   TANGENTIAL

OBLIQUE

Figure 10.3 Visualization of axial, tangential and oblique room modes. From *The Master Handbook of Acoustics* (p.88) by A Everest, 1989, Blue Ridge Summit: TAB BOOKS, Copyright 1989 by TAB BOOKS. Reprinted by permission

floor carpet is installed in a room, room modes are prominent because tile and carpet are poor absorbers of low frequency sound. Speech intelligibility will be affected more by room modes if enclosures are small than if they are large. This is because small rooms have higher frequency room modes, which in turn interfere with higher frequency speech energies. The frequency band affected includes the fundamental (pitch) and first formant frequencies (Berg, 1993). Fortunately, room modes do not affect high frequency energies of speech where most speech intelligibility is contributed. Special classrooms for students who are hearing-impaired typically are small, and therefore their modes may degrade speech intelligibility more than in regular classrooms. Rooms in most homes are also typically small and therefore particularly subject to room modal interference (Everest, 1989).

Echoes

Speech intelligibility within rooms may also be degraded by reflective characteristics of room surfaces. Too much or inadequately controlled reflection can be disastrous as described by a contributor to a book on designing learning environments: "Buildings erected between 1915 and 1940 contained all the characteristics of poor acoustical treatment... Sound bounced disastrously from the many reflective surfaces, creating... an echo chamber... and making communication unintelligible" (Silverstone, 1982, p. 79).

An echo may be defined as a reflected wave of sufficient amplitude and delay to make it distinct from the sound giving rise to it, such as a reflection of a yodel from a mountainside or a slap back of amplified music from a large auditorium surface. Figure 10.4 is a schematic of direct and reflected or delayed sound energy in a room and shows three significantly intense reflections or echoes.

Echoes with short delays must be much stronger to be heard than echoes with long delays. Echoes are incipient when we are conscious of their presence but do not perceive them as discrete. In classrooms, speech echoes are not usually heard as discrete phenomena, but they influence the apparent level, quality, and intelligibility of the sound. Whether echoes are audible or incipient, they still may be seen as distinct spikes on a time energy display (Figure 10.4). When two opposite reflective room surfaces are very close together, a repetitive or flutter echo may occur. For example, flutter echo may occur in a small hard-surfaced room or a hard-surfaced corridor of a large room. In either instance, when a person facing one of these surfaces speaks, or amplified sound from a loudspeaker facing one of these surfaces is delivered, flutter echo may be heard. This audible echo sounds like a high frequency ringing or buzzing. Flutter echo is seen as small

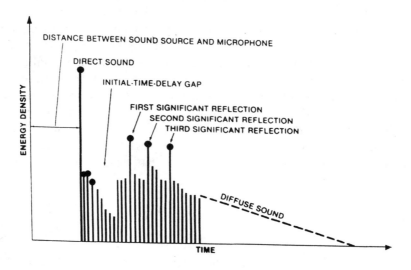

Figure 10.4 Schematic of time energy display showing three loud reflections within the reverberant field. From *Sound System Engineering* (p.220) by D. Davis and C. Davis, 1987. Indianapolis: Howard W. Sams. Copyright 1987 by Howard W. Sams. Reprinted by permission

repetitive spikes on a sound decay curve and degrades speech intelligibility.

Reverberation

In school classrooms, direct and reflected sound transmission causes the build-up (e.g., when someone slams the door) and decay of semi-reverberant sound fields (Figure 10.5). A semi-reverberant sound field is a semi-reflective enclosed space; it has at least some acoustic absorption. A reverberant sound field is a completely reflective enclosed space with essentially no acoustic absorption. Reverberation is simply defined as prolongation or repeated reflection of sound. In its pure form, it consists of many, very closely packed or diffuse reflections that decay over a long time when a sound source ceases. The time taken for the sound to decay from a certain intensity level to a sound intensity 60 dB lower (e.g., from 90 dB to 30 dB) is called the reverberation time (RT). A 60 dB decay is a decrease in sound intensity of one million times, or of sound pressure of one thousand times.

The RTs of school classrooms vary from 0.3 seconds to greater than 1.5 seconds (Berg, Blair, and Benson, 1996). This translates from relatively absorptive to relatively reflective room surfaces, respectively. A completely absorptive room would have a 0.0 second RT. A completely

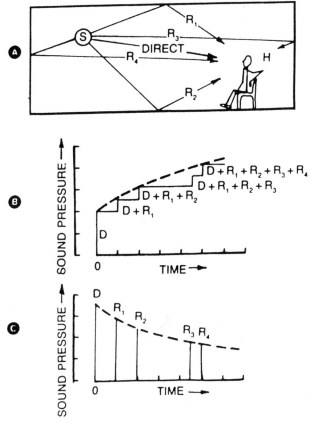

Figure 10.5 Illustration of room reflections, sound build-up, and sound decay in a room. From *The Master Handbook of Acoustics* (p.113) by A. Everest, 1989, Blue Ridge Summit, PA: TAB BOOKS. Copyright 1989 by TAB BOOKS. Reprinted by permission

reflective room (echo chamber) could have greater than a 10 second RT. Rooms in homes tend to have higher RTs than school classrooms. The RT of a kitchen or bathroom may be 2 seconds or longer while the RT of a living room or a bedroom may be about one second. In a kitchen, all surfaces typically are hard except for curtains on one wall. In a living room or a bedroom, all surfaces typically are hard except for a carpeted floor, which is relatively larger and somewhat more absorbent than most curtains.

The primary effect of excessive room reverberation is that the vowels of speech will mask the consonants of speech and thus degrade speech intelligibility. This is illustrated in Figure 10.6, which shows the masking effect of "ba" on hearing "ck" in the word "back", when the RT is 1.5 seconds as compared with 0.5 seconds. The "ba" intensity begins 25 dB higher than the "ck" intensity begins. When "ba" decays over

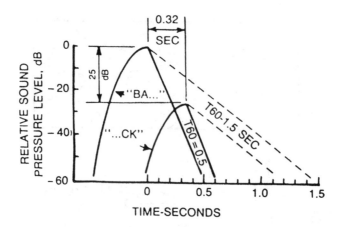

Figure 10.6 Illustration of the effects of reverberation on the masking of speech. From *The Master Handbook of Acoustics* (p.127) by A. Everest, 1989, Blue Ridge Summit, PA: TAB BOOKS. Copyright 1989 by TAB BOOKS. Reprinted by permission

0.5 second, it does not mask the "ck", but when it decays over 1.5 seconds, the "ba" completely covers the "ck" (Everest, 1989).

The writer takes exception to the specific effect of a 0.5 second RT. Vowels are typically 10–15 dB more intense than consonants. Therefore, masking can still degrade speech when RTs are 0.5 second or even less.

Noise competition

A final acoustical problem in schools and homes is excessive noise. Noise is unwanted or unintended sound that interferes or competes with speech transmission. Classroom noise levels typically are 30–35 dBA at night, or over a weekend, 40–50 dBA when the heating and air conditioning (HVAC) system is turned on, and 55–75 dBA when a teacher and 25 or more students are occupants. Unoccupied noise levels in homes are similar to unoccupied noise levels in schools. Occupied noise levels in homes may be lower or higher than occupied noise levels in schools. It is well known that excessive noise masks or renders inaudible wanted sound energies that carry information to listeners, which are called speech signals or just signals.

The sound levels of occupied rooms are combinations of signal and noise levels. During part of a school day when no children are present, just noise or unwanted sound exists in a classroom. When a teacher and children occupy the classroom, the signal, or wanted sound, is added to the unoccupied room noise. The signal is usually the teacher talking, but it can also be students talking at the teacher's request.

The highest sound levels often occur in occupied classrooms when teachers lose control of class behaviour. This happens when, for example, a student talks, and another student talks, and then two or more students are talking. Soon students are talking louder and louder, and the teacher has to talk even more loudly, or even shout, to be heard. At the same time, students may be creating other types of noise by dropping pencils, moving chairs, and shuffling feet. Also contributing to high noise levels are a myriad of other unwanted sounds from within and outside the classroom.

Children may be exposed to high sound levels throughout most of a day. Figure 10.7, for example, shows the sound levels a 13 year old boy experienced from the time he got up one school day to the time he went to bed. The recorded sound intensity levels exceeded 60 dBA the great majority of the time and 90 dBA at times. A dosimeter/sound level meter was worn by the boy. Measurements were taken automatically every 3 minutes. The horizontal bars are hourly averages. The readings were from signals and noises produced by the boy and other persons and by noise sources in and out of school and home. Note particularly the intense sound levels on the school bus, in the lunchroom, and in a science class. Note also that the intensity levels typically exceeded 70 dBA after the boy got home from school. It is important to guard against the assumption that home is necessarily a friendly acoustic environment.

The difference between the signal level in dB and the noise level in dB is commonly called the signal to noise (S/N) ratio and sometimes called the speech to competition (S/C) ratio. In a classroom, for example, if the noise level averages 60 dBA, and the teacher's speech level averages 60 dBA in the area where students are seated, the S/N ratio averages 0 dB at the students' seats. If the speech level is kept at 60 dBA, and the noise level lowered to 50 dBA, the S/N ratio is +10 dB. With speech at 60 dBA and noise raised to 70 dBA, the S/N ratio is –10 dB.

Finitzo-Hieber and Tilman (1978) studied the effects of noise and reverberation time (RT) on the speech recognition scores of students in

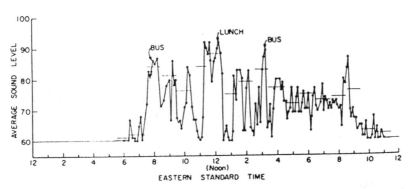

Figure 10.7 Dosimeter/sound level measures on a 13 year old boy during a school day. From *Why is the noise dose of humans important?* by D. Johnson. Unpublished presentation. Dayton, OH: Wright Patterson Air Force Base, Aerospace Medical Research Laboratory, 1979. Reprinted by permission

a classroom. The effects are illustrated in Table 10.1, which presents speech recognition scores of students who have normal hearing and who are hard of hearing, under several noise and reverberation conditions. Recognition scores are compared at 0.4 and 1.2 second RTs and with S/N ratios of 0, +6, and +12 dB, to simulate various classroom conditions. The students of normal hearing ability had mean speech recognition scores of 95%, and the students with hearing impairment had mean speech recognition scores of 83%, when tested in an audiometric test booth with negligible noise and reverberation.

The 0.4 and 1.2 second RTs simulate classrooms with considerable and minimal absorptive treatment, respectively. The +12 dB S/N ratio is commonly considered minimally acceptable for a student with hearing impairment in a classroom. The +6 and 0 dB S/N ratios are more typical of school classrooms. The scores shown in Table 10.1 reveal that even students with normal hearing cannot recognise speech optimally in a typically noisy school classroom, even when the RT is reduced to 0.4 second. Perusal of the data indicates that both noise and reverberation deleteriously affect speech recognition, and that the combination of both is especially detrimental. These scores were obtained at a distance of 12 feet, simulating class instruction.

Table 10.1 Average speech recognition scores of 12 students with normal hearing, and 12 students who are hard of hearing under RTs and S/N ratios simulating various school classroom conditions

Reverberation time (T, in sec)	S/N ratio (dB)	Scores of normal-hearing children	Scores of hard-of-hearing children with hearing aids
0.4	+12	83%	60%
	+6	71%	52%
	0	48%	28%
1.2	+12	70%	41%
	+6	54%	27%
	0	30%	11%

From "Classroom Acoustics" by T Finitzo-Hieber in *Auditory Disorders in School Children* (p260) edited by R Roeser and M Downs (1981) New York: Thieme Stratton. Copyright 1988 by Thieme Medical. Reprinted by permission.

Noise Control

Introduction

It is critically important that learning environments be designed or modified so that noise levels are low enough not to interfere with listening. Teachers of the deaf should be familiar with how to control noise in school and at home. Basic topics to consider are: actual and recommended noise levels; noise types; noise transmission and reduction principles; noise and vibration management; measurements and a formula; and a noise control plan. The discussion that follows will describe noise control in schools and then in homes.

Actual and recommended noise levels

The noise levels of many unoccupied and occupied school classrooms exceed recommended values for the quiet conditions in which children learn best. The noise level for an unoccupied classroom during school time should not exceed 35 to 40 dBA, and for an occupied classroom 40 to 50 dBA. In contrast, unoccupied classroom noise during school times is typically 40–50 dBA, and occupied classroom noise typically 55–75 dBA, depending on number of students and teachers.

When occupied classroom noise levels exceed 50 dBA, it is increasingly difficult for the teacher to teach and listen and for students to listen. The problem is exacerbated when students are school beginners or have learning disability or hearing impairment. To solve or alleviate excessive noise in classrooms, neither hearing aids nor FM systems are completely adequate solutions. The reasons for this will be described in the signal control section of this chapter. The most direct solution to the noise problem is to isolate or remove specific noises that contribute to excessive noise levels in a classroom.

School noise

In a classroom there are many specific noises that are present to varying extents during a school day. Each of these noises varies in overall dBA level from moment to moment, and is mixed with other noises. Noises that cover the same frequency range as speech signals have the greatest masking effect on teacher talk. However, because there is also an upward effect to masking, noises lower in frequency than speech signals also cause teacher talk to be less audible. Table 10.2 includes sound pressure levels in dB at octave intervals from 63 Hz to 8 kHz for various sounds that can occur inside and outside school. It shows that occupied classroom noise covers a broad range of frequencies. The dB values are 66, 72, 77, 74, 68, 60, and 50 at 125 Hz, 250 Hz, 500 Hz, 1 kHz, 2 kHz, 4 kHz and 8 kHz, respectively. Occupied classroom noise masks not only the low frequency vowel sounds of conversational speech that are relatively intense, but also the high frequency consonants that are relatively weak but contribute most to speech intelligibility. By comparison, the dB values of conversational speech given in Table 10.2 are only 57, 62, 63, 57, 48, and 40 at 125 Hz, 250 Hz, 500 Hz, 1 kHz, 2 kHz and 4 kHz.

Table 10.2 Sound pressure levels at octave band centre frequencies for sounds that can occur inside and outside school

Sound	63	125	250	500	1000	2000	4000	8000	dBA
Aircraft (turbofan) at 1 mile	77	82	82	78	70	56	-	-	79
Audiovisual room (occupied)	85	89	92	90	89	87	85	80	94
Auditorium (applause)	60	68	75	79	85	84	75	65	88
Classroom (occupied)	60	66	72	77	74	68	60	50	78
Conversational speech at 3ft	-	57	62	63	57	48	40	-	63
Dog barking at 50ft.	-	50	58	68	70	64	52	48	72
Gymnasium (occupied)	72	78	84	89	86	80	72	64	90
Laboratory (occupied)	65	70	73	75	72	69	65	61	77
Library (occupied)	60	63	66	67	64	58	50	40	68
Motorcycle at 50 ft (full throttle)	95	95	91	91	91	87	87	85	95
Mechanical equipment room	87	86	85	84	83	82	80	78	88
Window air-conditioning unit	64	64	65	56	53	48	44	37	59

Modified from *Architectural Acoustics* (p34) by D. Egan (1988) New York: McGraw Hill. Copyright 1988 by McGraw Hill. Adapted by permission.

When these dBA values for low and high frequencies are plotted and joined, detailed curves of noise values emerge. Each curve can be drawn directly on a graph that already includes a series of standard or noise criteria (NC) curves, which correspond to very quiet, quiet, moderately noisy, noisy, and very noisy listening conditions (Figure 10.8). The value of each noise curve is determined by the NC curve it intersects. The noise curve is then given the value of that NC curve. NC values vary from 20 to 70 in steps of five. An NC value of 20 is highly desirable and an NC value of 70 is highly undesirable. Ordinarily, the NC value is somewhat less than the dBA value of a given noise. For example, a noise level of 60 dBA ordinarily corresponds to an NC 50 or 55. Figure 10.8 shows unoccupied and occupied NC curves for an open classroom. The first has an NC value of 30 and the second an NC value of 65. If students are going to listen optimally, the NC value of an occupied classroom during school time should not exceed 30 to 35, which constitutes a quiet listening and learning environment.

There are three types of school noise: background, intruding, and internally generated. Background noise is fairly steady state and comes from vehicular traffic; heating, ventilating, and cooling systems; gymnasiums and cafeterias; and classroom projectors and fans. Intruding noise is more sudden or temporary. Examples include a jet plane overhead, yells on the playground, footsteps in the hallway, or a school buzzer. Internally generated noise includes students' and teachers' talking, chairs and tables sliding and shoes shuffling. The intensity and spectral composition of each type of noise varies constantly within each school classroom.

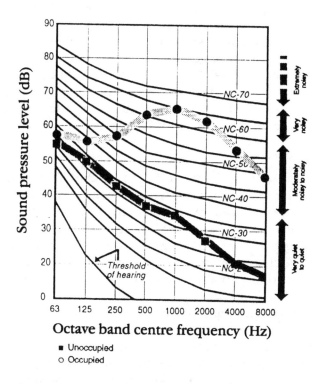

Figure 10.8 Noise criteria (NC) curves for an open classroom under unoccupied and occupied conditions. From *Architectural Acoustics* (p.235) by D. Egan, 1988, New York: McGraw-Hill. Copyright 1988 by McGraw Hill. Adapted by permission

Noise transmission and reduction

School noises are propagated from their sources through the air or through the structure of the school building into school classrooms and other learning environments. Community and playground noise frequently is transmitted into the school building through outside walls, windows, and doors. Heating, ventilating and air conditioning (HVAC) system noises reach a classroom airborne through ducts, or structure-borne through the equipment frame and housing, isolation mounts, and floor. Intruding or impact noises, such as footsteps, 'clicks', 'thuds' and 'bangs', can be transmitted into school classrooms through building structure. Noise can also be transmitted as vibration through walls, windows, and doors. The greater the weight of a wall, for example, the smaller the vibration, and the less noise is transmitted into a building or classroom.

The noise reduction (NR) from one side of a partition to the other side is largely dependent on the sound transmission loss (STL) of that wall, but also the area of the transmitting wall and absorption in the receiving room. The STL values at low, middle, and high frequencies for common building materials are shown in Table 10.3. When a 'weaker' element, such as a window or door, is included in a wall, the composite STL for the combination is usually closer to the STL of the weaker element than to the 'stronger'. When the receiving (inside) room has highly absorptive surfaces, NR is much greater, especially for mid and high frequency sounds, which are important for speech recognition. If the inside room has reflective surfaces, the NR is much less for the same STL of the wall and ceiling (Egan, 1988).

Vibration protection

One area of noise control is the protection of the school from structure-borne vibration, which can be felt and heard, and if uncontrolled, becomes excessive and annoying. Structure-borne vibrations in a school usually originate with machinery, pipes and ducts, footsteps, and dropped things. Such vibrations are transmitted through the concrete structure of a school building at high speeds and very low attenuation. They are converted into airborne noise and radiated into a classroom through a wall or floor.

Machinery vibration and noise are produced by mechanical equipment located outside or within a school as part of a HVAC system. Included are large centrifugal fans, refrigeration compressors, boilers, cooling towers, water pumps, and transformers. This equipment is often located in a machinery room inside a school. Rigid supports, flexible connections, expansion joints, and mufflers can be used to prevent or absorb vibrations of mechanical equipment components.

Water pipe hammering and air duct vibration can be kept out of a building structure by using ceiling hangers, pipe clamps with glass fibre or floor-mounted supports. Clicks from footsteps can be cushioned with carpeting and resilient rubber floors. Thuds from things dropped may require elaborate constructions, such as concrete slabs with suspended ceiling and floors.

Noise isolation

Another area of noise control for a school is the isolation of airborne noise. This requires consideration of noise sources, noise paths, and listener locations. Noise sources and paths can be outside a school, within a school, or within classrooms or other areas where listeners are located. The paths may be broad or narrow and still effectively carry noise. Outside an enclosure, airborne noise will propagate outward in all directions. Inside an enclosure when propagated noise meets a partition (wall, ceiling, or floor) or room barrier, it is affected in several ways. Part of the noise is absorbed, part is reflected, part passes through (is transmitted), and, with a barrier, part is diffracted, or bent around it. The softer the partition or barrier surface, the more sound will be absorbed.

Table 10.3 Sound transmission loss (STL) and sound transmission class (STC) ratings in dB for common building materials

Material	Total thickness		Frequency (Hz)						STC rating
	inch	cm	125	250	500	1k	2k	4k	
Walls									
Solid concrete	3	8	35	40	44	52	59	64	47
Concrete (6;15), layers of plaster	7	18	39	42	50	58	64	66	53
Solid concrete blocks, layers of plaster	16	41	50	54	59	65	71	68	63
Brick ($4\frac{1}{2}$;11), layers of plaster	$5\frac{1}{2}$	14	34	34	41	50	56	58	42
Brick (9;23), layers of plaster	10	25	41	43	49	55	57	59	52
Stone (24;61), layers of plaster	25	64	50	53	52	58	61	68	56
Hollow concrete block	6	15	32	33	40	48	51	48	43
Cinder block (4;10), layers of plaster	$5\frac{1}{4}$	13	36	37	44	51	55	62	46
Hollow gypsum block (3;8), layers of plaster	4	10	39	34	38	43	48	46	40
Double brick ($4\frac{1}{2}$;11) wall, cavity (2;5), layers of plaster	12	31	37	41	48	60	60	61	49
Double brick ($4\frac{1}{2}$;11) wall, cavity (6;15), layers of plaster	18	46	48	54	58	64	69	75	62
Solid sanded gypsum plaster	2	5	36	28	35	39	48	52	36
Solid gypsum core moveable partition	$2\frac{1}{4}$	6	34	34	37	38	39	45	36
Floor–ceiling									
Reinforced concrete slab	4	10	48	42	45	55	57	66	44
Reinforced concrete as above + carpeting and pad	$4\frac{1}{2}$	11	48	42	45	55	57	66	44
Concrete ($4\frac{1}{2}$;11), wood flooring, layer of plaster	7	18	35	37	42	49	58	62	46
Concrete ($4\frac{3}{8}$;11), screed, suspended plaster ceiling	10	25	38	41	45	52	57	59	48
Concrete (6;15), wood, battens floating on glass wool, layer of plaster	$9\frac{1}{2}$	24	38	44	52	55	60	65	55
Wooden joists (8;20), floor gypsum wallboard	$9\frac{1}{2}$	24	19	24	31	35	45	42	34
Wooden joists (7;18), wood + linoleum, reeds + plaster	$9\frac{1}{2}$	24	24	27	35	44	52	58	39
Windows									
Double window	$\frac{3}{8}$	1.0	21	22	19	24	25	33	24
Double window sealed	$\frac{3}{8}$	1.0	20	25	20	30	34	34	28
Double window with cracks	$\frac{3}{8}$	1.0	18	21	19	20	22	30	20
Doors									
Solid core wood, weather strip	$1\frac{3}{4}$	4.0	21	27	30	26	25	29	27
Hollow core wood, weather strip	$1\frac{3}{4}$	4.0	14	15	17	18	22	29	20

From "Principles of Noise Control" by A Nabalek and I Nabalek in *Noise in Audiology* (pp 59-79) edited by D Lipscomb (1978) Baltimore: University Park Press. Copyright 1985 by PRO-ED inc. Reprinted by permission.

The harder the surface, the more sound will be reflected. The less dense the partition or barrier, the more sound will be transmitted. The further away and lower the barrier, the more sound will be diffracted.

When propagated noise comes to a small obstacle in its path it bends around it, or when propagated noise comes to a small boundary opening it passes through it. Unless completely blocked, noise will reflect or bend around corners and pass through partitions and windows, under doors, and the like. Airborne noise is also easily propagated in both directions through water pipes or HVAC ducts from multiple sources. The noise level, however, dissipates as noise propagates from its source.

First line of defence

The first line of defence in a noise isolation programme is to keep community and playground noise out of a school. Community noise has increased with the advent of motorised equipment, larger road vehicles, and more powerful jet aircraft. Consequently, many schools that were originally built in quiet environments are now located in environments with noise levels exceeding 80 dBA. Playground noise has been a problem all along. At school boundaries, various intense noises will set into vibration any exterior walls that are tuned to the frequencies of the noises and which lack the mass and density to damp vibration. School administrators can establish policies restricting the use of motorcycles, power mowers, and similar noisy equipment to before and after school hours. A wall barrier can isolate a school from a heavily travelled road. Communities can monitor jet aircraft whine on take-off. Exterior windows and doors can be kept closed during playground activities. Careful inspection and repair of the school exterior can ensure that cracks are sealed. Doors with threshold gaps can be replaced.

Second line of defence

The second line of defence in a noise isolation programme is to keep school noises out of classrooms or other learning areas. This can be done by (1) reducing noise intensity levels in rooms where they originate, (2) reducing noise intensities within school pathways to classrooms, and (3) isolating and sealing learning areas from school noises. Within schools airborne noises exceeding 80 dBA may exist in audiovisual rooms, auditoriums, cafeterias, gymnasiums, hallways, mechanical equipment rooms, music practice rooms, wood and machine shops, and swimming pool areas.

Enclosure or room isolation

An area within a room or the room itself can isolate the sound source. Machinery enclosures are manufactured by the Industrial Acoustics

Company to contain intense machinery noises within specific locations (Hirschorn, 1989). Egan (1988) illustrated the principles of sound isolation with a door bell, sound absorbent fuzz, and a half inch thick, airtight, plywood enclosure. Firstly, he surrounded the bell with fuzz, decreasing its sound intensity 3 dB, or from 70 dB to 67 dB. Secondly, he surrounded the bell with the enclosure, decreasing the sound intensity 20 dB, or from 70 dB to 50 dB. Lastly, he surrounded the bell with the enclosure and fuzz, decreasing the sound intensity 27 dB, or from 70 dB to 43 dB.

Absorptive treatment can also be added to room surfaces to prevent noise build-up and to reduce airborne noise transmission. Figure 10.9 shows two types of absorbent materials mounted on walls and suspended from a ceiling in a gymnasium: SONEX plastic baffles and Varitone steel modules. Both materials have relatively high absorption characteristics between 250 Hz and 4 kHz, the frequency range critical for speech intelligibility. They both also meet rigid fire resistant requirements.

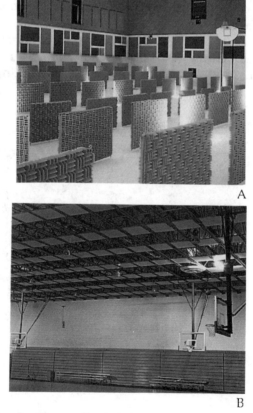

A

B

Figure 10.9 Wall and ceiling applications in gymnasiums. (A) Sonex noise baffles. Courtesy of Illbruck. (B) Varitone sound absorption system. Courtesy of Industrial Acoustics Company

Sound paths

There are many paths by which sound produced in one room of a building is transmitted into other rooms of the same building. Figure 10.10 shows direct transmission, flanking transmission, transmission via acoustic leaks, and transmission via adjacent rooms (Measurements in Building Acoustics, 1988). Sound is directly transmitted from one room to another room by setting into vibration their common walls. Sound is also transmitted within common or flanking walls, or enters directly through various wall openings or sound leaks. A one inch square hole in a 100-square foot gypsum board partition can transmit as much energy as the rest of the partition. This problem can only be prevented by sealing holes and similar openings, and even cracks, with caulking and insulation. Electrical outlets, for example, are potential locations for sound leaks and need to be carefully plugged. School classroom doors are often leaky. Such openings as louvres and gaps at thresholds have a sound transmission loss (STL) of 0 dB, and can seriously reduce the STL of doors. To provide maximum STL, doors should be solid-core wood or fibre-filled hollow metal and be gasketed around the entire perimeter to ensure a seal when closed.

Windows in doors or walls allow sound to be directly transmitted into classrooms. Often they do not provide as much STL as a classroom wall. Sound transmission class (STC) ratings for window constructions may vary from 26 to 43. STC is a single-number rating of

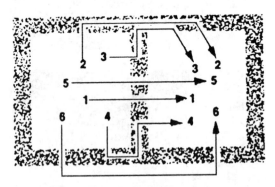

1 Direct Transmission

2–3 and 4 Flanking Transmission

5 Transmission via acoustic "leaks"

6 Transmission via adjacent Rooms

Figure 10.10 Paths of sound transmission between two rooms in a building. From *Measurements in Building Acoustics* (p.28), 1988, Naerum, Denmark: Bruel & Kjaer Instruments. Reprinted by permission

transmission loss performance for a construction element tested over a standard frequency range. The highest STC is gained with double-glazed construction with wide spacing between panes of different thickness.

The school HVAC system provides several pathways for noise transmission into classrooms as noted in Figure 10.11. Noise sources include equipment vibration and fans, ducts and plenums, and diffusers, registers, and dampers. Design and installation procedures for a comfortable, quiet HVAC system are not closely followed in many school installations. The resultant noise includes high intensity, very low frequency rumble caused by air turbulence buffeting the duct walls, low frequency fan rumble in supply and return ducts, mid frequency airflow noise in ducts and plenums, and high frequency outlet noise at diffusers, registers, and dampers. These noises from various locations travel through ducts into classrooms independent of airflow direction. Structure-borne elements of these noises do not dissipate with distance.

Stringent noise abatement requirements need to be met by HVAC designers and installers. When duct-borne noises are too intense, one or more of the following steps can be taken: (1) increase duct cross-sections, (2) smooth duct turns, transitions in size, and branch take-offs, (3) round ducts or if rectangular, increase ratio of depth to height, (4) increase number or size of outlets, (5) locate dampers away from outlets, (6) use glass fibre linings,(7) install mufflers, silencers, or sound traps, and (8) carefully align air outlets and diffusers in classrooms.

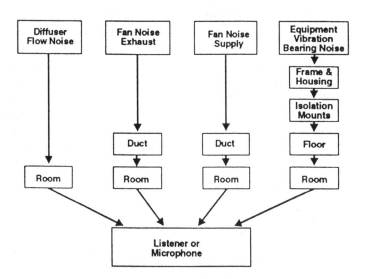

Figure 10.11 Typical paths by which HVAC noise can reach sound sensitive rooms. From "Common Factors in All Audio Rooms" by A. Everest in *Handbook For Sound Engineers* (p.97) edited by G.Ballou, 1991. Indianapolis: SAMS. Copyright 1991 by SAMS. Reprinted by permission

Final line of defence

The final line of defence in a noise isolation programme is keeping noise generated within the classroom from exceeding 50 dBA, when occupied by teacher and students. Typically, the sound level increases from 40–50 dBA with the HVAC system to 55–75 dB with the teacher and 25 students added, and the sound spectrum becomes relatively more loaded with high frequency energy. In an open plan teaching area with several teachers and up to 100 students, the noise is about 10 dB more intense than in a traditional classroom. In a smaller classroom occupied by one teacher and a small class of deaf children, the sound level may be 10 dB less intense if non-classroom generated noise can be controlled. To reduce classroom generated noise the classroom floor can be covered with carpet and padding, noisy equipment can be repaired or replaced, students can be required not to talk out of turn, and the teacher can maintain order.

In an open plan school, sounds from various sources are spread throughout the wings of buildings rather than restricted to small learning spaces. The acoustical demands of an open plan classroom involve the following: (1) freedom to teach a given group of students without other students listening, (2) freedom from distracting intruding speech noises, and (3) ensuring a quiet environment for face-to-face conversations of less than 6 feet. The level of background noise in an open plan classroom is critical. If it is too high, it will mask teachers' voices throughout the room. If it is too low, speech communication within one group will interfere with speech communication within adjacent groups.

Egan (1988) recommends introducing an electronic background masking noise into an open plan space if a very low noise level exists in the area. If this situation arises in a classroom, which is unlikely, the electronic noise covers up intruding speech noises. This masking noise must be uniformly distributed throughout the space and be less than 50 dBA in intensity. The sound level should fall-off 3–6 dB per octave at mid and high frequencies. The pleasant 'hushing' or 'whooshing' effect of the electronic noise is usually unobjectionable to most listeners.

Measurements and formulas

Each teacher of the deaf should have a sound level meter to monitor signal and noise levels in the classroom. Figure 10.12 shows the Realistic sound level meter, which is very inexpensive. It will measure overall sound intensities from 50 to 126 dBA, or 50 to 126 dBC. A dBA reading is obtained with the sound level meter weighting switch set at A, filtering out low audio-frequency noise. In contrast, a dBC measure is obtained with the meter weighting switch set at C, providing the meter with a much flatter frequency response to incoming sound.

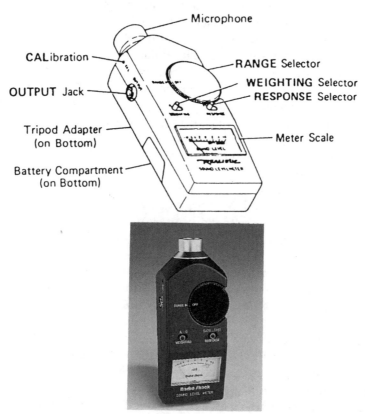

Figure 10.12 Realistic sound level meter. Courtesy of Radio Shack

Because this sound level meter will read as low as 50 dBA or 50 dBC, it is a practical device for occupied classroom measurements of signal and noise levels and for unoccupied classroom measurements of noise. The A weighting should be used for occupied classroom measurements if we consider the practical lower limit of classroom noise to be 50 dBA. The C weighting should be used for unoccupied classroom measurements because it provides greater sensitivity. In an unoccupied classroom, the noise is concentrated in the low audio-frequency range, with a 50 dBC measurement equivalent to a much lower (possibly 37) dBA measurement. It is important to obtain unoccupied noise levels as well as occupied noise levels of a classroom, since the unoccupied noise level provides a baseline to which occupied classroom noise is added. Achieving an unoccupied noise level of 50 dBC should make it practical to keep the occupied noise level down to 50 dBA in a regular classroom. Sound level meter readings of 50 dBC and 50 dBA will indicate that each of these criteria is being achieved in a classroom.

Other sound level meters with greater capabilities should also be available to an educational programme for deaf children. The Quest

2400 sound level meter will read sound intensities from 30–140 dBA or dBC. The Larson-Davis 710 dosimeter/sound level meter will read sound intensities from 35–145 dB. A special feature of the 710 is a time history capability. The 710 will store sound level data in memory, process these data in various ways, and download them to a serial printer. The Bruel and Kjaer type 2230 precision integrating sound level meter will read from 30–150 dB. A special feature of the 2230 is its capability to measure sound levels at a series of octave intervals from 20 Hz to 20 kHz, enabling the user to generate NC curves.

A consulting engineer named Jim Fulmer (1990) told of a noise study he conducted in the Salt Lake City schools during the 1960s. In one of the schools, big cabinet heaters beneath classroom windows were turned on when it was cold. NC values varied dramatically from one side to the other side of the classrooms. After these data were given to the school administration, teachers reported that grades of students whose seats were distributed across the classroom conformed closely to NC value differences. For example, students seated closest to the heaters where NC values were greatest had received the lowest grades. Students seated farthest away where NC values were least had received the highest grades.

Teachers of the deaf who take a special interest in school acoustics may also want to become familiar with the noise reduction formula, which expresses the relationship between the noise reduction (NR) of a wall and its transmission loss (TL). NR = TL + 10 log absorption in sabins divided by the surface area of the wall in square feet. The NR and TL may be computed for frequencies at each octave interval. For example, if the transmission loss from outside to inside an exterior wall of a school is 40 dBA, the surface area 200 square feet, and the absorption of the inside surface 300 sabins (1 sabin is acoustically equivalent to 1 square ft of complete absorption) at 500 Hz, the NR at 500 Hz will be 40 + 10 log (300/200) = 40 + 10 log 1.5 = 40 + 10 (0.1761) = 41.8 dBA. If the noise level outside a school at 500 Hz is 90 dBA, the inside noise level at 500 Hz will be 90 – 41.8 = 48.2 dBA, provided noise is only coming into the building through vibration of the common wall. The same procedure should be followed in determining NR at other frequencies. Also, if figuring NR between two adjacent rooms in a school, the number of sabins used in the formula should total those of the source room and of the receiving room (Egan, 1988).

Home applications

The listening and learning environment of the home requires a noise control programme similar to that of the school. The noise level of an occupied dining room or living room, for example, should not exceed 50 dBA. Background, intruding, and internally generated noise in homes often prevents this criterion from being met. Protection from structure-borne noise and isolation from airborne noise are necessary. Lines of defence have to be set up to protect homes from outside noise such as motor vehicle traffic, protect listening and learning environments from sounds generated within homes such as yells of children, and protect desired speech from being masked by unwanted sounds generated within listening and learning areas such as HVAC noise.

Noise control plan

When sufficient noise data are available, a noise control plan (NCP) can be designated for a school or home. A NCP is aimed at isolating and reducing noise outside a building, inside a building, and within specific listening and learning environments. The NCP should describe current noise levels, general and specific objectives, persons responsible for implementing the plan, and evaluation procedures. A study team should be appointed to write the NCP. Team members might include at least a consulting engineer, an educational audiologist, a teacher of the deaf or a regular teacher, and the principal of the school or the parents within the home.

Signal Control

Introduction

It is important also that teachers of the deaf know how to establish signal control in school and home environments. Consideration must be given to S/N ratio, room surface treatments, and various measurements.

The +10 dB criterion

In school classrooms, teachers instruct children primarily through speech communication. Their speech is transmitted through direct and reflected airborne sound from various distances and in competition with noise. If classroom acoustics characteristics such as modes, echoes, and reverberation are not a problem, the S/N ratio of a classroom may be as low as +10 dB without degrading speech intelligibility. Room resonances and echoes will have little degrading effect on speech intelligibility if room dimensions do not reinforce speech or noise and if room surfaces are sufficiently absorbent or diffusive. Reverberation will not be a problem if room surfaces are sufficiently absorbent for both low and high frequency sounds.

Room surface treatments

Figure 10.13 illustrates how direct or incident sound is modified in time and space by absorptive, reflective, and diffusive surface treatments. The absorptive treatment results in an attenuated reflection; the reflective treatment, a strong specular reflection, and the diffusive treatment, a scattering of reflected sound energy. Effective architectural acoustic design of classrooms requires an appropriate combination of absorptive, reflective, and diffusive surfaces. The specific mix depends on whether the goal is to enhance the signal or to remove or contain competing noise. In this section, signal control is covered; in the prior section, noise control. Either absorbent or diffusive treatment curtails resonance, echo, and reverberation problems. Either will also help alleviate problems when a room has an unusual shape, such as two opposite walls that are relatively close together.

Room resonances, echoes, and reverberation are affected by class-room size and shape. For example, a classroom with a volume of 5,000 cubic feet will be more subject to degrading room resonances than a classroom with a volume of 10,000 cubic feet. The small classroom, however, will tend to have a shorter RT, provided it has proportionately as much sound absorbent treatment as the large classroom. A very narrow, rectangular classroom will induce flutter echo. A wide rectangular classroom with the same volume will not.

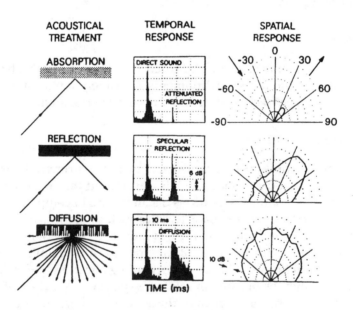

Figure 10.13 Temporal and spatial responses for absorption, reflection, and diffusion of sound. Courtesy of Peter D'Antonio, (1989) RPG Diffusor Systems, Largo, MD

Products

Various forms of absorptive and diffusive products can be used to fit the specific room surface treatment needs in a classroom. Sources of current acoustical materials for signal control and for noise control are described by the writer in his 1993 book, *Acoustics and Sound Systems in Schools*. Previously, Hedeen (1980) prepared an exhaustive description of various types of sound absorbers, laboratory methods of testing sound absorption, and absorption coefficients of many acoustic materials commercially available before 1980. Signal control is enhanced when absorption of sound in a room is uniform across the speech frequency range, 250 Hz to 4 kHz.

The efficiency of sound absorbing treatment can be greatly improved by partial as opposed to complete room surface coverage. This is exemplified in Figure 10.14, which shows that 25 panels of sound absorbing material, each 2 feet by 2 feet, will absorb more sound when applied partially to the entire wall in a checkerboard pattern than if applied fully to half of the wall. The improvement of efficiency is caused by the diffraction of sound energy around the perimeters of the spaced panels and by the added absorption of the exposed panel edges. The total absorption of the spaced panels in this example is only slightly less than if the entire 200-square foot surface was covered uniformly.

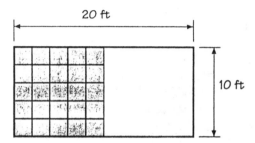

Figure 10.14 Checkerboard (above) and uniform (below) patterns of absorption treatment coverage. From *Architectural Acoustics* (p.59) by D. Egan, 1988, New York: McGraw Hill. Copyright 1988 by McGraw Hill. Reprinted by permission

A new generation of superior absorbing, diffusing, and reflecting products for signal control has been developed by Peter D'Antonio of RPG Diffusor Systems. One of his products, for example, is a fibreglass panel with a dense semi-rigid backing for lower frequency (250 Hz) absorption. Lower frequency absorption also increases progressively as air space is increased behind fibreglass wall panels. Less expensive Peabody fibreglass panels from Kinetics Noise Control provide sufficient absorption only down to 500 Hz.

Sound absorption is typically expressed as a coefficient. The absorption coefficient is the fraction of propagated sound energy absorbed at a surface, expressed as a value between 0 and 1. Sound absorption coefficients for common building materials are included in Table 10.4. Notice also that the absorption coefficients for each type of building material vary with frequency.

Diffusor products are many times as expensive as standard absorptive products and therefore out of reach of most school budgets. Such goods are used in recording studio control rooms or stereo sound rooms in homes. One RPG Diffusor Systems product to consider for school or home application is the Korner-Killer, which is placed in each corner of a room. A diffusive side is directed toward the room to control low frequency room modes, and two absorptive sides face the walls to control troublesome corner reflections. Another product to consider is Flutter Free, a hardwood moulding that eliminates flutter echo.

Brook (1991) states that most rooms meant for speech activities do not have a lot of need for sound diffusion. He says it is better to focus the available energy as useful reflections and to shift absorbent treatment from the room ceiling to the room floor.

A rule of thumb for rooms for speech is to make all surface areas that do not provide useful reflections absorbent and, conversely, not to cover any useful reflectors. The latter is widely violated. Almost all classrooms have absorbent ceilings and hard floors, yet the reverse would provide far better room acoustics. Carpet on the floor not only covers a useless reflective surface, it also greatly reduces audience noise. The elimination of footfall and chair- or desk-moving noises are an important contribution to quieter classrooms.

In large listening areas such as classrooms, the ceiling and side walls should be reflective to increase the signal level. The floor and rear wall are sources of harmful or useless reflections. The floor should be absorbent and the rear wall absorbent or diffusive.

A hard, sound-reflecting ceiling has the advantage of increasing the loudness and clarity of the teacher's speech. This is because the ceiling ordinarily is close enough to the teacher to reflect sound to students with minimum time delay, enabling the direct sound and its reflection to be heard as one sound according to the precedence or Haas Effect. This effect means that reflected sound arriving at the ear within 30 millisec-

Table 10.4 Sound absorption coefficients for building and absorbent treatment materials

Material	Frequency (Hz)						NRC rating
	125	250	500	1k	2k	4k	
Walls							
Brick	0.03	0.03	0.03	0.04	0.05	0.07	0.05
Concrete painted	0.10	0.05	0.06	0.07	0.09	0.08	0.05
Window glass	0.35	0.25	0.18	0.12	0.07	0.04	0.15
Marble	0.01	0.01	0.01	0.01	0.02	0.02	0.00
Plaster or concrete	0.12	0.09	0.07	0.05	0.05	0.04	0.05
Plywood	0.28	0.22	0.17	0.09	0.10	0.11	0.15
Concrete block, coarse	0.36	0.44	0.31	0.29	0.39	0.25	0.35
Heavyweight drapery	0.14	0.35	0.55	0.72	0.70	0.65	0.60
Fibreglass wall treatment, 1 inch (2.5 cm)	0.08	0.32	0.99	0.76	0.34	0.12	0.60
Fibreglass wall treatment, 7 inch (17.8 cm)	0.86	0.99	0.99	0.99	0.99	0.99	0.95
Wood panelling on glass fibre blanket	0.40	0.99	0.80	0.50	0.40	0.30	0.65
Floors							
Wood parquet on concrete	0.04	0.04	0.07	0.06	0.06	0.07	0.05
Linoleum	0.02	0.03	0.03	0.03	0.03	0.02	0.05
Carpet on concrete	0.02	0.06	0.14	0.37	0.60	0.65	0.30
Carpet on foam rubber padding	0.08	0.24	0.57	0.69	0.71	0.73	0.55
Ceilings							
Plaster, gypsum, or lime on lath	0.14	0.10	0.06	0.05	0.04	0.03	0.05
Acoustic tiles ⅝ inch (1.6 cm), suspended 16 inches (40.6 cm) from ceiling	0.25	0.28	0.46	0.71	0.86	0.93	0.60
Acoustic tiles ½ inch (1.2 cm), suspended 16 inches (40.6 cm) from ceiling	0.52	0.37	0.50	0.69	0.79	0.78	0.60
The same as above, but cemented directly to ceiling	0.10	0.22	0.61	0.66	0.74	0.72	0.55
High absorptive panels, 1 inch (2.5 cm), suspended 16 inches (40.6 cm) from ceiling	0.58	0.88	0.75	0.99	1.00	0.96	0.90
Others							
Upholstered seats	0.19	0.37	0.56	0.67	0.61	0.59	0.55
Audience in upholstered seats	0.39	0.57	0.80	0.94	0.92	0.87	0.80
Grass	0.11	0.26	0.60	0.69	0.92	0.99	0.61
Soil	0.15	0.25	0.40	0.55	0.60	0.60	0.45
Water surface	0.01	0.01	0.01	0.02	0.02	0.03	0.00

From *Noise in Audiology* edited by D Lipscomb (1978). Copyright PRO-ED. Reprinted by permission.

onds of the direct sound is integrated with the direct sound, resulting in increased apparent loudness, and a pleasant change in the character of the sound.

If the back wall reflects sound, however, the time delay of reflected sound energy at the ear of the listener will be greater than 30 milliseconds; therefore, loudness and clarity will not increase. If the time delay exceeds 62 milliseconds, a disturbing echo may be heard, particularly if teachers raise their voices too much. Either an absorptive or diffusive surface will prevent echoes and help reduce room reverberation to acceptable limits.

In small listening areas like special classrooms, the ceiling should be reflective to increase the signal level. The floor and walls are sources of harmful or useless reflections. The floor should be absorbent. The walls should include a mix of absorbent and diffusive materials. These recommendations are modified when sound field FM amplification is used.

Recommended reverberation

Recommended RTs for school children with normal hearing are about 0.5 second and for school children with hearing impairments, about 0.3 second. When the RT falls below about 0.3 second, it may be that useful sound energy is being absorbed when it should be redirected to enhance direct sound transmission.

Recommended RTs depend somewhat on the classroom size or volume. The larger the classroom size, the greater the RT, all else being the same. A simple formula for RT developed by Sabine shows this dependence: RT in seconds = 0.049 room volume (V) divided by total absorption (A) of the room surfaces in sabins. The volume (length × width × height) does not have as much influence on RT as surface absorption, since the volume is multiplied by a 0.049 constant.

The total absorption (A) of sound in any one frequency band of a room is the sum of all the separate absorption values of room surface materials within that frequency band. Each separate absorption value of a surface material within that frequency band is computed by multiplying its absorption coefficient by the area of that surface in square feet. Table 10.5 illustrates the relationship between the separate absorptions, the total absorption, and the RT of a classroom at each of a series of speech frequencies.

The RT should be reasonably uniform across the speech frequency range. Sound at 2 kHz, for example, should decay at about the same rate as sound at 500 Hz. For example, both RTs should be 0.4 second, rather than having the RT at 500 Hz be 0.6 second and the RT at 2 kHz be 0.2 second. Unfortunately, the RT of a school classroom typically varies widely from low to high speech frequencies because room surfaces have

Table 10.5 Absorption data for a hypothetical unfurnished classroom with a volume of approximately 10,000 cubic feet (38ft × 26.3 ft × 10 ft) RT = 0.49 V/A

Material	Area	Absorption coefficients (top) and Sabins (bottom)					
	sq.ft.	125Hz	250Hz	500Hz	1kHz	2kHz	4kHz
Floor carpet	1000	0.08	0.24	0.57	0.69	0.71	0.73
on foam rubber padding		80	240	570	690	710	730
Plaster ceiling	1000	0.14	0.10	0.06	0.05	0.04	0.03
		140	100	60	50	40	30
Wood panelling	526	0.40	0.99	0.80	0.50	0.40	0.30
on glass fibre blanket		210	521	421	263	210	159
Plastered walls	660	0.12	0.09	0.07	0.05	0.05	0.04
		79	59	46	33	33	26
Window glass	100	0.35	0.25	0.18	0.12	0.07	0.04
		35	25	18	12	7	4
Total area	3286						
Sabins		544	945	1115	1048	1000	949
RT in seconds		0.90	0.52	0.44	0.47	0.49	0.52

an inappropriate mix of absorbent materials. Not enough effort has been made to balance the absorption of room surfaces across frequency in classrooms. For example, commonly installed acoustic ceiling and carpet materials absorb high speech frequencies much more than they absorb low speech frequencies. The end result in such classrooms is degraded speech intelligibility.

School classrooms with RTs of less than 0.7 second may not be proper environments for using the Sabine formula. This is because the accuracy of a RT formula depends on statistical averages and presupposes a complete mixing of sound from numerous reflections in a room. When a classroom has a RT less than 0.7 second, relatively few reflections occur before sound dies down. In such semi-reverberant rooms, the statistical basis of the formula has been weakened.

There is also question whether talkers in occupied classrooms cause a reverberant sound field or echoes to develop that are above the noise level in such spaces. Sometimes the signal level is lower than the noise level, and often the signal level is only slightly higher than the noise level. In these instances, the effect of reverberation or echoes on speech intelligibility may be less than the effect of a negative or slightly positive S/N ratio on speech intelligibility.

Direct measurements

Various devices are available for direct measurement of reverberation, echoes and resonances. Two particularly useful devices will be briefly described. The first is for measurement of reverberation. The second measures both echoes and resonances, and can also be used for measurement of reverberation.

The Communications Company RT60 Reverberation Timer is an example of a user-friendly reverberation meter. It measures the overall RT as well as the RT within seven octave bands centred at 125 Hz, 250 Hz, 500 Hz, 1 kHz, 2 kHz, 4 kHz and 8kHz. A .22-calibre starter revolver with blank cartridges, or even slapping two short boards together, can be used to introduce a brief intense sound into the room in order to measure its decay. The RT60 measures how long this sound takes to fall 20 dB and then multiplies that time by three to give a standard RT60 readout. Resolution is 0.01 second and RTs up to 9.9 seconds can be measured. The Timer is powered by two 9-volt alkaline batteries. Figure 10.15 shows the RT60 with upward extending microphone. It is reading a RT of 2.52 seconds.

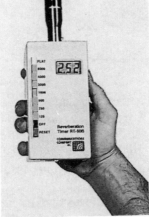

Figure 10.15 RT60 Reverberation Timer. Courtesy of Communications Company

The Techron Time-Energy-Frequency (TEF) Analyzer (Figure 10.16) is an extremely versatile, multi-purpose measurement system coupled to a PC or Macintosh computer. A sweep frequency signal generated within the console is transmitted from one or more loudspeakers placed in the front of the room where a teacher might be. For each echo measurement, the loudspeaker is directed toward a different room object or surface. The sound reaching the object or surface is reflected back to the microphone of the TEF Analyzer. Echoes or reflections are stored in computer memory and displayed on the computer monitor. Intensity is displayed vertically and time horizontally (time-energy display). A cursor is moved to any point along the time base to read the intensity of each reflection.

Distances from the loudspeaker to reflective surfaces can also be read for each cursor position. The relative intensities of the distances reveal which surfaces cause the greatest echo problems when a teacher is talking.

When using the TEF Analyzer to study room modes, keep in mind that all room modes terminate in the room corners. Therefore, the sweep frequency sound, or a varying low frequency sound from a separate audio oscillator, is transmitted from a loudspeaker placed in one low tricorner of the room facing the measurement or pick up microphone placed in the diagonal tricorner of the room. The frequency response of room resonances appears on the intensity–frequency display of the TEF Analyzer. When all room surfaces are hard and reflective, the prominent modes stand out like sharp spikes (Everest, 1989).

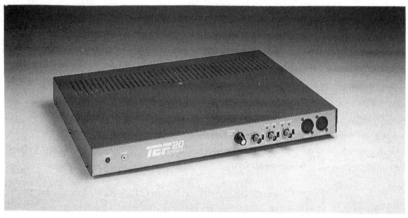

Figure 10.16 TEF 20 analyzer. Courtesy of Techron Division of Crown International

Speech intelligibility measurements

Speech intelligibility measures can also be obtained in classrooms. These scores will depend on room acoustics, where individual students are located, and the treatments used. Measures should be obtained in representative listener locations in classrooms. Measures can be obtained with word and sentence recognition lists, rating scales, and the TEF Analyzer.

Many word and sentence lists have been developed to assess speech recognition. Listeners in the classroom can be asked to repeat back or write down each item of a list after it is said by one or more selected talkers. The percentage of words or key words of sentences repeated or written correctly is computed. Equivalent forms of this type of test are given before and after the treatment. Each list takes 3–5 minutes to administer (Berg, 1987).

Word or sentence lists presented by a talker in a classroom can also be recorded in the ears of a manikin in various listener locations before and after a treatment. The recorded lists are later played back through earphones to individual listeners in an ideal listening environment, and their responses scored (Crandell, 1990). This procedure has been validated by comparing earphone listening scores with direct listening scores of a group of 30 students (Nordlund, Kihlman, and Lindblad, 1968).

Having students respond to a rating scale provides a fast estimate of the effect of a treatment on speech intelligibility in a classroom. An example of a procedure a teacher could use is: (1) talk to the students for one minute, (2) add the treatment, (3) talk to the students for another minute, and (4) ask them to rate how easy it was for them to listen after the treatment as compared with before. The following scale could be used: (1) much harder than before, (2) harder than before, (3) a little harder than before, (4) the same as before, (5) a little easier than before, (6) easier than before, (7) much easier than before.

Using the TEF Analyzer is a direct and rapid approach to assessment of speech intelligibility. An electronic signal similar to that of speech is transmitted from a loudspeaker, picked up by the microphone in various room locations, and speech transmission index (STI) scores read on the computer monitor. STI scores obtained by the TEF Analyzer are not affected by room background noise.

Amplification considerations

The TEF Analyzer can also be used to compare STI scores in various room locations with and without room amplification (Blair, 1995). This enables the effect of a sound field FM system in a room to be evaluated under different treatment conditions.

A sound field FM system will not function equally well in all rooms. It will compensate for considerable room noise, but does not tolerate reflective surfaces well if its loudspeakers face them, particularly in small rooms. Generally, a sound field FM system is deleteriously affected when a room reverberates or echoes, or has room modes at the same frequencies as the speech signal. It functions best (S/N ratio up to 10 dB or more) when a room is acoustically controlled (Berg, 1993). Wherever one or more loudspeakers project direct sound to a large surface, that surface needs to be absorbent or diffusive, or the initial reflected sound wave will prevent the teacher from turning up the system gain so that a desirable S/N ratio can be achieved.

A hearing aid will also not function equally well in all rooms. For example, if the S/N ratio in the room is unfavourable, it will be reflected in the output of the hearing aid. And if the room is reverberant or echoic, or has dead and live spots, these undesirable acoustics will adversely affect the hearing aid response (see Figure 10.17). In contrast, if the S/N ratio in a room is +10 dB or greater and room reflections are controlled, the hearing aid will provide considerable usable amplification for a child with hearing loss. It will also compensate for the deadening effect of adding absorbent treatment to the room; the more sound energy lost, the more the hearing aid gain can be increased.

In a room with a controlled acoustic environment, a sound field FM system can also be added, and its gain turned up enough to further enhance the S/N ratio. A sound field FM system is subject to less down time than a hearing aid or a personal FM system, which has the potential to allow the listener to hear better than when using just a hearing aid. All too often, however, a personal FM system does not perform up to its potential because of improper fitting and because of student carelessness or even sabotage. Chapter 4 includes an overview on individual amplification systems and their applications.

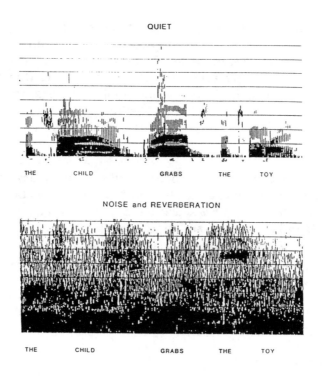

Figure 10.17 Spectrogram of the sentence "the child grabs the toy" in quiet (upper panel) and in noise and reverberation (lower panel). The S/N ratio was +6 db and the reverberation time was 0.8 second. From "An Introduction to Unilateral Sensorineural Hearing Loss in Children" by F. Bess and A. Tharpe in Ear and Hearing 7(1), 1986. Baltimore: Williams and Wilkins. Copyright 1986 by Williams and Wilkins. Reprinted by permission

Home applications

A signal control programme should also be conducted in a home. An attempt should be made to control echoes, reverberation, and modes in at least some of the rooms in which children are expected to listen and learn. The kitchen, for example, is a place where many families spend a lot of time and conduct a lot of business. It also may be the best location in the home for parents to help very young children develop language skills. The many activities associated with meals and snacks provide numerous opportunities for parent–child communication (Simmons, 1967). However, the kitchen often has the least desirable acoustics of any large listening and learning environment in the entire home. All surfaces of a kitchen, except for curtains, typically are highly reflective. More of its surfaces should be acoustically treated to reduce its very high RT and make it less subject to echoes.

Other applications

There are many other highly reflective areas that degrade communication and learning among children, particularly those with hearing loss. Gymnasiums, cafeterias, shops, and hallways can be particularly troublesome. Sport and shopping centres, traffic crossings, MacDonald equivalents, playgrounds, and swimming pools are also fraught with reverberation and echo as well as with noise.

Signal control plan

When sufficient data on room echoes, reverberation, modes, and speech intelligibility are available, a signal control plan (SCP) can be designated for a school or home. A SCP is aimed at increasing signal level and controlling reverberation, echoes, and modes inside rooms for listening and learning. The SCP should describe current signal and noise levels in the room, room surface treatments, and speech intelligibility scores at various locations. Like a noise control plan, the SCP should also describe general and specific objectives, persons responsible for implementing the plan, evaluation procedures, and the study team and its responsibilities.

Summary

There are formidable acoustical problems faced by students with hearing impairment. Many of these problems are largely unrecognised or misunderstood. This chapter has been written to help teachers of the deaf collaborate with other specialists and educators in resolving these problems through noise and signal control. If this is done, children with hearing impairments as well as children with normal hearing will listen and learn more effectively, and teachers and parents will find teaching easier and more effective. Acoustical problems and their resolution apply to listening and learning environments in schools and homes.

References

Berg F (1987) Facilitating Classroom Listening: A handbook for teachers of normal hearing and hard of hearing students. Austin, TX: PRO ED.

Berg F (1993) Acoustics and Sound Systems in Schools. San Diego: Singular Publishing Group.

Berg F, Blair J, Benson PV (1996) Classroom acoustics: The problem, impact, and solution. Language, Speech, and Hearing Services in Schools 27(1): 16-20.

Blair J (1995) Capabilities of TEF analyzer. Personal communication. Logan: Utah State University.

Brook R (1991) Rooms for speech and music. In Ballou G (Ed) Handbook for Sound Engineers. Indianapolis: Howard W Sams. pp 171-201.

Brook R, Uzzle T (1987) Rooms for speech, music, and cinema. In Ballou G (Ed) Handbook for Sound Engineers. Indianapolis: Howard W. Sams. pp 159-162.

Crandell C (1990) Effect of classroom acoustics on speech recognition in pediatric populations. In Berg F (Chair) Listening in Classrooms. Workshop conducted at Utah State University, Logan.

D'Antonio P (1989) Controlling sound reflections. Architecture 109: 112-137.

Davis R, Jones R (1989) Sound reinforcement handbook. Milwaukee: Hal Leonard.

Egan D (1988) Architectural acoustics. New York: McGraw Hill.

Everest A (1989) The master handbook of acoustics (2nd Edition). Blue Ridge Summit, PA: TAB Books.

Finitzo-Hieber T , Tillman T (1978) Room acoustics effects on monosyllabic word discrimination ability by normal and hearing impaired children. Journal of Speech and Hearing Research 21: 440-458.

Fulmer J (1990) Noise criteria curves and room acoustics. In Berg F (Chair) Listening in Classrooms. Workshop conducted at Utah State University, Logan.

Hedeen R (1980) Compendium of materials for noise control. U.S. Department of Health, Education, and Welfare (National Institute for Occupational Safety and Health) publication. Chicago: ITT Research Institute.

Hirschorn M (1989) Noise Control Reference Handbook. Bronx, NY: Industrial Acoustics Company.

Johnson D (1979) Why is the noise dose of humans important? Unpublished Presentation. Dayton OH: Wright.

Leavitt R, Flexer C (1991) Speech degradation as measured by the Rapid Speech Transmission Index (RASTI). Ear and Hearing 12: 115-118.

Lipscomb D (1978) Noise in Audiology. Baltimore: University Park Press.

Measurements in Building Acoustics (1988). Naerum, Denmark: Bruel & Kjaer.

Norlund B, Kihlman T, Lindblad S (1968) Use of articulation tests in auditorium studies. Journal of the Acoustical Society of America 44(1): 148-156.

Ray H (1990) Beginning and validation of sound field FM in classrooms. In Berg F (Chair) Listening in Classrooms. Workshop conducted at Utah State University, Logan.

Silverstone D (1982) Considerations for listening and noise distraction. In Sleeman P, Rockwell D (Eds) Designing Learning Environments. New York: Longman. p 79.

Simmons A (1967) Home language stimulation for hearing impaired children. In Berg F, Fletcher S (Chairs) Characteristics and needs of hard of hearing children. Institute conducted at Utah State University, Logan.

Waterhouse R, Harris C (1979) Sound in enclosed spaces. In Harris C (Ed) Handbook of Noise Control. New York: McGraw Hill. pp 4-9.

Chapter 11
The Development of Listening Skills

G CARR

Photographs by R Peters

Introduction

As professionals in the field of audiology and the education of deaf children, we believe in the child's right to early and accurate diagnosis and to appropriate high-quality amplification through personal hearing aids with well-fitting earmoulds. We believe also in the benefits of using those additional devices such as auditory training units and radio systems which enhance auditory awareness and access to sound. Therefore we hold central the belief that by allowing the child to maximise residual hearing, we afford him the fullest opportunity to achieve successful developmental and learning outcomes.

This chapter begins by highlighting the difference between hearing and listening and goes on to outline normal development of auditory skills and attention control. It describes aspects of the development of pre-verbal communication skills and their importance in auditory learning, and considers how quality adult–child interaction promotes effective language development. Auditory training for hearing-impaired children is discussed with regard to:

* integrating listening skills into everyday life,
* delivering specific listening programmes,
* using music to develop listening and communication.

An example of one listening programme in practice is given, with details of its implementation and suggestions for useful resources and follow-up materials.

The chapter aims to illustrate how teachers of the deaf with good audiological practice and a knowledge of auditory and communication development can intervene with deaf children to maximise auditory potential and develop listening behaviour. Whilst auditory skills are considered here with regard to the development of spoken language in particular, it is stressed that listening and auditory perception are important for all deaf children, regardless of communication mode, in order to give maximum access to the environment and the meaningful experiences a rich soundscape can provide.

Hearing and listening

Hearing can be described as the reception of sound by the ear and its transmission to the central nervous system, whereas listening implies paying attention to what is heard with the object of interpreting its meaning (Sheridan, 1973). In other words, there are two developmental processes involved:

1 The underlying capability to detect sound.
2 The behavioural response to sound.

(Bamford and Saunders, 1991)

In order to plan for intervention to enhance listening skills, it is important to be able to recognise these responses and to understand their progressive development.

Early listening behaviour

It is known that normally hearing babies can react to sound in utero (Pappas, 1985, in Flexer, 1994), and that newborns react to sound by making reflex responses such as eye-blinks, startles, head-turns or limb movement (Bamford and Saunders, 1991). Studies using the 'high amplitude sucking' (HAS) method indicate that babies are able to perceive change in, show preference for, or exert control over an auditory environment by sucking harder and faster to some sound stimuli than to others. One HAS experiment by DeCasper and Fifer in 1980 (quoted in Shaffer, 1995) found that infants between 1 and 3 days old could recognise the voices of their own mothers, preferring the maternal voice to that of other females. In the same way, babies have been shown to have preferences for certain kinds of music, and by 2–3 months of age, could discriminate between specific phonemes and syllables. Other HAS studies (Butterfield and Siperstein 1972, quoted in Shaffer, 1995) showed that babies tried to avoid listening to non-rhythmic noise and chose to 'tune-out' from sounds which did not attract interest.

These earliest auditory behaviours can be categorised as either 'reflexive' or 'attentive' (Flexer, 1994). Reflexive behaviours give an indication of sound detection, although it should be noted that auditory behaviour studies primarily use stimuli of 80–90 dBSPL to elicit responses even in normally hearing children. Flexer maintains, however, that reflexive responses do not imply learning and cites the following as meaningful early indicators of a learning/listening process:

- Arousal.
- Quieting.
- Eye-widening.
- Searching with the eyes (head still).
- Localising (eyes).
- Searching with the head.
- Smiling.

Careful observation, recognition and understanding of these early responses are crucial in identifying auditory potential and listening behaviour, especially in very young hearing-impaired children. Such observations may be critically important with children with a multiplicity of special needs.

Listening responses develop to become more controlled and sophisticated, and changes in the auditory behaviour of children can be observed clearly during the first 12 months of life. In the normally hearing child, a great deal of hearing and active listening takes place before verbal language begins to form (Ling, 1989). At 1–2 months of age, a child will turn its head towards a speaker. At 2–3 months, a normally-hearing child can be observed to purposively attend to sound which is meaningful and to react to it (being soothed by a familiar voice without seeing its source, or recognising that the sound of spoon and dish indicates feeding time). From 4 months to about 8 months, the infant's ability to localise sound becomes more accurate and consistent, and by 8 months of age, the child will recognise and turn to his own name. From that time until 12 months and beyond, the child shows an increasing capacity to understand spoken language and recognises and responds to an ever-increasing number of familiar sounds. The key to this development is the child's growing ability to ascribe meaning to the sound, since an auditory stimulus is meaningless when it cannot be connected to a familiar object or concept (Pogrund, Fazzi and Lampert, 1992). For hearing-impaired children, there is obvious need for active direction to make these connections.

Attention control

The normal child's listening development shows clear progression as the skill of focusing on an auditory stimulus and decoding it grows. Therefore, underpinning the skill of listening is the development of attentional strategies. In the early stages, the two can be seen to go hand in hand. Vision too plays an important part, since it is a key motivater for activity (Pogrund, Fazzi and Lampert, 1992). Equally, tactile experience can be a useful focus for attention, promoting learning through exploration by touch and often drawing initial attention to the source of sound for a deaf child.

In the development of attention control, some clear stages can be identified (adapted from Reynell and Huntly, 1985):

1 - Disengaged

Under the age of 12 months or so, children have very fleeting attention control and exhibit extreme distractability. The focus of attention shifts and re-shifts as different stimuli become more prominent at different times.

2 - Single-channelled

The child can focus on one thing at a time and this is very often adult-directed. This develops so that although still single-channelled, the child can exhibit more flexible attention control, switching from an activity, to a speaker, and back again, with help.

3 - Spontaneous focus of attention

The child takes increasing control over his attention focus, but engaging in a task and listening still need to be alternated.

4 - Dual-channelled

Usually, by the age of 4 or 5 years, looking and listening can be integrated to some degree, although the attention span may still be short.

5 - Integrated attention

Attention control is usually sustained and well established, normally around 6 years of age. The ability to sustain concentration and attention continues to improve until maturity, and it is thought that this is due to some extent to maturational changes in the central nervous system (Shaffer, 1995). The ability to listen selectively becomes a sophisticated skill, and a number of different but related auditory skills and strategies are employed in being a good listener.

Speech perception

According to Pinker (1994), "When we listen to speech, the actual sounds go in one ear and out the other; what we perceive is language". Rost (1990) reinforces this idea of the 'wholeness' of speech when he suggests that people listen for a purpose and it is this purpose that drives the understanding process. Auditory and linguistic processes are closely allied and normally interdependent. Deafness, by affecting the auditory feedback mechanism and by restricting access to full acoustic information, impacts adversely on the development of these processes. Understanding something of how spoken language is perceived and processed, however, can enable teachers of the deaf to create the most favourable conditions for hearing-impaired children to access maximum auditory information.

Phonemes are the smallest units of sound, which in any particular language differentiate between one word and another (Bamford and Saunders, 1991). These phonemes are necessarily important in that unless a child can make sense of them, he will have difficulty both in understanding spoken language and in being understood when he himself speaks. Individual phonemes are not perceived sequentially however, and there are many more factors at play in the process of speech perception. As Rost (1990) points out, frequency and intensity are critical aspects in the decoding of speech, and sounds can also be distinguished through differences in length or time and quality. Suprasegmental aspects of speech – intonation, stress, rhythm and disjuncture – all add to the message carried by the phoneme combinations and mould the meaning. Of particular importance are rhythm and flow. In referring to speech as an illusion, Pinker (1994) highlights that "In the speech sound wave, one word runs into the next seamlessly; there are no little silences between spoken words the way there are white spaces between written words". Rhythm is a crucial contributor to intelligibility. Without it, speech can become incomprehensible, just as music without rhythm can become unrecognisable. There are evident implications here for the way in which spoken language is presented to deaf children.

Auditory processing and listenership

Erber (1982) categorises four stages of development in auditory skills:

1 Detection (awareness of sound or its absence).
2 Discrimination (perceiving differences in sounds).
3 Identification (recognising and labelling sound).
4 Comprehension (understanding the purpose of sound).

Bamford and Saunders (1991) identify the following additional component skills in auditory processing:

1 Auditory memory.
2 Auditory sequencing.

3   Discrimination of auditory figure-ground tasks (i.e., recognition of speech in noise).

Rost (1990) also proposes the importance of listenership and listenership cues. These cues indicate a listener's part in conversation and communication, and allow the listener to shape the discourse. Listenership cues involve:

- prompting the speaker,
- challenging the speaker,
- clarifying,
- signalling understanding.

Appropriate back-channelling ensures that a speaker knows his listener is actively listening, by providing both visual and auditory/spoken feedback. Listenership cues are significant in supporting and perpetuating shared communication. For a deaf child, a communication partner showing good back-channelling signals can be the motivation to continue. In turn, to have true discourse and dialogue with others, the hearing-impaired person needs to internalise and utilise the rules of listenership for himself.

Clearly it can be seen that listening is not a single skill, but a complex combination of auditory processes, operating on a variety of levels. Listening skills are not separate from learning, but are the means to learning (Flexer, 1994). Therefore it is essential to consider them not only in terms of auditory access, but in the much wider context of communication and the growth of language.

Developing communication

Communication begins long before spoken language emerges. Pre-verbal communication behaviours include:

- eye-contact,
- eye-gaze,
- turn-taking,
- copying,
- auditory awareness.

Babies have their first social communication in eye-to-eye contact (Sheridan, 1973) within the first few weeks of life. Shortly afterwards, the baby can be observed watching the mother's face intently when within close range, and a social smile along with responsive vocalisation appears between approximately 5 and 8 weeks of age. Bamford and Saunders (1991) quote: "Somewhat later, the child follows the adult's line of regard (Scaife and Bruner, 1975) and this leads to the use of gaze direction (Beattie, 1979) and to joint shared attention of other objects". These pre-speech behaviours are interactive and conversational in nature. Sachs (1989) refers to research by Jaffe, Stern and Perry (1973) which showed that the gaze-coupling between mothers and their 3 month old infants very much resembles conversational turn-taking in adults. Eye contact remains significant in communication and listening throughout, and is an expectation in adult conversation, since good eye contact is important for normal social interaction (Lynch and Cooper, 1991).

Vocalisation

Early vocalisation is represented firstly by crying. Around 1 month of age, the infant can be heard to produce cooing vowel-like sounds. Consonant sounds appear around 3 to 4 months and the babbling period begins. A wide range of pitch is used in the vocalisation and clear syllables emerge. Initially, babies often vocalise whilst being spoken to, but by 7 or 8 months they have developed the skill of turn-taking, being silent when spoken to and then vocalising in response. Babies are naturally sensitive to the responses of their conversation partner and react to the feedback they receive. Visual feedback is provided by eye movements, facial expression and body language, and normally – and importantly – it matches the auditory feedback the child receives. When a child is deaf however, the auditory feedback system is imperfect (Ling, 1976, 1989; Flexer, 1994). Hearing-impaired children of around 8 to 9 months old, having paralleled to an extent the early communication development of their hearing peers, do not go on to develop the tuneful and repetitive babble that precedes spoken words and responsiveness to the auditory environment. Auditory feedback allows the child both to experience his own voice (and therefore facilitates the vocal experimentation which infants exhibit) and also to develop the same speech characteristics of those around him. The early years are critical for the proper maturation and development of the central auditory system and therefore it is crucial that for the deaf child, early amplification and habilitation are provided to tap auditory potential.

Motherese

The way in which adults talk to babies and young children is also significant in the communication and language learning process. Known as motherese, it has particular characteristics which are easily identified:

- An emphasis on repetition and questioning.
- A presentation of language in rhythmic patterns.

- Higher than normal pitch.
- An exaggerated intonation pattern.

Motherese has a sing-song quality and appears to attract the attention of the child. In doing so, it establishes and reinforces eye contact and perpetuates communicative interaction between adult and child. Pinker (1994) describes it as having "interpretable melodies: a rise and fall contour for approving, a set of sharp staccato bursts for prohibiting, a rise pattern for directing attention, and smooth legato murmurs for comforting". It is therefore a rich interactive process which is at the heart of the development of language, listening and communication from the very earliest stages. It is known that mutual play, turn-taking and shared activities, where mother and child attend jointly to an activity and the language experience is jointly focused on it, influence language development much more so than any imitative behaviour on the child's part (Bruner, 1983; Wood et al., 1986; Shaffer, 1995). Through interaction, children learn about the pragmatics of language – the rules of communication in its social use and the sub-skills of conversation such as initiating, maintaining a topic and closing the discourse. Hearing-impaired children can also gain a great deal of information from language interaction on a pragmatic level which supports their listening and attending behaviour.

Auditory training and the deaf child

It is a fact that deaf children with the same residual hearing capacity experience varying degrees of success in terms of auditory discrimination and in achieving good levels of speech intelligibility. Some deaf children, however 'promising' their audiograms and even aided thresholds, do not achieve the auditory access to spoken language that might be expected. Others frequently surpass theoretical expectation. The reasons for this wide variety of outcomes are, of course, multi-factorial, but it seems reasonable to assume that positive, active use of residual hearing must make a considerable contribution.

What is auditory training?

There is long-standing and widespread appreciation of the value of actively developing listening behaviour in deaf children. Markides (1983) reports the practice of auditory training for the purpose of improving speech intelligibility as far back as the late nineteenth century. Ewing and Ewing (1964), however, had perhaps the greatest influence in promoting awareness that use of hearing rather than just level of hearing is crucial to the development of auditory discrimination. The term motherese was not in use at that time, but the Ewings advocated "natural talk-to-baby" and emphasised the need for deaf children to experience their own voices through hearing aids "whenever situations and their emotions" motivated them.

The word training in itself implies some form of systematic teaching, and those involved in the education of deaf children have differed as to whether auditory training means the delivery of a planned teaching programme, carried out at a certain time and place, or whether it permeates everyday life. It is, of course, both, and the linking of the two must be mutually supportive.

Quality audition in everyday life

Unless attending residential schools, all children spend a good deal of time in the home. In the early years, this time is naturally at its greatest, and a stimulating home environment offers rich opportunity for childhood learning. The teacher of the deaf supporting in the home can advise parents and carers in facilitating language development and in creating a positive auditory environment or soundscape for the child, so that he can maximise his audition and use it in his learning. Accurate assessment, together with the provision of appropriate amplification, provide the basis of access for the child to his auditory environment. Careful ongoing observation of the child's auditory behaviour is then vital in order to:

- Plan purposefully for progress on a developmental level.
- Support the fine tuning of amplification to the child's needs.

The soundscape

Audiologists advise that the extent of signal to noise (S/N) ratio is probably the most important factor in the auditory recognition of speech and therefore it is crucial for the development of speech and language for a deaf child. It is also known that the S/N ratio disadvantage for hearing-impaired people is at its greatest when the competing noise is speech. There are clear implications here for the conditions in the home, especially where there are other young children also needing and deserving communication and interaction with their parents. Right from the beginning, the environment should be controlled for noise as far as possible. Flexer (1994) refers to the need to alter the auditory background for the child, since the amplification of sounds previously not heard may lead to the child's resistance to wearing hearing aids in the early days.

The home environment offers endless opportunity for exposure to sound which is significant for the child's social as well as auditory learning: the door knocker or bell heralding someone's arrival, the telephone signifying a communication contact, kitchen implements and garden equipment with their identifying noises, hairdryers, toilets flushing, the list goes on. However, the soundscape must not be chaotic; it is vital to order it so as not to swamp the child with sound which may be meaningless and confusing because its source cannot be identified. It is important therefore that parents and carers know what constitutes a positive listening environment for auditory learning. This can be summarised as one in which:

- The signal to noise ratio is favourable, i.e., the desired sound or speech signal is clearly louder than the background noise. Flexer (1994) cites a desirable S/N ratio of +20 dB, supported by findings by Finitzo-Hieber and Tillman (1978) and Hawkins (1984).
- The child, through systematic and planned exposure facilitated by an adult, can connect sound with its source.
- A wide range of meaningful auditory experiences (both in the home and outside it) is available to enable the child to learn through audition.
- Good quality language interaction takes place.

Particularly in the early stages, it is important to highlight auditory stimuli which one is reasonably sure the child can hear, so confidence is developed in both child and parents. Flexer (1994) also stresses the need for parents to be given realistic and concrete knowledge on which to structure initial learning experiences for the child. Such information can be regularly updated as the child's auditory responses become clearer and more consistent. Close co-operation between parents, teacher of the deaf and those responsible for audiological provision is central in formulating this.

Facilitating language development

An environment rich in communicative interaction is crucially beneficial for the learning, listening and language development of all children. For deaf children, adults need to actively facilitate natural and meaningful opportunities for this development to take place.

Drawing on a knowledge of listening and communication development, the teacher of the deaf can support parents in:

- Recognising and responding appropriately to early non-verbal communicative behaviour such as eye-gaze. With deaf children who will go on to rely on their ability to lip read to support listening skills, establishing good and lasting eye-contact may have heightened significance.
- Being aware of the importance of auditory feedback and therefore understanding and engaging in frequent vocal play. The parents need

encouragement to continue talking to the child, even when there seems to be little response.
* Making sure they give time for the child to make a response.
* Encouraging turn-taking in play situations.
* Patterning their language well, using motherese.
* Making positive use of an auditory training unit.

Early interaction might involve singing, games like peek-a-boo and finger rhymes. Later, toys might be shared and talked about (shape sorters, stacking toys) and pre-school musical instruments that have a quality sound can be a good focus of shared attention. It is important to choose age-appropriate toys and facilitate games that are suitable for non-deaf children of the same age. What is important is that adult and child jointly focus attention upon them and the language experience too is jointly focused. Everyday activities such as bathing, dressing, cleaning and mealtimes also provide opportunity for shared looking, listening and talking. The child however needs to be genuinely interested in the task in order for his attention to be truly caught. As McCracken and Sutherland (1991) advise: "Let your child control and focus your interest, then you can offer him your time, involvement and language".

The development of auditory training programmes

The work of Father A. van Uden of the residential school for the deaf at Sint Michielsgestel, Holland, has been crucial in the shaping of the development and practice of auditory training programmes. Van Uden's methods stress rhythm as a key factor in a wide range of speech, language and listening skills: rhythm within words, within phrase groupings, in breathing and in memory processes. Describing conversation as a 'duet', he claims also that music and dance are central to training "the basic functions of speech and language" and advocates that deaf children should have "a total rhythmic education from childhood ... the method of which must use sound perception to its fullest extent...".

In the Sint Michielsgestel listening programmes, emphasis was laid on the play-song which focused on the integration of rhythmic speech and language with musical interpretation. This was developed by taking as a focus conversational language, marking it with a flowing 'rhythm-curve' which indicated the stress pattern, and then performing it on blow organs and in rhythmic speech. Van Uden maintains that words are often remembered by their rhythm rather than by their constituent phonemes (the number of syllables and stress pattern being the more important factors in retrieving a forgotten word) and therefore that rhythm is crucial to auditory memory and growing language competence. For a more detailed consideration, the interested reader is referred to van Uden (1977).

The success of the work in Holland in positively affecting the development of listening and language skills inspired the establishing of auditory training groups in Britain in the 1970s. Known as Aurhythmics, these programmes focused on rhythmic movement to music and drew also on traditional auditory training strategies to combine with van Uden's innovations. Although Bamford (1981) found little hard evidence that auditory training actively improved the discrimination skills of the deaf person, he suggests (Bamford and Saunders, 1991) that by enhancing attention and auditory awareness, auditory training might improve selective listening, especially since there are many qualitative reports of its success. Today there are many programmes in action in a wide range of educational contexts across various countries. Each programme has its own emphasis and organisational structure in keeping with the needs of its hearing-impaired population and the type of local educational provision. What is common to all the programmes however is the aim of encouraging good use of hearing aids, establishing active listening and fulfilling auditory potential. To do so, they take account of what is normal sequential development, understanding the child's abilities on a variety of levels, behavioural and physiological.

Music and musical experience

Music is a world-wide activity; anthropologists have yet to identify a civilisation that did not include an engagement with music as one of its attributes (Ellis, 1995). Making and sharing in music is also a social activity and as such it has a significant contribution to make to social development. Equally if not more importantly, music is unique in the way it can communicate feelings and ideas without any other language and so has a special place in attempts to develop listening, communication and creative skills (Withers, Mendonca and Annear, 1995).

Music also has many aspects in common with spoken language. It has already been noted that motherese has a musical cadence and repeated patterns which can be likened to a refrain, and the crucial function of rhythm in carrying meaning has also been highlighted. Furthermore, it is significant that the fields of music and linguistics share so many technical terms, for duration, pitch, articulation, phrasing, tempo and timbre are amongst key features in both. For a deaf child, music may be one of the earliest auditory experiences. It can be amplified well. It can present clear rhythms and patterns and cause vibration – not only in floors, speakers and the instruments themselves, but also in the body. High fidelity systems can provide rich acoustic information free of distortion and across a wide spectrum of frequency.

It is also possible to give children first-hand access to quality musical instruments, thereby allowing them to use all their senses to perceive the properties of the instruments and the sounds they make, to support the stimulation of audition. Through active involvement with music, deaf children can:

- feel sound through vibration,
- focus attention and develop concentration,
- learn to discriminate different sounds,
- develop an understanding of turn-taking,
- express emotion,
- take the initiative in communicative interaction,
- relax, enjoy and have fun.

Musical experience in the early years

Singing is one of the easiest ways of sharing musical experience with a child (Figure 11.1). Whether using voice alone or singing along to a pre-recorded tape, it gains the child's interest and attention and supports the development of eye-gaze. Finger rhymes, songs involving actions and those with repetitive phrases all increase involvement and interaction. Research carried out with pre-school deaf children into the benefits of singing (Tait, 1985) showed a number of advantages over ordinary conversation, including increased eye-contact and vocalisation, better rhythm and breath control, improved intonation and increased understanding and auditory memory.

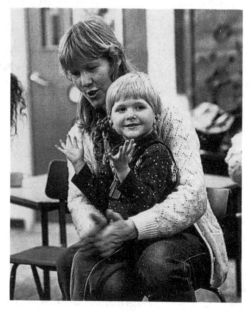

Figure 11.1

Very young children also enjoy making music, and through it can discover the difference between sound and silence, rhythms and patterns and sounds of different qualities. Musical instruments can be makeshift, or commercially produced. Instruments which can be played in a variety of ways (shaken, beaten with the hands, played with a beater, banged together or blown) provide rich opportunity for exploration and learning. For parents and teachers who are not musically confident, there are also some excellent commercial resources available which include taped music and ideas for activities which encourage the development of visual, tactile and motor skills as well as auditory awareness.

Music in the school curriculum

Whatever and wherever the educational placement, but especially if it is in mainstream provision, deaf children encounter music as part of the curriculum. The common requirements of the music National Curriculum in England and Wales state that children should have "appropriate provision" in order to access its content. It highlights the areas of performing and composing and listening and appraising. In detailing these, the National Curriculum describes those very aspects that have been identified with regard to developing auditory and discrimination skills for language learning: responding to sound, and recognising the elements of pitch, duration, dynamics, tempo, timbre, texture and structure. It goes on to outline a wide range of activities both within performing and composing and listening and appraising which would support the aims of teachers and parents in enhancing communication skills in deaf children, certainly within the key stage one programme of study. If teachers of the deaf liaise closely and sensitively with specialist music teachers to ensure maximum access to National Curriculum music, it can be an immensely positive experience for the hearing-impaired child which can enrich other areas of development.

Very special music

Music technology has made immense steps forward in recent years and has opened up hitherto denied avenues of expressive musical experience for deaf youngsters with additional or complex learning difficulties. Through music, special needs children can show self-expression and signal communication. Their experiences can enhance their perception about how they feel and it allows them to experiment and to discover cause and effect. Musical experience gives an increased sense of being functioning independent people with a capacity for aesthetic response (Ellis, 1995). Ellis also observes that when engaged in musical activity, concentration span is often lengthened and attention sustained for extended periods.

Special musical equipment includes technology such as synthesisers which can be played in a variety of innovative ways, computers which can create sound with simple triggering mechanisms, and a development called 'Soundbeam', which has associated vibrotactile adaptations such as 'Soundbox' and 'Soundbed'. Soundbeam was originally designed so that dancers could shape sound as they moved in and out of an ultrasonic field. It is sensitive to all kinds of physical movement and allows a child to learn through experimentation, conscious or otherwise, that he can control the musical reaction and shape the musical response. The sounds produced are rich, varied and interesting, and the possibilities for creativity are almost boundless. The Soundbox and Soundbed resonators can also be used with other amplified music.

The 'Magic Organ' is another development which allows access to musical sounds. The organ is about 3 feet long and can be placed on the floor or on a table. It can be played easily, with light body contact on coloured discs which activate the sound. Different cassettes can be attached so that the sounds produced can vary from musical in nature (piano, orchestra, opera or percussion) to human or animal noises, bells and horns. The organ itself is robust, attractive and brightly coloured to stimulate visual interest.

Other specialist equipment, although not technological, can include musical instruments from other countries and those which create special effects, such as surf-drums. The Remo Ocean drum, for example, is a professional quality frame drum which creates the sounds of crashing waves, offers opportunity to explore rhythm and is visually interesting. Covered in underwater design fabric, it has small metal balls enclosed inside and can be gently manipulated for the sensation of rolling waves, shaken for a 'stormier' effect or gently struck with a fabric covered beater to create other 'water' music. Such developments show the enormous scope that music-making can give, and that only lack of awareness and opportunity can set limits on the musical experience that hearing-impaired and complex needs children can enjoy. Information on all the instruments described here is given in Appendix E.

The Halle hearing-impaired project

The Halle orchestra is an internationally acclaimed orchestra based in Manchester, England. It began its outreach programme in 1990, with the stated aim being "to give hearing-impaired children the opportunity to create and share in music; to discover its dynamic, exciting and fun qualities with their peers, teachers and professional musicians". In practice, it is the direct involvement of children with real musicians that has marked this project as being special in making music-making accessible to deaf children. In its theory, and in its implementation, it supports music in the National Curriculum and the development of

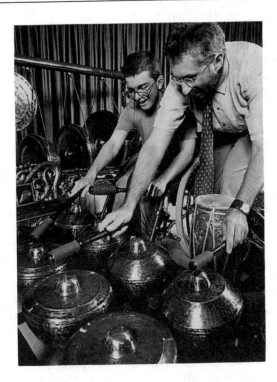

Figure 11.2

listening skills along the lines of what is described in the previous section on auditory training and in the next section on one programme in practice. It shares the same aims in developing listening skills, and adds the important element of music for relaxation. It encourages effective use of amplification and recognises the value of observing auditory behaviour emphasising rhythm and recognising the importance of patterns in both music and spoken language. The Halle also offers a Gamelan programme, which provides an original and unique type of aural group music-making which is immediately accessible to its participants, using over forty iron and brass instruments from central Java, Figure 11.2. Gamelan consists mainly of tuned percussion (gongs, metal and wooden xylophones, drums), but also includes vocals, flutes, fiddles and zithers. Its traditional role – as accompaniment for dance, theory and puppetry – leads naturally into multi-media and cross-arts projects (Withers, Mendonca and Annear, 1995). A contact address for the Gamelan is given in Appendix E of this book.

It is not possible here to give a detailed account of all the opportunities for deaf children's listening development which the Halle project might promote. These include conducting, graphic scores and repeating patterns as well as Gamelan. It is however important to focus on the aspect of conversations, for it is in this respect most of all that the project supports the idea of music for communication, as a language. Both adult and child have a musical instrument, usually of the same type. Together, reinforced by eye-contact, gaze and turn-taking, the players form a conversation, maybe revolving around contrast or perhaps one imitating the other. Sometimes a musician may play an instrument to a child and the conversation may be sustained by a vocal response by the child. The musician takes the cue from the child's response and vice versa. In the beginning, the musician or teacher will undoubtedly be in control of the structure of the conversation. In time, as the child's confidence grows and he focuses his listening, the control changes, and the child is structuring both the music and the conversation. The value to the communication process and to the development of attentive listening is clearly evident.

Access to such exciting, valuable and innovative programmes is not always easy. Neither is the acquisition of quality musical resources, especially of the technological kind. Teachers of the deaf should take the initiative in approaching local orchestras and music groups. Approaches for funding might be made to voluntary organisations to purchase musical instruments. Throughout the world, deaf people themselves are experiencing musical achievement and becoming music specialists; through their success and their talents, there is much to learn. In England 'Music and the Deaf' does much to promote musical access and performance for deaf people, and particularly encourages musical activity in deaf children. Such organisations can provide invaluable help to teachers of the deaf in maximising the value of music and musical experience.

One programme in practice

The particular programme described here is entitled auditory rhythmic training (A.R.T). It recognises as a central principle the importance of rhythm and the rhythmic elements of language in auditory perception, utilising van Uden's 'rhythm curve'. It is not musical in the same way as the Halle project, but it does include musical experience and emphasises the importance of singing. It draws also on traditional aspects of auditory training, and deems as essential that children are appropriately aided. To this extent, the programme is neither new, nor original. What may mark it as potentially different, however, is that it has been designed to be developmental, with a structured and graded progression intended to be successfully integrated into a peripatetic framework of support for deaf children and their families. In addition, it links closely to the audiological status of those children participating in the programme.

At all stages, close reference is made to available audiological information, and this is used in planning the activities for individual children. Sound levels are closely monitored, and information about children's responses is shared with the audiologist. In this way, audiological assessment and the auditory experiences within the programme are mutually supportive, enabling 'fine-tuning' of amplification based on actual experience of use, and the gauging of the volume and frequency of the sound stimuli in the programme sessions to encourage the child to listen at appropriate, and sometimes challenging, levels. The children's experiences in the programme have even influenced their behaviour in the audiology clinic: in addition to responding in pure-tone testing, children as young as 3 years old have also been telling the audiologist whether the tones are high or low and long or short! The programme is described here not only in terms of its content, but also with regard to the practicalities of organisation and implementation. Although these details may seem somewhat mundane, it is important to include them since the key to success for such a programme lies not only in the value of its content, but also in the effectiveness of its delivery.

Organisation and implementation

The programme has been developed to operate within the provision of the peripatetic service in Stockport, England, where it has been running successfully for some 8 years. The programme's co-ordinators have also introduced it to professionals and parent groups in several other regions of England and Scotland, where it has formed the basis for the setting up of similar programmes.

The Stockport Service is based in the centre of the town, which is easily accessed from the surrounding areas. The programme takes place at the service's base on two afternoons per week. Where families of pre-school children do not have transport to attend the sessions, it is provided. School-age children are also transported to the Centre. All the teachers of the deaf within the service are fully conversant with the aims and activities of the programme and since it is always important to generalise listening programmes into everyday contexts, they continue and extend the activities in their work with children, families and schools beyond the sessions. Teachers from the children's mainstream schools receive in-service training about the programme, so that they understand its aims and function and can then reinforce and build on progress on an ongoing basis. Some elements of A.R.T have also been adapted for work with children with multi-sensory special needs and also for those children with normal hearing who have poor listening skills and attention control.

An overview

Initially, the A.R.T programme emphasises the child's response to external sound stimuli through vibrotaction as well as through audition.

Parent and child work closely together as activities focus not only on physical and rhythmic movement to sound and music, but also on reinforcing early communication skills and listening behaviours in keeping with Erber's (1982) progression of auditory skills. The transfer from visual and tactile emphasis to auditory emphasis is facilitated by the gradual withdrawal of physical prompts, and as auditory awareness grows, alongside general maturation and development, more complex activities are introduced, including games and songs which encourage use of higher-level auditory skills and increased child–child interaction. The children focus on rhythm and characteristics within music, such as duration and pitch, and with these growing skills comes the opportunity to link these with the spoken word.

Firstly, the children look at the rhythm within their own familiar names. Games are based around the recognition of the rhythm patterns. The rhythm is shown by means of a 'rhythm curve' where height indicates stress. Later, simple words and phrases are studied, children being able to recognise them in accordance with their rhythm pattern. As the children progress still further, they acquire the skills of deciding for themselves upon rhythm and stress patterns for their own phrases, as well as for poems and songs, and also learn to discuss and debate aspects of music, speech and language.

The A.R.T programme is arranged into three broad stages. Stage one activities are generally aimed at the pre-school age range, although most of the activities can be modified for older children if they are late-comers to the programme or are at this level of development at an older age. Within stage one, there are usually two groups:

- Under threes.
- 3 to 4½ year olds.

Usually, children are moving on to stage two by the time they are entering school, but some pre-schoolers will have already 'graduated' and some school-age children may need further experience within stage one. Stage three children are usually between the ages of eight and eleven years, although again it should be stressed that the progression is developmental, not chronological.

Stage one

It is important to remember that some activities will demand a certain level of maturation in co-ordination and, therefore, the choice of activities for inclusion in a session will depend on the make-up of the group. In the early days of stage one, it is very much a parent–child partnership and initially, when a child cannot move rhythmically by himself, the parent does the moving for and with him. As the child matures and progresses, he achieves a growing level of independence within the activities. In practical terms, sessions last approximately 45 minutes. New activities are introduced carefully into already-familiar formats. As a general rule, only one or two new activities are introduced in any one half-term period (approximately 6 weeks). The running order of a session tends to be the same each week so that the children can develop anticipation within the session as a whole. The order of activities is not in itself vital, but should be chosen so as to ease the movement of one activity into the next. However, the sessions always begin with an attention-getting activity and end with a quiet close-contact activity.

The aims of stage one are:

- To develop awareness of sound (including vibration feeling), leading on to the development of auditory detection and discrimination.
- To achieve good eye-contact and visual attention.
- To encourage development of attention control.
- To increase body-awareness.
- To develop anticipation.
- To encourage awareness of others and turn-taking, leading to group co-operation and participation.
- To encourage the enjoyment of sound and music and making music for fun.
- To experience and develop rhythm.

Early activities might include:

- movement to music (slow swaying or lively bouncing on the parent's knee),
- responding to sound (kicking a skittle on the beat of a drum; throwing a bean bag on hearing an organ tone; coming out from behind a screen or from under a sheet when a sound is heard; playing Pass the Parcel),
- action rhymes and songs,
- exploring musical instruments through directed play.

As the children progress, and listening skills are clearly seen to be developing, some activities involving discrimination are introduced:

- Different music for running/skipping/marching etc.
- Music to act to and interpret – trains, racing cars etc.
- Discrimination between two different sounds (a different physical response to each).
- Discrimination between high/low, fast/slow (stretching up to high tones, crouching down to low ones: running to fast rhythms, slowly striding to slow beats).

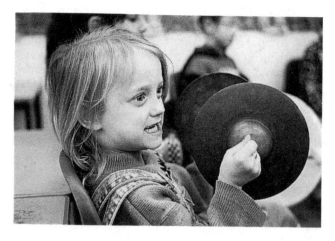

Figure 11.3

The children learn to recognise the rhythms of their own names (clapped or beaten out), and copy body rhythms and rhythmic patterns on musical instruments. Participation games with a greater emphasis on language are also introduced. A wide range of resources and props is used in the activities – hats, spiders on sticks, puppets, dressing-up clothes, skittles, musical instruments (mainly percussion) (Figure 11.3), bean bags – along with the inventiveness of parents and teachers. Excellent suggestions and detailed guidelines for activities at all stages of the programme (but of particular value at stage one) have been gleaned from published materials, which are listed in Appendix D.

Stage two

Stage two does not generally have parental involvement in the session. A session lasts some 40 minutes, the last five of which are spent reviewing the activities with the children themselves. Teachers do not need to be music specialists or even able to play an instrument or sing in tune, but it is important to have a well-developed sense of rhythm. Stage two assumes that the children are – or can be – listeners, that they have begun to develop rhythmically and that they can participate in group activities. Many of the aims in stage one will have been achieved, yet others will need to be consolidated.

The additional aims of stage two are:

- Improving breathing and breath control.
- Refining discriminatory abilities.
- Developing inner rhythm to a greater degree.
- Developing auditory memory and sequencing.

- Channelling knowledge and feeling for rhythm into language.
- Encouraging greater use of voice and participating in singing.

The 'rhythm curve' is introduced in its written form for the first time, initially on the children's own names, the rhythms of which they should already recognise. The rhythm curve indicates not only the number of syllables in utterances, but also the stress each one carries. The greater the stress, the higher the curve – for example,

banana   going home

The activities in stage two sessions can be broadly grouped into the following categories:

- Non-verbal (body) rhythmic movement (including dance).
- Rhythmic language activity.
- Singing.
- Listening and differentiating.
- Breathing.

The session always begins with the rhythmic name game, which serves as a familiar introduction to the session and emphasises eye-contact and turn-taking. The children sit around a drum, and each has on a card their name and its rhythm curve. When they are identified by the drum beat, they take over and beat out the name of another child. It continues in this way until all the children are identified and welcomed to the session. The session always ends with a musical listening game to exit on the same principles. Other activities are chosen as appropriate for the group. Generally speaking, each session contains one activity in each of the above categories.

Discrimination work at this stage extends further than in stage one. The children are encouraged to discriminate between long/short, quiet (soft)/loud, fast/slow, smooth/jerky, high/low (and middle), strong/weak (gentle). Work on localisation of sound also begins. Greater emphasis is put on language and rhythmic units of language and on using songs and stories to develop and extend auditory memory and sequencing skills. Sessions are generally intensive, yet fun. Stage two activities include the types of games described in the following paragraphs.

For rhythmic body movement:

- Body clapping (in front of the mirror children 'clap' in rhythm with hands on different parts of the body).
- 'Pass the Rhythm' extension of body clapping (chants are added when the clapping is good).
- Rowing to music.

- Country dancing (when steps are known and rhythm is good, words are added and songs are created).
- Simple Latin American dancing.

For rhythmic language work:

- The 'name-game' with the rhythm curve.
- Nursery rhymes, action songs.
- Indian drum rhythms (auditory memory/listening also – the children walk round a large drum, copying a rhythmic pattern initiated by the first child in the group).

For listening and discrimination:

- Musical chairs/statues.
- 'Match the sound' (using screen and hidden musical instruments).
- Various games discriminating between two, three and four different sounds (endless permutations).
- Organ work, using the set rhythms, varying tempos.
- Find the source of sound – hot/cold game. The other children in the group help the seeker find the hidden sound by shouting 'hot' when close and 'cold' when far away.

For breathing:

- The car game (children sing a tone to keep their car going along a track).
- Names and phrases played on the blow organ (melodion).
- Ping-pong target game, where children state where on a table top they will aim to blow the ball to and stop at a stated point.
- General relaxation and breathing techniques.

Stage three

Many of the aims of stage two are carried through, developed and extended at this stage, but the main emphasis of the work lies in the rhythm curve and its use in enhancing language skills and also in listening for comprehension. As in stage two, sessions last 40 minutes, including a 5 minute review. Whilst the musical and non-verbal rhythmic activities are carried out with the full group, children may be in pairs or even working individually for the language section.

Discrimination work at stage three involves considerable use of music, and the children respond to it in different ways, interpreting mood and feeling, deciding on beat and tempo, discussing use of instruments and the sounds they make. The children may interpret the music through movement and dance. Non-verbal and verbal rhythmic work is also continued to extend auditory memory further, and greater emphasis is laid on quality of speech and voice production through the use of tone bars (individual rosewood bars on a resonating case which amplifies and projects a clear tone, available across a range of notes). The use of tone bars was introduced to England by the Danish teacher of the deaf and music therapist Claus Bang in the late 1970s.

Each session contains four basic parts:

- A rhythmic activity.
- A musical / discrimination activity.
- Language / rhythm curve work.
- A listening activity, focusing on listening for rather than to something.

For working on the rhythm curve, the language may be a poem or song, something built around a spontaneous discussion or something prepared beforehand. It is written up on a flip chart. The children then discuss the number of syllables, not only in individual words but in phrase units and sentences. The stress pattern is discussed – children give their own opinions and debate them – and, when the final decision is made, the curve is marked on the chart.

The language is practised, chanted, sung, beaten out, in accordance with the rhythm curve. The children may use percussion instruments to help them. The rhythm curve can help to interpret intonation and also intensity, e.g.:

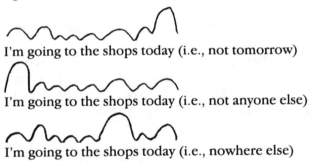

I'm going to the shops today (i.e., not tomorrow)

I'm going to the shops today (i.e., not anyone else)

I'm going to the shops today (i.e., nowhere else)

The children match rhythm curves to language, and create language to match rhythm curve patterns. When they are fully conversant with its use and purpose, they can use it at any time to aid pronunciation and understanding,

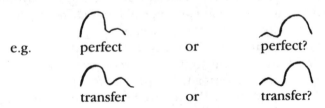

e.g.   perfect   or   perfect?

            transfer   or   transfer?

Examples of stage three activities are:

For musical discrimination work:

- Listening to pieces of music, discussing them and interpreting them physically.
- Writing and singing own words to fit musical accompaniment.
- Sound stories – discussing and producing sound effects.
- Discussing attributes of different instruments, listening and feeling, discussing the appropriate vocabulary.

For music activity:

- Complex body clapping.
- Complex Indian drum rhythms - copying by rhythm, not by counting beats.
- Dancing and singing.
- Extended activities from earlier stages.

For language/rhythm curve work:

- Poems, stories, songs – some made up by the children themselves.

For listening:

- Various activities involving picking out particular sounds from other background noise.
- Listening for spoken language – e.g., specific key words or phrases in sentences or paragraphs, spotting the deliberate mistake in stories, following a sequence of verbal instructions to complete pictures or puzzles.

For work on speech and voice quality:

- Tone bar work.
- Extended rhythm curve work using musical notation and organ for enhancing flow of speech and intonation.

The range of activities in listening programmes which the teacher of the deaf in partnership with parents and the children themselves might employ is limited only by imagination. Exciting pathways may be followed taking the lead from the children's responses, auditory and otherwise, and building on them. The underlying aims and principles of such programmes however should always be borne in mind. The teacher should continually be asking "What?", "Why?" and "Where next?". The "How?" should be purposeful, clearly-defined and, in addition, fun.

Summary

Whilst not having the scope to give in-depth consideration of the development of the full range of auditory skills, this chapter has shown how the teacher of the deaf might support the development of listening behaviour in hearing-impaired children through (a) having an understanding of the strategies involved in listening and attending, and (b) having a knowledge of speech perception and the development of communication.

The importance of the auditory environment has been highlighted, along with the positive influence of the use of music and structured listening programmes in enhancing listening ability. By outlining early developments in aurhythmics, aspects of the music National Curriculum, a professional music project with deaf children and one listening programme in practice, key features of auditory training have been emphasised and various strategies for promoting active listening have been suggested. Underpinning the presentation of listening activities is the belief that residual hearing can be maximised by providing high quality amplification, a favourable acoustic environment, and planned opportunity to actively develop raised auditory awareness.

References

Bamford JM (1981) Auditory training: What is it, what is it supposed to do and does it do it? British Journal of Audiology 15.

Bamford JM, Saunders E (1991) Hearing Impairment, Auditory Perception and Language Disability. London: Whurr.

Beattie GW (1979) Planning units in spontaneous speech: some evidence from hesitation in speech and speaker gaze direction in conversation. Linguistics 17: 61-78.

Bruner JS (1975) The ontogenisis of speech acts. Journal of Child Language 2: 1-19.

Butterfield EC, Sipersten GN (1972) Influence of contingent auditory stimulation upon non-nutritional suckle. In Bosma JS (Ed.) 3rd Symposium on Oral Sensation and Perception: The Mouth of the Infant. Springfield, Ilinois: Charles C. Thomas.

Carr G, Smith A, Wheeler C (1994) Auditory Rhythmic Training: a handbook. Stockport Service for Sensory Impaired Children.

DeCasper AJ, Fifer WP (1980) Of human bonding: Newborns prefer their mothers' voices. Science 208: 1174-1176.

Department for Education (1995) The National Curriculum. London: HMSO.

Ellis P (1995) Sound Therapy. Information Exchange No.45. Primary Music Today.

Erber N (1982) Auditory Training. Washington D.C.: The Alexander Graham Bell Association for the Deaf.

Ewing A, Ewing EC (1964) Teaching Deaf Children to Talk. Manchester: Manchester University Press.

Finitizo-Hieber T, Tillman TW (1978) Room acoustics effects on monosyllabic word discrimination ability for normal and hearing-impaired children. Journal of Speech and Hearing Research 21: 440-458

Flexer C (1994) Facilitating Hearing and Listening in Young Children. San Diego, CA: Singular Publishing Group Inc.

Hawkins DB (1984) Comparison of speech recognition in noise by mildly-to-moderately hearing-impaired children using hearing aids and FM systems. Journal of Speech and Hearing Disorders 49: 409-18.

Jaffe J, Stern D, Perry C (1973) "Conversational" coupling of gaze behaviour in pre-linguistic human development. Journal of Psycholinguistic Research 2: 321-330.

Ling D (1976) Speech and the Hearing Impaired Child: Theory and Practice. Washington D.C.: The Alexander Graham Bell Association for the Deaf.

Ling D (1989) Foundations of Spoken Language for Hearing Impaired Children. Washington D.C.: The Alexander Graham Bell Association for the Deaf.

Lynch C, Cooper J (1991) Early Communication Skills: The Manual. Bicester: Winslow Press.

McCracken W, Sutherland H (1991) Deaf-ability not Disability. Clevedon: Multilingual Matters.

Markides A (1983) The Speech of Hearing-Impaired Children. Manchester: Manchester University Press.

Pappas DG (1985) Diagnosis and Treatment of Hearing Impairment in Children: A clinical manual. San Diego: College-Hill Press.

Pinker S (1994) The Language Instinct. London: Penguin.

Pogrund L, Fazzi D, Lampert J (Eds) (1992) Early Focus. New York: American Foundation for the Blind.

Reynell J, Huntley M (1985) Reynell Developmental Language Scales Revised Edition. Windsor: NFER-Nelson.

Rost M (1990) Listening in Language Learning. New York: Longman.

Sachs J (1989) Communication Development in Infancy. In Gleason JB (Ed) The Development of Language. Columbus, Ohio: Merrill.

Scaife BK, Bruner JS (1975) The capacity for joint visual attention in the infant. Nature 253: 265-266.

Shaffer DR (1995) Developmental Psychology: Childhood and Adolescence. Pacific Grove, California: Brooks/Cole.

Sheridan MD (1973, reprinted 1993) From Birth to Five Years: Children's Developmental Progress. London: Routledge.

Tait M (1985) Reaching our Children Through Song. Nottingham: University of Nottingham.

van Uden A (1977) A World of Language for Deaf Children Part 1. Amsterdam: Swets and Zeitlinger BV.

Withers M, Mendonca M, Annear P (1995) Halle Education / BT Hearing Impaired Project. Manchester: Halle Education.

Wood DJ, Wood HA, Griffith AJ, Howarth CI (1986) Teaching and Talking with Deaf Children. London: John Wiley.

Appendices

Appendix A - Core book list

Bamford JM, Saunders E (1991) Hearing Impairment, Auditory Perception and Language Disability. London: Whurr.

Beazley S, Moore M (1995) Deaf Children, Their Families and Professionals: Dismantling Barriers. London: David Fulton

Berg F (1987) Facilitating Classroom Listening: A Handbook for Teachers of Normal Hearing and Hard of Hearing Students. Boston: College Hill Press/Little Brown.

Berg F (1993) Acoustics and Sound Systems in Schools. San Diego: Singular Publishing.

Bishop D, Mogford K (Eds) (1994) Language in Exceptional Circumstances. Hove: Lawrence Erlbaum Associates.

Denes PB, Pinson EN (1993) The Speech Chain. New York: WH Freeman Co.

Flexer C (1994) Facilitating Hearing and Listening in Young Children. San Diego: Singular Publishing.

McCormick B (Ed) (1993) Paediatric Audiology 0-5 Years. London: Whurr.

McCormick B, Archbold S and Sheppard S (Eds) (1994) Cochlear Implants for Young Children. London: Whurr.

Plant G, Spens K-E (Eds) (1995) Profound Deafness and Speech Communication. London: Whurr.

Pinker S (1994) The Language Instinct. London: Penguin.

Ross M (Ed) (1992) FM Auditory Training Systems: Characteristics, Selection and Use. Timomium, Maryland: York Press.

Appendix B – Speech perception

Appendix B1: The speech audiogram

More information is added to even simple speech tests by measuring the percentage of correct responses at a variety of different presentation levels. Thus in the McCormick toy test it can be useful to demonstrate the score achieved when a normal or quiet voice is employed. In tests such as the AB word lists, responses to a wider range of speech intensities can be recorded. A graph can then be presented as a speech curve displayed in audiogram format. The speech audiogram presents speech intensity level on the X-axis and the percentage scored on the Y-axis. Separation of the ears by headphone usage enables the speech curve for each ear to be plotted as shown below. Normal curves for test equipment and test material are obtained by testing a group with normal hearing and plotting the relative speech level against performance scored as a percentage. This allows for inter-subject comparisons.

The terms employed in speech audiometry have been summarised by the BSA (1981).

The speech detection threshold (SDT) is the level at which the listener can just detect that a stimulus is present without being able to recognise it. The **speech reception threshold (SRT)** is the speech intensity necessary for a score of 50% to be achieved. When speech curves have been measured it is usual to employ measures of the **half peak level (HPL)** rather than the SRT. This allows measurement of the speech intensity level when a 50% score is never achieved. The shift in the speech curve from the normal is termed the **half peak level elevation (HPLE)**. Its calculation is demonstrated in the Figure below.

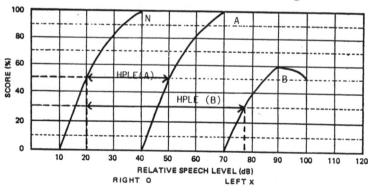

N = **Normal Curve**
A = **Example of Conductive Loss with HPLE of 30dB and MDS of 100%**
B = **Example of Sensory Loss with HPLE of 57dB and MDS of 60%**

The speech audiogram; format, terms and examples

The slope of the speech curve differs according to the material used, with high redundancy causing a steep rise after the SDT has been achieved. For this reason single level measures may be employed with more redundant material. Slight increase in the slope of the curve also occurs with age when AB lists are used with children (Markides, 1978).

Diagnostic use of speech audiometry

Confirming the degree of hearing impairment

Monosyllable speech tests are so devoid of linguistic cues that they accurately reflect the degree of hearing impairment. They thus have an important place in the assessment of children's hearing. The pure-tone thresholds averaged at 500, 1 kHz and 2 kHz correlate within 15 dB of the HPLE when AB word lists are employed (Markides, 1980). The HPLE is greater when there is a steep high frequency loss, but correction factors are available and with their use robustly measure the degree of impairment.

The correlation between the HPLE and the pure-tone thresholds is usefully employed as one test of non-organic hearing loss (NOHL). The presence of such a loss is usually apparent from the discrepancy between pure-tone thresholds and the informal hearing for speech. Such informal tests are always important. Although it is often assumed that it is too difficult to feign deafness on speech testing, Priede and Coles (1976) found that there was a degree of elevation of the HPLE in non-organic hearing loss, albeit less than would be predicted. Often the inaccuracy of the responses is transparent, with children tending to omit every other word, constantly replacing the initial phoneme or even substituting a word with the same meaning (for example, "ship" heard as "boat"). Aplin and Kane (1985) simulated NOHL in students, and once again they confirmed that whilst it was possible to demonstrate an unpredicted discrepancy between the pure-tone threshold and the speech audiogram, it was not possible to demonstrate unequivocally the presence of normal hearing. This was also noted by Baldwin and Watkin (1992) who found objective test methods more useful in NOHL.

Differential diagnosis

The speech curves also help to differentiate the type of hearing loss. Examples are illustrated on page 413. Curve 'A' is typical of a conductive loss. The curve is shifted to the right. A louder intensity is required for maximum discrimination, but when it is achieved the child can recognise the words clearly. Curve 'B' demonstrates the curve seen with a sensorineural loss. The Maximum Discrimination Score (MDS) is 60% at 90 dB with greater loss of discrimination above this. This roll-over confirms increased distortion of the speech signal at louder speech intensities. Speech audiometry in adults has been extensively used to differentiate sensory from neural losses (Priede and Coles, 1976), but this is rarely used in children, and electro-physiological and diagnostic imaging are more usefully employed if retrocochlear pathology is suspected.

References

Aplin DY, Kane JM (1985) Variables affecting pure tone and speech audiometry in experimentally simulated hearing loss. British Journal of Audiology 19: 219–228.

Baldwin M, Watkin PM (1992) The clinical application of otoacoustic emissions in paediatric audiological assessment. Journal of Laryngology and Otology 106: 301–306.

British Society of Audiology (1981) Speech audiometric terminology. British Journal of Audiology 21: 191–204.

Markides A (1980) The relationship between hearing loss for pure tones and hearing loss for speech among hearing impaired children. British Journal of Audiology 14: 115–121.

Priede VM, Coles RRA (1976) Speech discrimination tests in investigation of sensorineural hearing loss. British Journal of Audiology 90: 1081–1092.

Appendix B2: Tests of speech perception

From: The Pediatric Working Group of the Conference on Amplification for Children with Auditory Deficits, 1996. Used with permission.

Common speech recognition materials used with children

Test name	Investigator(s)	Material	Number of Lists	Items Per List	Response Format	Response Task	Age Range	Degree of HL
1. PBK-50	Haskins (1949)	Monosyllables	4	50	Open set	Verbal	6–9 years	Mild to moderate
2. Word intelligibility by picture identification (WIPI)	Ross and Lerman (1970)	Monosyllables	4	25	Closed set (6-picture matrix)	Psycho-motor	3–6 years	Mild to severe
3. Sound effects recognition test (SERT)	Finitzo-Hieber, Gertin, Matkin, Cherow-Skalka (1980)	Environmental Sounds	3	10	Closed set (4-picture matrix)	Psycho-motor	3 years and over	Severe to profound
4. Spondee recognition test	Erber(1974)	Spondees	1	25	Closed set	Written	8–16 years	Severe to profound
5. Six-sound test	Ling (1978); Ling (1989)	Vowels /oo/ar/ /ee/s/sh/m/	1	6	Open set	Psycho-motor	Infant/children	Moderate to profound
6. Glendonald auditory screening procedure (GASP)	Erber (1982)	Phonemes Words Sentences	1 1 1	10 12 10	Closed Set	Psycho-motor and verbal	6–13 years	Moderate to profound

(contd)

Appendix B2 (contd)

Test name	Investigator(s)	Material	Number of Lists	Items Per List	Response Format	Response Task	Age Range	Degree of HL
7. Children's perception of speech (NUCHIPS)	Katz and Elliott (1978)	Monosyllables	4 (randomisations)	50	Closed set	Psycho-motor	3 years and over	Mild to moderate
8. Discrimination by the identification of pictures (DIP)	Siegenthaler and Haspiel (1966)	Monosyllables	3	48	Closed set (2-picture matrix)	Psycho-motor	3–8 years	Mild to severe
9. BKB sentences	Bench, Koval and Bamford (1979)	Sentences	21 11	16 16	Open set	Verbal	8–15 years	Mild to moderate
10. Auditory numbers test (ANT)	Erber (1980)	Numbers	1	5	Closed set	Psycho-motor	3–8 years	Severe to profound
11. Pediatric speech intelligibility test (PSI)	Jerger, Lewis, Hawkins and Jerger (1980)	Monosyllables Sentences	1 2	20 10	Closed set	Verbal	3–10 years	Mild to moderate
12. Hoosier auditory visual enhancement test (HAVE)	Renshaw, Robbins, Miyamoto, Osberger, and Pope (1988)	Monosyllables	1	40	Closed set	Verbal/ Sign	2 years and over	Mild to profound
13. Minimal pairs test	Robbins, Renshaw, Miyamoto, Osberger, and Pope (1988)	Monosyllables	2	80	Closed set	Psycho-motor	5 years and over	Mild to profound

Appendix B2 (contd)

Test name	Investigator(s)	Material	Number of Lists	Items Per List	Response Format	Response Task	Age Range	Degree of HL
14. Imitative tests of speech pattern contrast perception (IMSPAC)	Boothroyd (1996)	Syllables	4 (plus randomisations)	40	Auditors: Closed set	Child: Imitation	3 years and over	Mild to profound
15. Three interval forced choice test of speech pattern contrast perception (THRIFT)	Boothroyd (1995)	Syllables	1 (plus randomisations)	54 or 108	Choose odd one of 3	Pointing, button-press or verbal	7 years and over	Mild to profound
16. Arthur Boothroyd lists (AB lists)	Boothroyd (1968)	Phonemes in CVC words	15	30 phonemes	Open set	Verbal/written	4 years and over	Mild to profound

Common speech recognition materials used with children. Adult list.

Test name	Investigators	Material	Number of Lists	Items Per List	Response Format	Response Task	Age Range	Degree of HL
1. Northwestern University auditory test No. 6 (NU-6)	Tillman and Carhart (1966)	Monosyllables	4	50	Open set	Verbal/written	9 years and over	Mild to moderate
2. Central Institute for the Deaf W-22 (CID W-22)	Hirsch et al. (1952)	Mono-syllables	20	50	Open set	Verbal/written	7 years and over	Mild to moderate
3. Nonsense syllable test (NST)	Levitt and Resnick (1978)	Syllables	16 (7 subtests within a list)	62	Closed set	Written	6 years and over	Mild to moderate

References

Bench J, Koval A, Bamford J (1979) The BKB (Bamford-Koval-Bench) sentence lists for partially-hearing children. British Journal of Audiology 13: 108-112.

Boothroyd A (1968) Developments of speech audiometry. Sound 2: 3-10.

Boothroyd A (1995) Speech perception tests and hearing-impaired children. In Plant G, Spens CE (Eds) Speech Communication and Profound Deafness. London: Whurr Publishers.

Boothroyd A (1996) Speech perception and production in hearing-impaired children. In Bess FH, Gravel JS, Tharpe AM (Eds) Amplification for Children with Auditory Deficits. Nashville, TN: Bill Wilkerson Center Press.

Erber NP (1974) Pure-tone thresholds and word-recognition abilities of hearing-impaired children. Journal of Speech and Hearing Research 17: 194-202.

Erber N (1980) Use of the auditory numbers test to evaluate speech perception abilities of hearing-impaired children. Journal of Speech and Hearing Disorders 45: 527-532.

Erber NP (1982) Auditory Training. Washington, D.C.: Alexander Graham Bell Association for the Deaf.

Finitzo-Hieber T, Gerlin IJ, Matkin N, Cherow-Skalka E (1980) A sound effects recognition test for the pediatric audiological evaluation. Ear and Hearing 1: 271-276.

Haskins H (1949) A phonetically balanced test of speech discrimination for children (unpublished Master's thesis). Northwestern University.

Hirsch IJ, Davis H, Silverman SR, Reynolds EG, Eldert E, Benson RW (1952) Development of materials for speech audiometry. Journal of Speech and Hearing Disorders 17: 321-337.

Jerger S, Lewis S, Hawkins J, Jerger J (1980) Pediatric speech intelligibility test: I - Generation of test materials. International Journal of Pediatric Otorhinolaryngology 2: 217-230.

Katz D, Elliott L (1978) Development of a new children's speech discrimination test. Paper presented at American Speech and Hearing Association Convention.

Levitt H, Resnick SB (1978) Speech reception by the hearing impaired: Methods of testing and the development of new test. Scandinavian Audiology 6, 107S-130S.

Ling D (1978) Auditory coding and reading: An analysis of training procedures for hearing impaired children. In Ross M, Giolas TG (Eds) Auditory Management of Hearing-Impaired Children. Baltimore, MD: University Park Press. pp 181-218.

Ling D (1989) Foundations of Spoken Language for Hearing-Impaired Children. Washington, D.C.: Alexander Graham Bell Association for the Deaf.

Renshaw J, Robbins AM, Miyamoto R, Osberger MJ, Pope M (1988) Hoosier Auditory Visual Enhancement Test (HAVE). Indianapolis, IN: Indiana University School of Medicine, Department of Otolaryngology-Head and Neck Surgery.

Ross M, Lerman J (1970) A picture identification test for hearing-impaired children. Journal of Speech and Hearing Research 13: 61-66.

Siegenthaler B, Haspiel B (1966) Development of two standardized measures of hearing for speech by children. Co-operative Research Program, Project No. 2372, United States Office of Education, Washington, DC.

Tillman TW, Carhart R (1966) An expanded test for speech discrimination utilizing CNC monosyllabic words: Northwestern University Auditory Test No. 6. Technical report no. SAM-TR-66-55. USAF School of Aerospace Medicine, Brooks Air Force Base, TX.

Appendix B3: The hierarchy of increasing redundancy for different speech tests used within the UK

Type of test/Test	Materials	Response	Scoring
Feature Perception Nonsense Syllables			
Monosyllabic Words			
McCormick toy	Six pairs of toys	Closed pointing	Word
Kendall toy	Three sets of 10 toys	Closed pointing	Word
Manchester picture	Eight lists of 10 pictures	Closed pointing	Word error types
Two-alternative picture	24 minimal word pairs + noise	Closed pointing	Word
Four-alternative auditory feature	20 sets of four CVC words +/– noise	Closed	Phonemes error types
Manchester junior word	Four lists of 25 CVC words	Open	Words
Fry word	Ten lists of 35 words	Open	Phonemes
Arthur Boothroyd (AB) Word	15 lists of 10 words	Open	Phonemes
Sentences			
Bench, Koval, Bamford (BKB)	21 lists of 16 sentences +50 key words	Open	Key words
Sentence identification in noise	BKB lists + noise	Open	Key words
Audio-visual			
BKB audio visual	BKB lists + video	Open	Key words
Four-alternative disability and Speechreading	FAAF lists + video of speaker	Closed	Phonemes error types

Appendix B4: Resources - Speech tests materials

Audio cassettes

***Auditory perception of alphabet letters:** cassette version with scoring sheets and clear plastic easel for pointing. Auditec.

***Minimal auditory capability battery:** standardised on adventitously deafened adults, only parts of this test battery are suitable for children. Auditec.

***NUCHIPS:** cassette version including 2 picture books, instructions and scoring forms included. Auditec.

Sound effects capability battery: cassette, picture book and scoring form. Auditec.

Word intelligibility by picture identification: cassette available, pictures, test booklet and scoring forms included. Auditec.
Auditec, 2515 S. Big Bend Boulevard, St. Louis, Missouri, 63143, USA. Tel (314) 781-8890.
*Denotes that test materials were not standardised on deaf children. Only available in American English.

Test of auditory comprehension: standardised on a national sample of children, 4 to 17 years old, with mild to profound hearing losses. Test results give a profile of performance on a continuum of auditory tests. Ten subtests. Administration time approximately 30 mins. A Spanish version of TAC is in preparation. Foreworks.
Foreworks, Box 82289, Portland, Oregon, 97282, USA. Tel (503) 653-2614. Fax: (503) 786-2492, E-mail: ejbagai@teleport.com

Early speech perception test: a test battery designed for children from 3 years, profoundly deaf. Two versions are included, standard and low verbal. Administration time approx. 20 mins. Test includes manual, scoring forms, toy materials, pictures and a cassette. Central Institute for the Deaf.
Central Institute for the Deaf, 818 South Euclid Ave., St Louis, Missouri, 63110, USA. Tel: (314) 652-3200.

Meaningful auditory integration scale: questionnaire/interview approach involving parents/carers. Considers three aspects: acceptance of device, alerting to sound and deriving meaning from auditory signals. Robbins AM, Renshaw JJ, Berry SW (1991) Evaluating meaningful auditory integration in profoundly hearing-impaired children. American Journal of Otology 12: 144S-150S.

Glendonald auditory screening procedure (GASP): designed for children ranging from 6 to 13 years, moderate to profound hearing loss. Three sections: phoneme detection, word identification and sentence comprehension. Erber N (1982) In Auditory Training. Washington DC: Alexander Graham Bell Association for the Deaf.

Three interval forced choice test (THRIFT): consists of nine subtests involving speech pattern contrasts. The audio digital approach THRIFT for Windows requires 4Mb RAM, hard disk with 12.5Mb free, sound card, headphones, external speakers, Microsoft Windows version 3.1 or later and a mouse. Designed to minimise the effects of linguistic and world knowledge. Suitable for children from 8 years, moderate to profound hearing loss.

Appendix C:
The Hearing Aid Check (post-aural hearing aids)

(adapted by permission of the Educational Services for Hearing Impaired Children, Shropshire)

You will need your hearing aid kit which should include:

The stetoclip and attenuator (stenoset).
Spare tubing.
Spare batteries.
Spare tone hooks.

The Earmould

LOOK	ACTION
Is it beginning to crack? Is it chipped or rough?	Arrange urgent earmould appointment. Contact teacher of the deaf or hospital about possible smoothing down of edges pro tem; replace with spare earmould pro tem.
Is it blocked with wax? Is it clean?	Remove wax carefully. Immerse earmould in earmould cleaning solution overnight or clean gently in a little warm soapy water using a soft toothbrush if necessary. Dry thoroughly in a warm environment, taking care to get rid of any remaining moisture with the air puffer.
Is the tubing turning yellow? Is the tubing hard?	Change the tubing immediately.
Is there condensation or moisture in the tubing?	Use the air blower or puffer to get rid of this; if you are finding this to be a persistent problem then mention it to your teacher of the deaf and audiologist.

The hearing aid (post-aural)

LOOK	ACTION
Are the casing or switches damaged?	Use replacement aid and alert teacher of the deaf.
Are the switches in appropriate position?	Set aid appropriately.
Is the tone hook cracked?	Replace tone hook.
Is the tone hook free from any water or particles of wax or any other debris?	Use air blower, remove debris carefully or, if this is not possible, replace tone hook.
Is the battery correctly fitted?	Re-insert as necessary.
Is the battery compartment clean?	Clean gently with soft toothbrush.
Gently shake the aid to make sure no components have become loose internally	Contact the teacher of the deaf or audiologist; check and use spare aid.

Batteries (post-aural aids)

It is important that you store batteries and follow the battery regime as advised by your teacher of the deaf.
The agreed days that you will change batteries are:

_____and_____

Do not be lulled into a false sense of security however. Batteries can fail at any time. When in doubt check your child's aid and change the battery.

The Listening Check (post-aural hearing aids)

Do this at least once per day, before your child puts the hearing aid in for the day. Recheck at any time that you feel the aid may have had a knock or if your child appears less responsive. Try and involve your child in this routine whenever possible. Remember to do the morning testing routine in a similar acoustic environment with as little background noise as possible so that it is easier for you to be alerted.

1 Detach the earmould.
2 Attach the stetoclip to the tone hook (sometimes called the elbow) of the hearing aid.
3 Switch the aid on.
4 * If you have been given a stetoclip with an attenuator: Turn the aid gradually up to the child's user setting. For your child this is volume
   _____.

   * Turn the aid up to a comfortable listening level for you. (Always try to turn the aid to a similar level each time you check this.)
   Teachers, please put a line through the instruction that does not apply.
5 Clearly but without exaggeration say the Ling six sounds:

   mm - oo - ee - ah - sh - s

   Do they all sound as clear as usual?
   If you have any doubts follow the instructions below ('What to do if an aid is not working properly').
6 Say a nursery poem or rhyme, listening-in to the aid carefully as you move it about – gently squeeze the casing; move the volume control backwards and forwards slightly. If the sound goes on and off or crackles, the aid should be taken off the child. Follow the instructions 'What to do if an aid is not working properly'.
7 If the aid is working appropriately re-attach the earmould and follow the listening check procedure again from step 3 to step 5, but now for the whole system as the child will be wearing it. Any problems you identify now will be directly related to the earmould or its tubing.
8 Check the aid when the child is wearing it. Is the volume setting at the desired level? Is there any feedback from the earmould? Is the microphone position appropriate?

What to do if an aid is not working properly

1 Change the battery. Retest.
2 Change the tone hook. Retest.
3 If the aid is still not functioning: Put the spare hearing aid on the
                                           child.
                                           Ring the contact number for the
                                           teacher of the deaf to inform
                                           him/her. They will advise as to the
                                           quickest way to arrange for a
                                           repair and for a further spare
                                           hearing aid to be supplied to you.

The contact number for your teacher of the deaf is _____.

Checking a Body Worn Aid

(adapted by permission of Oxfordshire Sensory Impairment Service)

Visual check

Damage and dirt	e.g. Cracked case. Broken switches. Food or dirt on the microphone.
Controls	1. Check the internal settings. 2. Mark and fix the external settings – for a quick check.
Receiver	Know the coding – check you always replace with the same type. Is the washer in place?
Baby cover	Check that it is clean, secure and not obstructing the sound.
Bone vibrator (if used)	Check for visible damage.
Harness	Check that it is comfortable and holds aid securely. The optimum position is up on the chest in appropriate position for maximum amplification of the child's voice and well spaced for directional cues.
Earmould	1. Clean each day – make it a daily fun routine. 2. Blow through the earmould to check it is not blocked. 3. Check for perforations or cracks. 4. Check the tip is smooth, not chipped or chewed. 5. Check the ring clip is secure and flush with the receiver.
Battery	Is it a battery changing day? Battery changing days are _____ and _____ . Are the battery compartment contacts clean? Is the battery inserted correctly?

The listening check

1 Connect the hearing aid and receiver to the stetoclip. Make sure that you have the attenuator connected between the receiver and the stetoclip.
2 Switch on the hearing aid, gradually increasing the volume to your child's setting.
   Use the Ling six sounds to check the aid functioning
              mm - oo - ee - ah - sh - s
   Does the sound quality and loudness appear as usual?

N.B. Remember that you should not listen-in to the aid at this volume level if for some reason you do not have an attenuator. In this case you should turn the volume up to a comfortable listening level for you.

3 Increase and decrease the volume level slightly, whilst reciting a nursery rhyme or poem. Is the change in volume smooth and without crackles?
4 'Wiggle' leads about particularly near to all connection points — is the sound in any way interrupted?
5 Reconnect the earmould and carry out steps 1 and 2 again.
6 Place aids on child with harness appropriately worn. Recheck that switches/volume control are in appropriate position and have not been disturbed by this process.

Remember if you identify a fault but cannot resolve it (see fault finding) do not put the suspect aid on your child. Use the spare hearing aid and contact the support teacher immediately.

Fault finding - body worn aids

No Sound

1	Not switched on	Check.
2	Battery fault	Insert correctly or replace.
3	Lead broken/ frayed	Replace.
4	Lead placed in wrong socket or incorrectly in socket	Check/ re-insert.
5	Connection junction sockets	Call support teacher.
6	Earmould blocked	Wash/ blow through.

Intermittent

1	Switches poor	Remove aid/ inform support teacher.
2	Poor battery contact	Clean if necessary/ contact support teacher/temporarily hold in place.
3	Lead junction points	Remove aid/ inform support teacher.
4	Lead	Replace.
5	Lead to receiver	Push in fully/ replace if fault persists.
6	Cord bent over/ under stress	Re-insert so that lead travels straight up.

Feedback

1	Poor earmould seal with receiver	Is the washer still present? Replace washer with 'Blu-Tack' if necessary.
2	Poor seal in the ear	Check earmould correctly inserted; is volume setting correct? Contact hospital for earmould impression and middle ear check.
3	Perforated earmould	Arrange for new impressions to be taken/spare earmould to be used.

Poor sound quality

1	Weak battery	Replace.
2	Damaged/dirty microphone	Clean as demonstrated by support teacher; replace microphone if necessary.
3	Check switch positions	Alter as required.
4	Dirty or partially blocked earmould	Clean.
5	Receiver	Change receiver.
6	Internal fault	Replace hearing aid; contact support teacher.

Remember to inform the support teacher if you use any of the hearing aid or FM spares in your kit so that he/ she can replenish them on the next home/ school visit.

The cochlear implant - is it working?

As with all hearing aid systems you need to check at least once each day that the cochlear implant is working. These notes are intended to remind you of the procedure. Remember that if you have any doubt about the implant's functioning it is better to check it again, rather than leave it simply because you have checked it earlier.

It is not possible to check a cochlear implant via a listening test nor via a test box as in the case of your child's previous hearing aids. It is however possible to carry out a simple test routine that will allow you to broadly check the speech processor and the microphone functioning and the total system with your child.

Visual check: the speech processor

1 Check that there is no obvious damage to casing and switches that might affect the working of the processor.
2 Are the volume controls and settings set correctly? Check these against those given to you by the implant centre.
3 Is the system on?
4 Now repeat the 6 Ling sounds:

mm - oo - ee - ah - sh - s

Do the function lights flash for each of these sounds?
If the lights flash this suggests that the information across the frequency range is getting through. Wiggle the leads as you are talking (repeat the sounds above); if the lights' flashing is interrupted there may be an intermittent fault. If the function lights do not respond in the usual way, systematically change the lead, clean the contact, change the microphone and batteries and then recheck.
5 Get into the habit of playing a listening check game with your child either with the Ling sounds or other little phrase. Initially they may involve just reacting to the sounds — jumping, dropping a ball, imitating. Such games will help you to know whether sounds across the frequency range are getting through. If your child complains that the device sounds different, if you notice that the child's behaviour with the device is different or if the system function lights seem to flash erratically, contact your implant centre or teacher of the deaf for advice.

The radio aid check

(adapted by permission of Educational Services for Hearing Impaired Children, Shropshire, UK)

Check the child's personal behind the ear hearing aids or body worn aids first. Make sure they are working properly.

Visual check: the whole system

1 Check that the contact points on the personal hearing aids are clean and undamaged.
2 Check the casing of the FM receiver (the child's part) and the transmitter for splits, cracks or damage, loose screw and so on. Are the lead/ cord/ sockets clean?
3 *Remove the batteries
     or
   *Slide out the battery pack (*delete as appropriate*) from the transmitter and receiver. Check batteries for damage. Check the battery voltage with the battery tester. Replace if necessary.
4 Check battery contacts are clean, then re-insert batteries in radio aid ensuring the terminals match the label inside the battery compartment.
5 Check switches on receiver and transmitter are clean and unclogged (clean with alcohol swab if necessary). Check switches are not damaged (send for repair if they are).
   Where appropriate: volume control or balance wheel – check this is unclogged and moves smoothly to distinct settings.

Listening check: the radio aid

1 Use the radio aid listening stick to check the radio itself is working. First attach the stetoclip to the receiver and then switch it on. The battery light should glow momentarily. Switch on the transmitter. The battery light should glow momentarily.
2 Give the transmitter to another person and ask them to stand outside the room. Ask them to talk to you, e.g., say a nursery rhyme.
3 Listen carefully to the receiver and check that the sound is smooth and not crackly. If there is a problem, first replace the transmitter microphone and listen again; then change the aerial. If there is still a problem contact your teacher of the deaf.
   If the radio aid is working, now connect it to the hearing aids, taking care that the connecting lead is inserted correctly both to the radio aid and to the hearing aid.

Linking the systems: post-aural hearing aids

1 Look carefully at the connection to the shoe and at the point at which the shoe connects to the hearing aid so that you are sure that the shoe and the contact points are connecting.
2 Switch on the hearing aid and ask the child/adult to leave the room again and talk into the transmitter again. Listen carefully to the hearing aid; wiggle the lead, particularly at the weak points where the sound links into the receiver and shoe, to make sure that the sound is not intermittent.
3 Repeat for the other hearing aid. Continue to listen whilst gently shaking the receiver. Then ask the person who is holding the transmitter to shake it gently and wiggle the aerial.

If there is an uninterrupted good quality signal then the aid is ready to wear.

Faults

If the radio aid and the hearing aid were working well before you connected them then the fault must lie with the connections between them. Change the lead, shoe and contact points (if you have been given these). If the system is still not working contact your teacher of the deaf immediately.

Linking the system: body worn aids

1 Attach the connecting lead to the receiver and to the hearing aids. Remember if you are using a Y-lead then both hearing aids must be connected to it before you start to test.
2 Look carefully at the point at which the lead connects to the hearing aid and the radio aid so that you are sure that the lead is inserted properly.
3 Switch on the hearing aid and ask the child/adult to leave the room again and talk into the transmitter again.
4 Listen carefully to the hearing aid; wiggle the lead, particularly at the weak points where the lead links into the receiver and hearing aid to make sure that the sound is not intermittent.
5 Repeat for the other hearing aid. Continue to listen whilst gently shaking the receiver. Then ask the person who is holding the transmitter to shake gently that and wiggle the aerial.
6 If there is an uninterrupted good quality signal then the aid is ready to wear.

Faults

1 No transmission — check that the transmitter is switched on appropriately.

2 If the sound received from the radio aid transmitter is intermittent or
   of very poor quality, first check the input sockets to check they are
   clean, and clean if necessary. Retest.
3 If the fault continues, change the lead. Retest.
4 If the fault continues, recheck the radio aid transmitter.

Still doubts? Contact the teacher of the deaf. The contact number for
your teacher of the deaf is _____

Procedure for using a hearing aid test box

The service has a number of portable test boxes available, all of which have slightly different operating procedures. It is important that before you use the test box you familiarise yourself with its controls and discover whether the test box is pre-set to test at certain inputs and to carry out certain procedures. If those are not the procedures that you need to carry out or if there is no pre-set programme, then you need to know the following:

> how to vary the input level
> how to vary the input frequency
> how to measure distortion (THD)
> where the hearing aid or transmitter microphone needs to be placed in the sound chamber
> how to connect a body worn aid to the coupler and sound level meter
> how to connect a post-aural aid to the coupler and sound level meter
> how to connect an earmould and hearing aid to the coupler and sound level meter
> whether the test box is automatically levelled when the test box is switched on or whether this has to be done by you.

Please also note when the test box was last calibrated externally.

Procedure: aids that have been newly fitted

N.B. a listening and visual check should always be carried out on hearing and radio aids before test box measurements are attempted.

When an aid is new, back from repair or settings have been amended you need to obtain baseline graphs and figures to compare with the manufacturer's specification sheets. It is important that you do this using inputs and settings as described in the manufacturer's data. You may well have to adjust the aid's internal settings to do so and should always be careful to return the settings to the child's recommended ones.

Baseline data obtained in comparison with manufacturer's specifications are entered directly in the child's file. These should include details as to maximum gain, maximum output, frequency response, Total Harmonic Distortion and internal noise. If the data obtained is within 3 dBSPL of the manufacturer's specifications then details of maximum gain and output should also be entered onto the child's 'Hearing and Radio aid check' form and the aid accepted as functioning appropriately.

Reset the aid to the child's user settings and volume level. Measure the frequency response and output at this setting using an input of

65db. If the test box does not automatically print out the distortion figures at this level select the option for checking THD and test also using an input of 65dBSPL. Place a copy of these print-outs in the child's file and on the child's hearing and radio aid check form.

Measure the maximum output at this level using an input of 90db. Check that this does not exceed the child's known tolerance levels. File this in the child's audiology file but also record maximum output on the child's hearing and radio aid check form.

Monthly and weekly checks

According to the listening level of the child, you will be carrying out electro-acoustic test on aids at weekly, fortnightly or monthly intervals, to support the daily subjective visual and listening tests. It is not necessary to check the aid against the manufacturer's specifications unless you find a discrepancy against the baseline user settings. Any discrepancy of more than +3dB should be responded to for further investigation. Growth in distortion levels should be reacted to quickly.

Potentially faulty aids should not be left on children's ears. Aids which are under-performing, but not necessarily distorting also need careful investigation.

The regular electro-acoustic testing of the hearing aids should involve:

1 An initial visual and listening check of the systems.
2 Using a 65db input, run the hearing aids through the test box at user setting to determine that the frequency response, THD and output at this setting are still comparable with the baseline measures. Run the aid through the test box with the earmould attached to check for any major effect of the earmould on the amplification configuration.
3 Using an input of 90db to check the SSPL or maximum output still compares with the SSPL on the baseline measures.
4 If any of these measures differ significantly, try and replicate the curve or graph. Systematically change any components such as batteries, tone hooks, leads and receivers as applicable. If the fault or under-powering persists, return the aid to HQ and give the child a spare that is working within the desired parameters.

Test box procedures for fitting and balancing radio aids

All radio aids must be checked daily by a visual and listening check; the balancing of the radio aid and hearing aid (Type II systems) must be checked whenever the hearing aid is run through the test box. Radio systems and hearing aids must always be rebalanced when either comes back from repair or when the child's settings are adjusted.

If a child is given a spare hearing aid or a spare FM transmitter or receiver the systems will need to be rebalanced. The procedure for balancing the two systems is basically the same whether the child wears a body worn or post aural/ITE aid:

1 First carry out visual and listening checks of the hearing aid and radio aid systems independently and when connected.
2 Connect each hearing aid in turn to the test box coupler and obtain a print-out of the output at user settings using an input level of 65 dB for post-aural and ITE aids; use an input of 60 dB for body worn aids. Note the output at 1000Hz.
3 Connect the radio aid to the hearing aids. Keep both aids connected to the system. This is particularly important for body worn aids. Place the hearing aid and coupler outside the test box ; place only the radio aid transmitter microphone inside the test box and if possible at the spot that the hearing aid microphone was placed. This may be difficult if the microphone used is integral to the transmitter. In this case place the whole transmitter in the test box, taking care that the microphone is directed towards the sound source and as close to the desired spot as possible.
4 Switch on the coupled hearing aid, the FM transmitter and FM receiver.
5 Change the input level on the test box to 75 dB. Rotate the balance wheel or screw on the FM receiver until the figure for output at 1000 Hz is similar to that for the hearing aid user setting curve at 1000 Hz.
6 Check the output and harmonic distortion across the frequency range and adjust further the balance screw or wheel until the closest match across the frequencies is found. N.B. This should be a match within +3dB across the frequencies and one which affects the frequency response curve and harmonic distortion figures minimally if at all.
7 Check that the balance is also suitable for the other hearing aid by following the procedure again. Sometimes you will have to find a compromise fitting to suit two radically different aids but if the result is significantly different to the child's desired amplification configuration you must consult the audiologist.

The 'good' balance should be printed off and kept with the child's hearing and radio aid check form for regular comparison.

Neck loops

Although neck loops should only rarely be used with children — direct input being infinitely preferable — there are some pupils who are able to manage them effectively or who will not wear a direct input facility.

The procedure for fitting, balancing and testing the system is similar to that described above. The location of the aid within the neck loop is however critical. Wherever possible the aid should be attached to the coupler and then replaced on the user's ear so that it is to the most consistent signal that the child is exposed to that the two systems are balanced. In the absence of this, then place the coupled hearing aid on your own ear when performing these measurements.

Appendix D: Video Resources

Educational audiology demonstrations on video cassette:

Berg Technologies, 516 E. Summit Creek Drive, Smithfield, Utah, 84335, (801) 563-5733

I Listening Problems In The Classroom (37.10 Minutes)

1 Imposing a hearing loss on yourself
2 Impedance meter and tympanometer
3 Identifying symptoms of hearing and auditory perceptual problems
4 Speech check
5 Audiometer and audiograms
6 Five-sound test
7 Listening test
8 Calculating reverberation time
9 Measuring signal and noise
10 Preventive servicing of hearing aids
11 Personal FM
12 Sound field FM

II Educational Audiology (59.55 Minutes)

1 Local delivery model
2 Listening and speech materials
3 Developmental Approach to Successful Listening (DASL)*
4 Listening Handbook tests and tasks
5 Sound level meter options
6 Reverberation determination
7 Obtaining insertion gain of hearing aid
8 Hearing aid management kit
9 Determining speech recognition
10 FM equipment options
11 Sound field FM equipment management
12 Personal FM receiver options

III Acoustical Problems In School Classrooms (34.18 Minutes)

1 School classrooms are acoustically hostile listening environments
2 Sound level meter measurement in a school
3 Sound transmission loss measurements in a school
4 Measuring room volume with an ultrasonic device
5 Measuring reverberation time of a classroom
6 Placement of loudspeakers in a classroom
7 Measuring the Rapid Speech Transmission Index (RASTI) with a Bruel and Kjaer Speech Transmission Meter

8 Measuring RASTI with a TEF 20 Sound Lab
9 Obtaining minute-by-minute graph of sound levels in a classroom
10 Measuring audio and electrical spectra of amplifiers and loudspeakers
11 Selecting from Acoustical Palate of RPG Systems
12 Selecting and installing sound field FM Systems
13 Connecting amplifiers and loudspeakers
14 Matching impedance of amplifiers and loudspeakers

Phone Resource Point, (800) 688 8788 for information on obtaining a copy of the DASL II manual.

Video material

1 Practical Ways to Help Deaf Children in Mainstream Classrooms
   Designed as a support video for schools and services for hearing-impaired children, for mainstream teachers, and for trainee teachers of hearing-impaired children.
2 Collaborating for Successful Integration
   A support video designed for use in all primary school contexts where teachers of hearing-impaired children and mainstream teachers work together.
3 Working with Hearing-Impaired Students in Mainstream Colleges
   The video is designed for both mainstream and college staff as an introduction to the subject and as a support video for schools and colleges, or services for hearing-impaired young people.
4 Do Radio Aids Really Help?
   Designed for all those involved in using radio aids with hearing-impaired children.
5 Fitting and Balancing Radio Hearing Aids
   A video designed for trainee and qualified teachers of hearing-impaired children who require an update and the large number of experienced teachers who are ultimately responsible for ensuring quality and efficacy of the individual child's amplification system.

Videos available from:
Ewing Foundation, CAEDSP,
University of Manchester
Oxford Road
Manchester M13 9PL
U.K.
Tel. 00 44 (0) 161 - 275 3367

Appendix E: Resources - Learning to listen

1- For A.R.T:

- A vibrating sound box (very useful but not essential). Commercial ones are available, and although sophisticated, can be expensive (see below). It is possible to make a basic version by placing speakers inside a large rectangular wooden box, or alternatively a disco-quality speaker may be used, provided that it is large enough for children to sit or lie on and clamber over.
- An electronic keyboard or organ, with a good amplification system.
- A quality cassette player, with good amplification and large speakers which do not distort.
- A range of percussion instruments which can be played in a variety of ways, with at least one large drum.
- Blow organs (melodions).
- Tone bars.
- Various hand puppets, bean bags, baskets, skittles, soft toys, dressing-up clothes and other home-made props.
- Wall mirrors.
- A selection of music with strong rhythm; brass band music and Latin American music has proven particularly useful, as have pre-recorded tapes of pre-school songs.
- "Early Communication Skills" by Charlotte Lynch and Julia Cooper, available from Winslow Press, Telford Rd., Bicester, Oxon, OX6 OTS.
- "Early Listening Skills" by Diana Williams, also available from Winslow Press.
- "Body and Voice" by Carrie Leonard, available from Galt Educational, Culvert St, Oldham, Lancs OL4 2ST.

2 - For music:

- "Carousel: Primary Music" by Joan Child, Richard Crozier and Ken Storry: a complete music programme, available from Ginn and Co. Ltd., Prebendel House, Parson's Fee, Aylesbury, Bucks, HP20 2QY.
- "Move and Relax with Music" by Monika and Ralph Schneider, available from Galt Educational (address above).
- Soundbeam, Soundbox, Soundbed and Magic Organ are all available from SpaceKraft Ltd., Crowgill St., Rosse St., Shipley, West Yorks., BD18 3SW (information about Soundbeam/box/bed is also available from Tim Swingler, 463 Earlham Rd., Norwich NR4 7HL).
- The Remo Ocean drum is available through the Yorkshire Purchasing Organisation, 41 Industrial Park, Wakefield, Yorkshire WF2 0XE.

3 - For assessment and monitoring development of pre-verbal skills:

- "The Preverbal Assessment Intervention Profile" by P. Connard. Available from Pro-Ed, 8700 Shoal Creek Boulevard, Austin, Texas 78757, USA.
- "Profiles of Development", by Alec and Valerie Webster, available from Avec Designs Ltd., PO Box 709, Bristol BS99 1GE.

Contacts and addresses

- For information regarding Claus Bang and Tone Bar/Music therapy work: The Beethoven Trust for Deaf Children, 2 Queensmead, St. John's Wood, London NW8 6RE.
- For details regarding the Halle Project and Gamelan: M Withers, Halle Education, Heron House, Albert Square, Manchester M2 5HD.
- Music and the Deaf: Paul Whittaker, 39 Grasmere Rd., Gledholt, Huddersfield, West Yorks HD1 4LH.

Index